Introduction to Exercise Science

Introduction to Exercise Science

EDITORS

Terry J. Housh

University of Nebraska–Lincoln

Dona J. Housh

University of Nebraska Medical Center

Allyn and Bacon

Boston ■ London ■ Toronto ■ Sydney ■ Tokyo ■ Singapore

Editor in Chief: *Paul A. Smith*
Publisher: *Joseph Burns*
Editorial Assistant: *Tanja Eise*
Executive Marketing Manager: *Lisa Kimball*
Editorial Production Service: *Bernadine Richey Publishing Services*
Manufacturing Buyer: *David Repetto*
Cover Administrator: *Jennifer Hart*
Electronic Composition: *Omegatype Typography, Inc.*

A Pearson Education Company
160 Gould Street
Needham Heights, MA 02494

Internet: www.abacon.com

Between the time web site information is gathered and published, some sites may have closed. Also, the transcription of URLs can result in typographical errors. The publisher would appreciate notification where these occur so that they may be corrected in subsequent editions.

Library of Congress Cataloging-in-Publication Data

Introduction to exercise science / Terry J. Housh, Dona J. Housh, editors
     p.   cm.
   Includes bibliographical references and index.
   ISBN 0-205-29168-6 (pbk.)
   1. Exercise—Physiological aspects.   2. Sports—Physiological aspects.   3. Sports sciences.
I. Housh, Terry J.   II. Housh, Dona J.
QP301.I65 1999
612'.044—dc21

99-047827
CIP

Printed in the United States of America
10 9 8 7 6 5 4 3 2 1   04 03 02 01 00 99

CONTENTS

Contributors   vii

Preface   ix

PART ONE   Introduction   1

1 An Introduction to Exercise Science   1

Terry J. Housh and Dona J. Housh

2 History of Exercise Science   12

Herbert A. deVries

PART TWO   Areas of Study in Exercise Science   36

3 Anatomy   36

Glen O. Johnson

4 Athletic Training: The Profession   69

Ronald P. Pfeiffer

5 Biomechanics   98

Daniel J. Blanke and Nick Stergiou

6 Exercise Physiology   122

Joseph P. Weir

7 **Exercise and Sport Nutrition**   157

Joan M. Eckerson

8 **Exercise and Sport Psychology**   203

Richard J. Schmidt

9 **Measurement in Exercise Science**   226

Dale P. Mood

10 **Motor Control and Motor Learning**   252

David E. Sherwood

Index   277

CONTRIBUTORS

Daniel J. Blanke
School of Health, Physical Education, and
 Recreation
University of Nebraska-Omaha
Omaha, NE

Herbert A. deVries
Emeritus Professor
Department of Physical Education
University of Southern California
Los Angeles, CA

Joan M. Eckerson
Exercise Science Department
Creighton University
Omaha, NE

Dona J. Housh
Department of Oral Biology
College of Dentistry
University of Nebraska Medical Center
Lincoln, NE

Terry J. Housh
Department of Health and Human
 Performance
University of Nebraska-Lincoln
Lincoln, NE

Glen O. Johnson
Department of Health and Human
 Performance
University of Nebraska–Lincoln
Lincoln, NE

Dale P. Mood
Department of Kinesiology
University of Colorado-Boulder
Boulder, CO

Ronald P. Pfeiffer
Department of Health, Physical Education,
 and Recreation
Boise State University
Boise, ID

Richard J. Schmidt
Department of Health and Human
 Performance
University of Nebraska-Lincoln
Lincoln, NE

David E. Sherwood
Department of Kinesiology
University of Colorado-Boulder
Boulder, CO

Nick Stergiou
School of Health, Physical, Education, and
 Recreation
University of Nebraska-Omaha
Omaha, NE

Joseph P. Weir
Program in Physical Therapy
Osteopathic Medical Center
Des Moines University
Des Moines, IA

PREFACE

Introduction to Exercise Science is designed to introduce undergraduate students to such aspects of the discipline as the areas of study, technology, certifications, professional associations, and career opportunities. It also helps students develop an appreciation for the history, as well as current and future trends in exercise science. This textbook is not designed as an in-depth exposure to the individual areas of study (i.e., anatomy, biomechanics etc.) within exercise science and, therefore, each chapter identifies prominent and timely lines of inquiry without exhaustive reviews of the primary literature.

This textbook is divided into two parts: Introduction and Areas of Study in Exercise Science. Part I includes chapters entitled An Introduction to Exercise Science and History of Exercise Science, while Part II includes chapters on Anatomy, Athletic Training: The Profession, Biomechanics, Exercise Physiology, Exercise and Sport Nutrition, Exercise and Sport Psychology, Measurement in Exercise Science, and Motor Control and Motor Learning. Each chapter in Part II provides information on the specific area of study including a brief history, health and sports performance-related issues, technology, professional associations, employment opportunities, glossary of terms, study questions, an abstract of research, and suggested readings.

Chapter 1: An Introduction to Exercise Science

Chapter 1 provides basic information about exercise science. It defines exercise and science and provides a working definition of exercise science as "how and why the human body responds to physical activity." It also describes the coursework typically included in an undergraduate major in exercise science and provides examples from four universities presently involved in training undergraduate exercise science students. Furthermore, this chapter synopsizes the Basic Standards for the Professional Preparation in Exercise Science 1995 prepared by the Applied Exercise Science Council of the National Association for Sport and Physical Education (NASPE) of the American Alliance for Health, Physical Education, Recreation, and Dance (AAHPERD).

Chapter 2: History of Exercise Science

In Chapter 2, Herbert deVries provides a historical foundation for the understanding of exercise science. To fully appreciate the current and future trends in the field it is important to know how exercise science developed. Chapter 2 discusses the influence of medical doctors as pioneers in exercise science as well as factors that contributed to the emergence of exercise science as a unique field of study. This chapter also identifies important scientists from the United States and Europe who influenced the development of exercise science and describes selected classic research studies which added to our understanding of the effects of exercise training. Finally, Dr. deVries provides a perspective on the divergence between exercise science and the applied, professional area of physical education pedagogy (teacher training).

Chapter 3: Anatomy

An understanding of human anatomy is essential to the development of knowledge in exercise science. In Chapter 3, Glen Johnson discusses the basic science area of anatomy. This chapter provides a brief history of anatomy and defines the subspecialties of gross anatomy, cytology, histology, comparative anatomy, developmental anatomy, and pathological anatomy. Furthermore, Dr. Johnson ties the study of anatomy to exercise science by relating it to research in growth and development, body composition, and the cellular adaptations to training.

Chapter 4: Athletic Training: The Profession

Chapter 4 addresses issues in Athletic Training. In this chapter, Ronald Pfeiffer includes a description of the profession, the National Athletic Trainer's Association (NATA) Board of Certification examination, and employment opportunities. Athletic training provides a unique opportunity for exercise science professionals to combine work in the area of sports performance with health-related, clinical careers. The national certification process is highly structured and Dr. Pfeiffer outlines the expectations for professionals in athletic training.

Chapter 5: Biomechanics

Chapter 5 on biomechanics is co-authored by Daniel Blanke and Nick Stergiou from the University of Nebraska-Omaha. Biomechanics has many applications in exercise science and this chapter outlines various sports performance and health-related aspects. In addition, a number of new technologies are discussed in Chapter 5 which are used for in-depth analyses of human movement. Furthermore, as the chapter indicates, there are many interesting employment opportunities for students with knowledge and skills in biomechanics.

Chapter 6: Exercise Physiology

Exercise physiology is central to an understanding of exercise science. In Chapter 6, Joseph Weir describes many areas of basic and applied research. Exercise physiologists have a number of employment opportunities in academia as well as the private sector. Furthermore, professional organizations such as the American College of Sports Medicine (ACSM) and National Strength and Conditioning Association (NSCA) provide certifications that include topics in exercise physiology which supplement the formal college and university training for exercise science students.

Chapter 7: Exercise and Sport Nutrition

Proper nutrition is important for optimal health as well as successful sports performance. In Chapter 7, Joan Eckerson includes information about nutrition as it relates to chronic disease and athletic performance. In addition, nutritional supplements as ergogenic aids are discussed. In terms of employment opportunities, there is a growing trend towards combining formal training in nutrition with exercise science to meet the needs of health clubs and wellness centers.

Chapter 8: Exercise and Sport Psychology

In Chapter 8, Richard Schmidt provides information regarding various aspects of exercise and sport psychology. Exercise psychology deals with factors related to motivation, exercise initiation, adherence, and compliance as well as the psychological changes associated with exercise training. Sport psychology includes factors which limit as well as enhance the ability to perform athletic events. Dr. Schmidt also discusses ways in which sports participation can enhance psychological growth and development.

Chapter 9: Measurement in Exercise Science

Measurement theory and procedures have many applications in exercise science. In Chapter 9, Dale Mood explores the roles of measurement in exercise science. In addition to the assessment of cognitive, physical, and psychological aspects of human performance, measurement also includes issues related to statistical procedures and computer applications.

Chapter 10: Motor Control and Motor Learning

In Chapter 10, David Sherwood provides basic information concerning the psychological and neurological theories underlying motor control and motor learning. The applications of these theories have implications for health-related fields such as physical therapy and rehabilitation as well as sports performance. Basic knowledge of motor learning and control is valuable for allied health professionals as well as athletes.

This textbook includes contributions from four generations of exercise scientists. Herbert A. deVries, Emeritus Professor at the University of Southern California, is truly a pioneer in the study of exercise and its relationship to sports performance and health across the life span. In 1986, we were at Portland State University, Portland, Oregon. A faculty member, Mike Tichy asked whether we would be interested in helping with a research project organized by Herb at PSU. It turned out that Mike and Herb attended undergraduate school together at East Stroudsburg University in Pennsylvania and were lifelong friends. It was to our great benefit to have the opportunity to assist Herb with that initial project. Since then, we have remained friends and Herb comes to the University of Nebraska-Lincoln periodically to continue our research on electromyography and muscle fatigue. We were very fortunate to be in the right place at the right time in 1986 and it has been our personal and professional pleasure to work with Dr. deVries for over 12 years now.

Glen O. Johnson, and Dale P. Mood attended graduate school together at the University of Iowa in the late 1960s. They have continued their friendships over the years, and we were fortunate to persuade them to contribute to this textbook. We were also fortunate to have Glen as a doctoral advisor at the University of Nebraska-Lincoln. It was through Glen that we were introduced to Dale and have greatly enjoyed attending professional conferences together such as the annual meeting of the American Alliance for Health, Physical Education, Recreation and Dance (AAHPERD).

Joan M. Eckerson and Joseph P. Weir earned their doctoral degrees at the University of Nebraska-Lincoln in the early 1990s. Glen O. Johnson, Terry J. Housh and Richard J. Schmidt were doctoral advisors for Joan and Joe and the succession of exercise scientists will continue with their students.

Editing this textbook has also given us the opportunity to further develop existing friendships as well as make new ones. In this regard, it has been our pleasure to work with Daniel J. Blanke and Nick Stergiou from the University of Nebraska-Omaha, Ronald P. Pfeiffer from Boise State University, and David E. Sherwood from the University of Colorado-Boulder.

One of the true joys of academic life is the long-term associations with students and colleagues who have similar professional interests. It is our hope that the collective insights of the four generations of exercise scientists represented in this textbook will contribute to the professional development of future generations of exercise scientists.

We thank the following reviewers for their helpful suggestions: John Hauth, East Stroudsburg University; Gary Liguori, University of Wyoming; Lori Dewald, Shippensburg University; Andrew Kozar, University of Tennessee–Knoxville; Robert Behnke, Indiana State University; B. Sue Graves, Florida Atlantic University; and Susan Barnd, University of Wisconsin–LaCrosse.

Introduction to Exercise Science

1

An Introduction to Exercise Science

TERRY J. HOUSH

DONA J. HOUSH

What Is Exercise Science?

What Do Exercise Scientists Study?

Academic Programs in Exercise Science
Emergence of Academic Programs
Growth of Academic Programs
The Curriculum

Professional Standards for Exercise Science Programs
Foundational Core
Exercise Prescription for Normal
  and Special Populations
Health Promotion

Administrative Tasks
Human Relations
Professional Development
Practical Experience

Summary

Study Questions

Glossary

Suggested Readings

References

What Is Exercise Science?

Exercise is defined as "the performance of any physical activity for the purpose of conditioning the body, improving health, or maintaining fitness, or as a means of therapy for correcting a deformity or restoring the organs and bodily functions to a state of health" (13). *Science* is "a systematic attempt to establish theories to explain observed phenomena and the knowledge obtained through these efforts" (13). Simply stated, *exercise science* is concerned with how and why the human body responds to physical activity. From this generic description, it is clear that exercise science is a very diverse field of study that encompasses many areas of inquiry. For example, the simple act of walking can be viewed from many different perspectives. An anatomist can describe the muscles involved in walking. An exercise physiologist may study how the systems of the body respond to the stress of walking, and a biomechanist can apply the laws of physics to examine the efficiency of each stride. An exercise psychologist may be interested in what motivates the subject to walk, and a sports nutritionist can describe how the food that we eat is used to supply the energy for the walk.

Furthermore, each of these exercise scientists can study how we respond during an exercise bout (acute responses to exercise) or how we adapt to exercise training (chronic responses to exercise). For example, an exercise physiologist may find that as we begin to walk our cardiovascular and pulmonary systems respond to the demands of the activity by increasing our heart rates and ventilatory rates. These are examples of acute responses to exercise. On the other hand, if we change from a sedentary life-style and begin to walk regularly, our cardiovascular and pulmonary systems become more efficient, which results in reduced heart rates and ventilatory responses to exercise. These improvements in physical fitness are examples of chronic responses to exercise. It is likely that as a student of exercise science, you will discover that even simple acts of physical activity, such as walking, can be more complex and thought provoking than they initially appear. This, however, is the exciting challenge of studying exercise science and learning how and why the human body responds to physical activity.

What Do Exercise Scientists Study?

Two primary areas of inquiry for exercise scientists are (1) the health-related aspects of physical activity and (2) sports performance. Recent research has provided valuable information concerning various aspects of the relationship between physical activity and health (4–6, 8–12, 14–16, 18). For example, exercise epidemiologists have found compelling evidence to suggest that an active life-style reduces the risk of developing diseases such as coronary heart disease (CHD) and some forms of cancer (4, 6, 9). Furthermore, studies indicate that disease risk factors can be favorably modified with appropriate exercise and dietary interventions (3, 5, 15, 18). Recent studies have also found that exercise can affect the immune system and potentially influence the risk of developing infectious diseases (11, 14). The total picture regarding the health-related benefits of physical activity, however, is far from complete. For example, perhaps the greatest public impact from exercise science research is the study of how low to moderate levels of exercise improve health and well-being throughout the life-span (2, 3, 8, 15, 18). We still know very little about how much exercise is needed to reduce the risk of developing specific diseases. Thus, with our present level of knowledge we are limited in the ability to provide "safe and effective" exercise prescriptions for various age groups (4). Future generations of exercise scientists will carry on these important lines of research.

Exercise scientists also study factors related to the improvement of sports performance. The study of sports performance includes a wide range of diverse areas, such as (but not limited to) the growth and development of young athletes, the nutritional needs of adult athletes, biomechanical analysis of Olympic athletes, and the psychological characteristics of Masters age-group athletes. Applied research involving the development and application of training techniques for athletes is a primary interest of strength and conditioning coaches associated with universities and professional teams. In addition, athletic trainers often study methods of preventing athletic injuries and rehabilitating athletes injured in competition or practice. Clearly, there are many opportunities for exercise scientists with regard to the development and application of knowledge related to sports performance.

Academic Programs in Exercise Science

Most current academic programs in exercise science in colleges and universities grew out of the applied, professional discipline of physical education, which in the 1960s encompassed various aspects of sports, fitness, and physical activity (17). Today, however, physical education majors are usually preparing to teach in elementary and secondary schools. On the other hand, exercise science is normally a nonteaching option. At many universities, exercise science has replaced physical education teacher preparation as the largest undergraduate major in departments such as Kinesiology, Health and Human Performance, and Health, Physical Education, and Recreation (17).

Emergence of Academic Programs

Many academic programs in exercise science emerged in response to public concerns about our society's lack of physical fitness and the aerobic fitness movement of the 1960s and 1970s. Even with this increased interest in exercise, a number of studies have shown that people today are generally not very fit or active, which increases the risk of developing a number of diseases (18). This, combined with the results of other studies that have shown that we can improve our health and quality of life through regular physical activity (5, 6, 15), has sparked an interest in understanding the responses of the body to exercise. As the role of exercise in maintaining fitness and healthy life-styles has become better understood, researchers have been able to obtain government as well as private funding to study the health-related aspects of exercise. The increased funding has been, in part, responsible for the development and continuation of programs in exercise science in postsecondary institutions.

Growth of Academic Programs

Initially, many students are drawn to the undergraduate major in exercise science because they enjoyed athletic participation during childhood and adolescence. The opportunity to study the scientific bases of sport performance is often appealing. Some students also find it interesting to apply the knowledge gained to their own training for competitive athletics or to work with athletes in various settings. Other students major in exercise science because the rigorous scientific coursework prepares them for future careers. The dramatic growth in exercise science programs in colleges and universities in recent years is also due to the diversity of career opportunities available to graduates (Table 1.1).

Undergraduate exercise science programs are frequently used as the foundation for attending professional schools in medicine, physical therapy, chiropractic, occupational therapy, and dentistry, as well as other *allied health* fields. In addition, an exercise science degree is valuable for careers in *corporate or agency fitness* (YMCA, YWCA, Jewish Community Centers, and the like) and in **private consulting,** such as for health clubs. The

TABLE 1.1   Potential Career Options for Students in Exercise Science

Agency and Corporate Fitness

Young Men's Christian Association (YMCA)
Young Women's Christian Association (YWCA)
Jewish community center
Corporate-sponsored fitness and wellness centers

Clinical Rehabilitation

Cardiac rehabilitation
Pulmonary rehabilitation
Athletic trainer

Preprofessional Schools

Medicine: allopathic (M.D.) and osteopathic (D.O.)
Physical therapy
Occupational therapy
Physician's assistant
Dentistry
Chiropractic
Optometry

Private Sector

Corporate employee or consultant, such as athletic shoe manufacturer or athletic
    equipment design
Ergonomics consultant, such as insurance claims for worksite injuries
Health club employee or owner
Personal trainer
Strength and conditioning coach for professional team

Teacher, Researcher, and/or Coach

University, college, or community college professor
University or college strength and conditioning coach
Athletic team coach
Researcher for institution, such as the Cooper Institute or Olympic Training Center

expansion of fitness facilities by corporations has been driven not only by a desire to provide a valued fringe benefit for employees, but also by research that indicates that the company can benefit economically through reduced health insurance costs and absenteeism
when their work force is physically fit and active (7). The need for qualified managers of
such facilities has led to the development of exercise science majors at colleges and universities, as well as certification programs through professional organizations such as the
American College of Sports Medicine (**ACSM**) and the National Strength and Conditioning Association (NSCA).

The combination of a degree in exercise science and certification from a reputable
professional organization increases the likelihood of success in the job market. Another
career option for undergraduate exercise science students is to attend graduate school.

Generally, the graduate school options involve advanced preparation for students interested in corporate or agency fitness, specialized training in clinical aspects of exercise science, such as cardiac rehabilitation, or the development of research skills for those interested in teaching and conducting research in university settings.

The Curriculum

The typical undergraduate exercise science curriculum includes a foundation in the basic sciences, followed by a series of courses related to exercise. Table 1.2 includes examples from Boise State University, Creighton University, University of Colorado–Boulder, and the University of Nebraska–Lincoln. Although there are differences among curricula from various institutions, they generally follow a similar format. For example, the science core usually includes courses in anatomy, biology, chemistry, and physiology. The exercise-related courses often include biomechanics, exercise physiology, laboratory techniques, and sports nutrition.

The philosophy underlying the undergraduate exercise science curriculum is that there is a knowledge base that all students should have. In general, this knowledge base is important for all specialized areas of interest, whether it be cardiac rehabilitation, corporate and agency fitness, physical therapy, or medicine. There is also an underlying concept that, in addition to core courses, students should develop the skills and knowledge associated with their specialized area of interest in many ways, including elective courses, practicum experiences, volunteer noncredit activities, work experiences, and/or special training from professional certification programs during their undergraduate preparation. Many students also specialize through postbaccalaureate experiences, such as professional school (physical therapy, medicine, chiropractic, and the like) or graduate school.

Professional Standards for Exercise Science Programs

The Ad Hoc Committee on Program Accreditation of the Southeast Regional Chapter of the American College of Sports Medicine has developed a document entitled *Guidelines for Professional Preparation in Exercise Science* (available at www.dlu.edu). These guidelines describe the "knowledge, skills, and abilities needed by professionals to function in settings in which exercise is used in prevention of or as a nonpharmacological treatment for various health-related problems" and provide a "minimum foundation upon which other educational/curricular objectives for training Exercise Science professionals can be based." At the undergraduate level (e.g., bachelor's degree), the suggested content areas include Anatomy/Physiology, Biomechanics, Kinesiology, Statistics, Physiology of Exercise, Nutrition/Weight Control, Behavioral Change, Exercise Testing for Normal and Special Populations, Exercise Prescription for Normal and Special Populations, First Aid/Athletic Training (including emergency and safety procedures for facilities), Exercise Leadership for Facilities, Practicum Experience, and Computer Proficiency. In addition to demonstrating competency in the undergraduate content areas, the recommended graduate level (e.g., master's degree) content areas include Research Design and Statistics, Advanced or Clinical

TABLE 1.2 Examples of Undergraduate Exercise Science Curricula

Example 1

Undergraduate Exercise Science Emphasis,
Department of Health, Physical Education, and
Recreation, Boise State University, Boise, ID

Basic Science Courses
Human Anatomy and Physiology
Human Physiology
Foundations of Physical Science or
    General Physics
Cell Biology
College Chemistry
College Chemistry Laboratory
Organic Chemistry
Organic Chemistry Laboratory
Nutrition

Exercise-related Courses
Health Education
Foundations of Physical Education
Rhythmic Skills and Dance
Fitness Foundations
Standard First Aid and CPR
Applied Anatomy
Microcomputers in Physical Education
Internship I
Human Growth and Motor Learning
Evaluation in Physical Education
Exercise Physiology
Conditioning Procedures
Kinesiology
Psychological and Sociological Aspects of Activity
Health Promotion
Adapted Physical Education
Internship II
Sport and Fitness Activity
Electives

Example 2

Undergraduate Exercise Science Curriculum,
    Exercise Science Department, Creighton
    University, Omaha, NE

Basic Science Courses
General Biology I
General Chemistry
Human Anatomy

Exercise-related Courses
Beginning Swimming
First Aid

Introduction to Athletic Training
Personalized Weight Training
Aerobic Dance
Beginning Tennis or Beginning Racquetball
Designing a Personalized Fitness Program
Nutrition for Health and Sports Performance
Biomechanics
Exercise Physiology
Exercise Prescriptions: Their Design and Evaluation
Basic Statistics and Research Design
Laboratory Methods and Procedures
Exercise Leadership and Program Administration
Directed Independent Study
Exercise Sciences Practicum

Specialty Tracks
Corporate, Community, and Commercial Fitness
Business Ethics
Marketing
Education
Management
Legal Environment
Business Law

Athletic Training
Practicum I–IV
Modalities and Rehabilitation
Selected Topics
Physiology
Athletic Training Independent Study

Physical Therapy
Chemistry
Biology
Physics
Physiology
Philosophy

Personal Training
Certification Independent Study
All Courses in the Corporate, Community, and
    Commercial Fitness Track
Strength and Conditioning
Certification Independent Study

Cardiac Rehabilitation
Psychology II
Psychology III
Education
Clinical Exercise Testing and Electrocardiogram
    Interpretation

Example 3

Undergraduate Kinesiology Curriculum,
Department of Kinesiology, University
of Colorado–Boulder, Boulder, CO

Basic Science Courses
Biology I
Biology I Laboratory
Biology II
Biology II Laboratory
Chemistry I
Chemistry II
Physics I
Physics II
Human Anatomy
Human Physiology
Psychology I
Psychology II
Calculus

Exercise-related Courses
Introduction to Kinesiology
Introduction to Statistics and Research
    in Kinesiology
Mechanical Kinesiology
Neuromuscular Kinesiology
Psychological Kinesiology
Physiological Kinesiology

Electives
Introduction to Scientific Writing in Kinesiology
Nutrition, Health, and Performance
Theory and Practical Applications of Resistance
    Exercise and Conditioning Programs
Scientific Writing in Kinesiology
Colloquium in Kinesiology
Selected Topics in Exercise Physiology
Advanced Laboratory Techniques in
    Motor Behavior

Motor Control
Critical Thinking in Motor Behavior
Independent Study
Honors Thesis
Internship

Example 4

Undergraduate Exercise Science Curriculum,
    Department of Health and Human Performance,
    University of Nebraska–Lincoln, Lincoln, NE

Basic Science Courses
General Biology
General Biology Laboratory
General Chemistry I
General Chemistry II
Organic Chemistry I
Organic Chemistry I Laboratory
Organic Chemistry II
Organic Chemistry II Laboratory
Elements of Biochemistry
Elementary Physics
Introduction to Nutrition
Advanced Nutrition
Human Anatomy
Human Physiology

Exercise-related Courses
Healthy Life-Styles
First Aid and Care of Athletes
Emergency Health Care
Biomechanics
Physiology of Exercise
Exercise Testing and Programs
Statistical Methods
Exercise Science Practicum
Electives

Exercise Physiology, Epidemiology of Exercise and Disease Prevention, Advanced Exercise Testing and Prescription for Normal and Special Populations, Behavioral Changes in Special Populations, Pharmacology, Computer Applications for Exercise Science, and Internship.

The National Association for Sport and Physical Education (**NASPE**) is an association of the American Alliance for Health, Physical Education, Recreation and Dance (**AAHPERD**). The Applied Exercise Science Council of NASPE has developed a document called ***Basic Standards for the Professional Preparation in Exercise Science*** (1), which was designed to provide guidance for curricular development for college and university programs that prepare undergraduate students for careers in exercise science. Basic standards are included in the major areas of Foundational Core, Exercise Prescription for Normal and Special Populations, Health Promotion, Administrative Tasks, Human Relations, Professional Development, and Practical Experience. Each area also includes specific behavioral objectives related to the knowledge and skills expected of entry-level exercise science professionals.

Foundational Core

The behavioral objectives associated with the Foundational Core indicate that exercise science students should have basic knowledge in the scientific areas of human anatomy, human physiology, exercise physiology, biomechanics, first aid, and the care and prevention of fitness-related injuries. Furthermore, students should maintain cardiopulmonary resuscitation (CPR) certification and be able to discuss and implement emergency and safety procedures for exercise settings.

Exercise Prescription for Normal and Special Populations

Entry-level exercise science professionals should be able to administer field and laboratory tests for evaluating cardiovascular endurance, body composition, muscular strength, muscular endurance, and flexibility and to develop safe and effective exercise prescriptions based on the results of these tests. Furthermore, exercise scientists should be able to modify exercise prescriptions for participation under various environmental conditions and by different populations, including the elderly. In addition to exercise prescription, it is important to be able to provide leadership for the implementation of aerobic, strength, and flexibility programs.

Health Promotion

Exercise scientists must be knowledgeable of factors related to nutrition and weight control, stress management, and substance abuse. Furthermore, it is important to have basic knowledge of available community referral services for individuals who need additional professional help with these issues.

Administrative Tasks

Exercise science professionals should have practical knowledge of (1) the equipment and facilities needed to develop and evaluate health and fitness programs, (2) trends related to health and fitness programming, (3) marketing strategies, and (4) legal and ethical issues involved in implementing health and fitness programs.

Human Relations

Entry-level exercise science professionals must possess sufficient verbal and written communications skills to speak clearly and concisely to individuals and groups and to prepare business letters, proposals, and technical reports. They must also demonstrate a basic knowledge of the motivational techniques related to exercise program adherence and retention.

Professional Development

It is important for exercise science professionals to understand the cultural environments and organizational structures within which fitness, wellness, and cardiac rehabilitation programs operate. Furthermore, exercise scientists should have knowledge of the professional organizations and publications related to their discipline and be able to articulate career planning strategies.

Practical Experience

Practical, hands-on experience is integral to the preparation of exercise science professionals. In this regard, students should have at least one observation experience at a worksite and develop, with the site supervisor and university supervisor, a contractual agreement that includes specific learning experiences for an internship.

Summary

Exercise science, as an academic area of study, is growing, as evidenced by the increasing number of undergraduate and graduate programs available to students. At many institutions, more students are now enrolled in the nonteaching option in exercise science than the traditional physical education teacher preparation major. The diversity of career options in areas such as agency and corporate fitness, **clinical rehabilitation,** allied health, consulting for the private sector, and **higher education** attract many students to the exercise science major. Furthermore, the strong background in the basic sciences (such as anatomy, biology, and chemistry) associated with most undergraduate exercise science programs provides a solid foundation for students to meet the entrance requirements of many professional schools. In addition to the basic sciences, exercise science graduates are well grounded in the application of theory to practice from exercise-related courses and practical hands-on experiences such as practicums and internships.

STUDY QUESTIONS

1. Define exercise science.

2. Name and describe the two primary areas of inquiry for exercise scientists.

3. Discuss the career opportunities of an exercise scientist.

4. Discuss the skills that an entry-level exercise scientist should possess in order to prescribe exercise programs for normal and special populations.

5. Exercise science degrees are often used as a foundation for:

   a. Attending a professional school in medicine.
   b. A career in corporate, or agency, fitness.
   c. Specialized training in cardiac rehabilitation.
   d. Teaching and/or conducting research at a university.
   e. All of the above.

6. Which of the following would be considered health-related aspects of physical activity?

   a. The biomechanical analysis of a high jumper jumping.
   b. The relationship between an active life-style and a reduction in coronary heart disease risk.
   c. The psychological characteristics of an athlete.
   d. None of the above.

7. In order to promote a healthy life-style, exercise scientists must be knowledgeable of factors related to:

   a. Nutrition.
   b. Weight control.
   c. Stress management.
   d. Substance abuse.
   e. All of the above.

GLOSSARY

AAHPERD   American Alliance for Health, Physical Education, Recreation, and Dance.

ACSM   American College of Sports Medicine.

Allied health   A field of study and practice that includes hospital and other clinical settings that promote a positive state of well-being. These settings provide a number of employment opportunities for the exercise scientist.

Basic Standards for the Professional Preparation in Exercise Science   A document developed by the Applied Exercise Science Council of NASPE. It was designed to provide guidance for curricular development for colleges and university programs that prepare undergraduate students for careers in exercise science.

Clinical rehabilitation   A career opportunity that involves an exercise scientist working in a hospital or other clinical setting and using exercise as the primary mode for rehabilitating patients following disease, injury, or surgery.

Corporate (or agency) fitness   An exercise science career opportunity that involves developing and/or supervising fitness programs in various workplaces and community centers.

Exercise   The performance of any physical activity for the purpose of conditioning the body, improving health, or maintaining fitness or as a means of therapy for correcting a deformity or restoring the organs and bodily functions to a state of health.

Exercise science   The study of how and why the human body responds to physical activity.

Higher education   An exercise science career opportunity that usually involves teaching and/or research at the college or university level.

NASPE   National Association for Sport and Physical Education. This is an association of the American Alliance for Health, Physical Education, Recreation, and Dance.

Private consulting   A career opportunity that involves sharing one's expertise in exercise science with others (law firms, hospitals, fitness centers, private individuals) so that they can benefit from the information.

Science   A systematic attempt to establish theories to explain observed phenomena and the knowledge obtained through these efforts.

SUGGESTED READINGS

Bouchard, C., R. J. Shephard, T. Stephens, J. R. Sutton, and B. D. McPherson (Eds.). *Exercise, Fitness, and Health: A Consensus of Current Knowledge.* Champaign, IL: Human Kinetics, 1990.

Shephard, R. J. *Aerobic Fitness and Health.* Champaign, IL: Human Kinetics, 1994.

Watson, R. R., and M. Eisinger (Eds.). *Exercise and Disease.* Boca Raton, FL: CRC Press, 1992.

REFERENCES

1. American Alliance for Health, Physical Education, Recreation, and Dance. *Basic Standards for the Pro-fessional Preparation in Exercise Science 1995.* Reston, VA: AAHPERD, 1995.

2. American College of Sports Medicine. *Guidelines for Exercise Testing and Prescription.* Baltimore: Williams and Wilkins, 1995.

3. Blair, S. N. *Living with Exercise: Improving Your Health through Moderate Physical Activity.* Dallas, TX: American Health Publishing Company, 1991.

4. Blair, S. N. Physical activity, fitness, and coronary heart disease. In: *Physical Activity, Fitness, and Health: International Proceedings and Consensus Statement,* C. Bouchard, R. J. Shephard, and T. Stephens (Eds.). Champaign, IL: Human Kinetics, 1994, pp. 579–590.

5. Blair, S. N., H. W. Kohl, C. E. Barlow, R. S. Paffenbarger, L. W. Gibbons, and C. A. Macera. Changes in physical fitness and all-cause mortality: A prospective study of healthy and unhealthy men. *J.A.M.A.* 273:1093–1098, 1995.

6. Blair, S. N., H. W. Kohl, R. S. Paffenbarger, D. G. Clark, K. H. Cooper, and L. W. Gibbons. Physical fitness and all-cause mortality: A prospective study of healthy men and women. *J.A.M.A.* 262:2395–2401, 1989.

7. Kaman, R. L., and R. W. Patton. Cost and benefits of an active versus an inactive society. In: *Physical Activity, Fitness, and Health: International Proceedings and Consensus Statement,* C. Bouchard, R. J. Shephard, and T. Stephens (Eds.). Campaign, IL: Human Kinetics, 1994, pp. 134–144.

8. Kaplan, G. A., T. E. Seeman, R. D. Cohen, L. P. Knudsen, and J. Guralnik. Mortality among the elderly in the Alameda County Study: Behavioral and demographic risk factors. *Am. J. Public Health* 77:307–312, 1987.

9. Lee, I.-M. Physical activity, fitness, and cancer. In: *Physical Activity, Fitness, and Health: International Proceedings and Consensus Statement,* C. Bouchard, R. J. Shephard, and T. Stephens (Eds.). Champaign, IL: Human Kinetics, 1994, pp. 814–831.

10. Linsted, K. D., S. Tonstad, and J. W. Kuzma. Self-report of physical activity and patterns of mortality in Seventh-Day Adventist men. *J. Clin. Epidemiol.* 44:355–364, 1991.

11. Mackinnon, L. T. *Exercise and Immunology.* Champaign, IL: Human Kinetics, 1992.

12. Morris, J. N., D. G. Clayton, M. G. Everitt, A. M. Semmence, and E. H. Burgess. Exercise in leisure time, coronary attack and death rates. *Br. Heart J.* 63:325–334, 1990.

13. *Mosby's Pocket Dictionary of Medicine, Nursing, and Allied Health.* St. Louis, MO: C. V. Mosby, 1990.

14. Nieman, D.C. Physical activity, fitness, and infection. In: *Physical Activity, Fitness, and Health: International Proceedings and Consensus Statement,* C. Bouchard, R. J. Shephard, and T. Stephens (Eds.). Champaign, IL: Human Kinetics, 1994, pp. 796–813.

15. Paffenbarger, R. S., R. T. Hyde, A. L. Wing, I.-M. Lee, D. L. Jung, and J. B. Kampert. The association of changes in physical activity level and other lifestyle characteristics with mortality among men. *New Engl. J.Med.* 328:538–545, 1993.

16. Rowland, T. W. *Exercise and Children's Health.* Champaign, IL: Human Kinetics, 1990.

17. Siedentop, D. *Introduction to Physical Education, Fitness, and Sport, 2nd ed.* Mountain View, CA: Mayfield Publishing Company, 1994.

18. U.S. Department of Health and Human Services. *Physical Activity and Health: A Report of the Surgeon General.* Atlanta, GA: U.S. Department of Health and Human Services, Centers for Disease Control and Prevention, National Center for Chronic Disease Prevention and Health Promotion, 1996.

CHAPTER

2 History of Exercise Science

HERBERT A. deVRIES

Evolution of Exercise Science
  Physiology
  Anatomy
  Kinesiology
  Health and Fitness
  American College of Sports Medicine

**Impetus for the Emergence of Modern
Exercise Science**
  Need for Science-based Principles for Exercise
  Need for Correction of Myths
    Regarding Exercise
  Need for Methodology for Training Athletes
  Need for Methodology for the Development
    of Optimal Health and Fitness

History of Exercise Science in the United States
  Important Figures in the Emergence
    of Exercise Science

Contributions of YMCA Leaders
    to Exercise Science
Important U.S. Leadership by Scientists
    Trained Abroad
Exponential Growth of Leaders in Exercise
    Science in Contemporary Times

History of Exercise Science in Europe
  Important British Exercise Scientists
  Important German Exercise Scientists
  Important Scandinavian Exercise Scientists

Present and Future Trends in Exercise Science

Summary

Study Questions

Glossary

Suggested Reading

References

Exercise science as a structured body of knowledge has only existed since the early part of the nineteenth century. Although the value of exercise was recognized and interest taken in it by earlier civilizations (notably by the Greeks who were the progenitors of Olympic competition), the basic sciences were not yet sufficiently developed to allow use in such diverse fields as athletic competition, military conditioning, medical applications, and physical fitness. Methods for measuring human functions at rest were difficult in themselves; measurements in the course of activities such as walking, running, jumping, swimming, and cycling and during involvement in athletic activity or vigorous exercise had to wait for the future development of electronics, which did not occur in any practical sense until the twentieth century.

The purpose of this chapter is to describe the development of exercise science from a very small part of physical education that was built around pedagogical concerns to the situation that exists today. Now the divergent interests of those who will become physical educators and coaches and those who will develop academic interest in the scientific bases underlying all movement have necessitated a division of curricula in many of our universities into a physical education major versus a major in exercise science.

Evolution of Exercise Science

Physiology

It has been said that *physiology* is the meeting place of the sciences. This is so because understanding the function of biological systems requires an understanding of anatomy, biology, physics, and chemistry, as well as the mathematical principles undergirding the analysis of findings in the laboratory.

As our knowledge base increases in sophistication, we must add molecular biology to general biology. Some aspects of biology merge with physical principles to become biophysics. Biology merges with chemistry to become biochemistry, and chemistry, which started out as simple general inorganic and organic chemistry, now requires special applications of physics and mathematics to become physical chemistry. So it is easy to see how all the sciences contribute to our understanding of the functions of the human body. Furthermore, as sophistication progresses, our methods of measurement of human movement and exercise require at least a rudimentary knowledge of electronics to utilize the complex instrumentation in use today, and a thorough understanding of statistics and computer applications is needed to digest and report the findings of the laboratory.

Anatomy

Modern study of anatomy had its beginning in the 1500s as the gross study of organ structure and function. However, the study of cellular structure within the tissues of muscles and organs remained to be discovered after the invention of the microscope by Anton van Leeuwenhoek around 1660. Only then were muscle fibers identified as the cellular element of muscle tissue. *Histology,* the study of the anatomy of tissues and their cellular basis, opened the door to a much better understanding of organ structure and function for the medical profession, but a true understanding of how force was developed by muscle fibers through changes in molecular structure remained to be studied by the electron microscope, which was not developed until the 1950s.

A subdivision of anatomy, *embryology,* or developmental anatomy, developed largely in the 1800s as scientists studied the changes in form and structure of the embryo and fetus in chicks and pigs. This work was of great importance to physicians and especially to obstetricians in their applications to humans. Exercise scientists who deal with questions regarding exercise and pregnancy also benefit from this work.

Kinesiology

Kinesiology can be defined most simply as the study of human motion; indeed, in recent years some universities have used this term for their departments or schools of physical education. In the early days of physical education, when few activities were taught besides gymnastics and dance, the contents of a course in kinesiology were confined largely to functional anatomy. In any event, the unique contribution of kinesiology is that it selects from sciences such as anatomy, physiology, and physics the principles that are pertinent to human motion and systematizes their application. Gradually, as sports assumed a more important place in the physical education curriculum, the concept of kinesiology was broadened to include the study of mechanical principles that applied to sports techniques. The advent of the computer has resulted in highly technical analyses of human movement, and this area of study is frequently referred to as *biomechanics.*

Health and Fitness

The nature of the illnesses that beset the U.S. population in recent years has undergone a transition from a predominance of infectious diseases to the present predominance of degenerative diseases. This change represents the contribution of the medical profession, both in research and clinical practice, toward the virtual control and the imminent eradication of a large portion of the formerly dreaded infectious scourges.

The increase of such degenerative diseases as cardiovascular accidents (heart attacks and strokes), hypertension, neuroses, and malignancies offers a challenge not only to medicine, but to exercise science as well. It seems that as improvements in medical science allow us to escape decimation by such infectious diseases as tuberculosis, diphtheria, and poliomyelitis, we live longer only to fall prey to the degenerative diseases at a slightly later date. Whether this involvement with the degenerative problems follows from our living longer or is the result of our simultaneous change in life-style cannot yet be answered.

The influence of life-style on the health and illnesses of a lifetime has been suggested in the past, but hard, scientific evidence has only recently become available. In a survey of 6928 adults of Alameda County, California (4), individual health practices were related to health and also to mortality statistics. The health practices surveyed included (1) smoking, (2) weight in relation to desirable standards, (3) use of alcohol, (4) hours of sleep, (5) breakfast eating, (6) regularity of meals, and (7) physical activity. It was found that the average life expectancy of men age 45 who reported 6 or 7 "good" practices was more than 11 years greater than that of men reporting fewer than 4. For women, the difference in life expectancy was 7 years. It was also found that good health practices were reliably associated with positive health and that the relationship of the different health practices was cumulative; those who followed all the good practices, even though older, were in better health than those who failed to follow them. This association was found to be independent of age, gender, and economic status.

American College of Sports Medicine

It is not surprising that many of the pioneers in the development of exercise science were trained as medical doctors. The American College of Sports Medicine (ACSM) was formed in 1954 in recognition of the need to promote and integrate scientific research, education, and practical applications of sports medicine and exercise science to maintain and enhance physical performance, fitness, health, and quality of life. In 1954 there were only 11 charter members. Today that membership has grown to over 15,000, whose interests are divided into (1) Basic and Applied Sciences, (2) Medicine, and (3) Education and Allied Health.

Impetus for the Emergence of Modern Exercise Science

Need for Science-based Principles for Exercise

More and more people, laymen as well as physicians and other health scientists, came to realize the potential health benefits derived from the pursuit of physical fitness. This interest in physical fitness was accelerated by the need for physically fit young men for the armed forces of World Wars I and II. Our leaders recognized the need to develop scientific bases for the conduct of exercise programs, whether directed toward health enhancement, physical fitness for work and play, sports performance, or rehabilitation after injury. That is, we needed to be guided by evidence developed from scientific experiments that were conducted under laboratory-controlled conditions wherever possible.

Need for Correction of Myths Regarding Exercise

Even as recently as the World War II years, there was very little scientific data by which exercise programs could be governed. To exemplify the problem, consider the following *myths,* which were widely accepted as fact until recently.

   1. Heavy exercise, such as weight training, resulted in becoming "muscle bound." This would slow the athlete and restrict range of motion. Consequently, athletic coaches of the 1930s and 1940s strictly forbade their athletes from lifting weights. Scientific research in the 1950s completely reversed this thinking and now weight rooms are necessities in any athletic program.

   2. "Athletes heart" was thought to result from heavy endurance training such as long-distance running and swimming. This myth resulted from the well-known fact that the hearts of well-trained athletes grew larger. In some types of heart disease, the heart also grows larger, but for very different reasons. In any event, cardiologists now recognize that endurance exercise programs are beneficial, not detrimental, for the normal individual.

   3. As recently as the 1950s, it was believed, even by many members of the medical profession, that older individuals (after 40 years of age) would not benefit from physical conditioning. They were no longer capable of the usual training response found in younger people. The present author is happy to have been among the pioneers who disproved this myth by bringing about significant training effects in men who averaged 70 years of age (10). In recent years this work has been extended to show that even in the 90s age group significant benefits occur through appropriate conditioning (13).

   4. Another myth of long standing has been corrected only in the last decade: "No pain, no gain" was the philosophy of many coaches and physical educators who worked their charges unmercifully to supramaximal efforts in the belief that anything less would be ineffective. Although this belief may have some merit when training champion athletes, it is definitely not a valid concept for the training of the general public interested in improvement of their fitness levels. For example, we now know that even walking constitutes a training challenge and elicits a beneficial response for the untrained individual and, especially, for the elderly.

Need for Methodology for Training Athletes

A major problem in developing scientific bases for exercise science lies in the great diversity of what lies in the realm of exercise. It is abundantly obvious that the exercise that will improve a distance runner will not be the method of choice for the shot putter or weight lifter. Then consider the many different sports and it is easy to see that, instead of a "cook book" for each conceivable activity, it would be far preferable to have scientifically based principles that can be applied to any given type of activity. For these reasons, textbooks in exercise physiology often break down into chapters organized by the element of performance involved, such as strength, endurance, or speed. deVries and Housh (11) have broken down the elements of performance as follows:

1. Strength
2. Endurance
3. Speed
4. Efficiency of movement
5. Flexibility
6. Muscle soreness (cause and treatment of)
7. Warming up and cooling down
8. Nutrition: effects on athletes
9. Special aids to performance
10. Gender differences

The research-based knowledge concerned with these elements of performance is already voluminous and is growing exponentially. Exercise science is now well on its way!

Need for Methodology for the Development of Optimal Health and Fitness

Over the past five decades, much evidence has been furnished that supports the value of exercise as a prophylactic and therapeutic measure. Although we can confidently say that the available evidence indicates that a vigorous life-style maintains optimum levels of health and well-being, we do not yet have all the answers as to how and why. The following areas are in need of further investigation.

1. Potential benefits of exercise
2. Definition of physical fitness

3. How do we go about testing physical fitness? Age differences? Gender differences?
4. Prevention of cardiovascular disease
5. Metabolism and weight control
6. Growth and development
7. Age and exercise
8. Fatigue
9. Exercise and immune function

At the rate at which scientific investigation has proceeded in these areas in the past five decades, it may not be unrealistic to expect the ultimate development of a "Pharmacopia of Exercise" in the next five decades.

History of Exercise Science in the United States

Important Figures in the Emergence of Exercise Science

Dudley Allen Sargent (1849–1924) was one of the pioneers of U.S. physical education and, since measurement is the essence of science, his system for measuring strength and power and for recording and evaluating anthropometric measurements makes him a pioneer in exercise science as well. Sargent attended Yale Medical School from 1875 to 1879, where he was awarded the M.D. degree. In 1879, he became the director of the Hemenway Gymnasium at Harvard University, where he remained until retirement in 1919.

Sargent made many important contributions to the pedagogical aspects of physical education, not least of which was his founding and development of the Sargent School for Physical Education, which became a normal school and which still survives as Boston University Sargent College of Allied Health Professions (14). However, his contribution to exercise science lies in his development of a comprehensive system for individual exercise programs. Sargent's program at Hemenway Gymnasium began with a complete physical examination and included measurements of strength in the various parts of the body as tested by dynamometers designed and/or developed by him. He also made comprehensive anthropometric measurements.

From these voluminous data, exercise prescriptions were made specifying the amount of work and the adjustment of the apparatus to be used, as well as other hygienic data. The testing procedures were repeated after 6 months, and the prescription was adjusted according to the recorded changes. His apparatus included chest expanders, leg machines, pulley weights, and hydraulic rowing machines. Based on his testing methods, he provided minimum fitness levels for admission to competition on the various varsity and intramural sports teams.

An interesting insight into his melding of science with athletics lies in his concept of a "fair physical test of a man," which is still in use and which we now call the *Sargent Jump Test.* It is calculated as follows: (weight × jump height)/height.

Sargent's measurement methods and charts were widely used in colleges and YMCAs, and his thinking has influenced exercise science to the present day. He must be considered one of the great pioneers in U.S. exercise science.

TABLE 2.1   Prominent Historical Figures in Exercise Science

Name	Date	Contribution
Important Figures in the Emergence of Exercise Science		
Dudley A. Sargent	1849–1924	Developed a comprehensive system for individual exercise programs at the Hemenway Gymnasium.
George W. Fitz	1860–1934	Established the first formal laboratory in physical education in the United States at Harvard University in 1891.
Lawrence J. Henderson	1878–1942	Established the Harvard Fatigue Laboratory in the School of Business Administration at Harvard University in 1927.
David B. Dill	1891–1986	Research director at the Harvard Fatigue Laboratory from 1927 to 1947.
Sid Robinson	1903–1981	Student of D. B. Dill who conducted classic research on the effects of aging on the heart and lungs (31).
Ancel Keys	1904–	Developed the Laboratory of Physiological Hygiene at the University of Minnesota.
Kenneth H. Cooper	1931–	Known as the father of aerobics for his many books on the subject and established the Cooper Institute in Dallas, Texas, for the study of exercise and health.
YMCA Leaders and Exercise Science		
Arthur H. Steinhaus	1897–1970	Established the YMCA-supported exercise physiology laboratory at George Williams College in 1923.
Peter V. Karpovich	1896–1975	Established the YWCA-supported exercise physiology laboratory at Springfield College in 1927.
Thomas K. Cureton	1901–1993	Professor at the University of Illinois and a leader in the physical fitness movement following World War II.
Important U.S. Leadership by Scientists Trained Abroad		
Bruno Balke	1907–1999	Professor at the University of Wisconsin–Madison who was influential in starting the American College of Sports Medicine and was the first editor in chief of the ACSM research journal *Medicine and Science in Sport.*
Ulrich Luft	1910–1991	Contemporary of Bruno Balke who became director of the Physiology Research Laboratory at the Lovelace Foundation in Albuquerque, New Mexico.
Ernst Simonson	1898–1974	Professor at the University of Minnesota who published classic work in the area of muscle fatigue (33).
Wilhelm Raab	1895–1970	Cardiologist at the University of Vermont whose research provided a scientific foundation for exercise in the prevention of ischemic heart disease (22, 29).

Name	Date	Contribution
Hans Kraus	1905–1996	Coauthor with Wilhelm Raab regarding the physical fitness of U. S. schoolchildren and the need for exercise to improve health (22).

Important British Exercise Scientists

Name	Date	Contribution
Archibald V. Hill	1886–1977	Shared the 1922 Nobel prize for physiology or medicine with Otto Meyerhof for research on energy metabolism (15, 16).
John S. Haldane	1860–1936	Studied the role of carbon dioxide in the control of breathing and developed a respiratory gas analyzer that bears his name.
Claude G. Douglas	1882–1963	Conducted pioneering research with J. S. Haldane on the role of oxygen and lactic acid in the control of breathing during exercise and developed the Douglas Bag for collecting respiratory gases.

Important German Exercise Scientists

Name	Date	Contribution
Christian Wilhelm Braune	1831–1892	Conducted early studies on human gait.
Otto Fischer	1861–1917	Coauthored pioneering studies with W. C. Braune on human gait.
Werner W. Siebert		First researcher to demonstrate experimentally that the increase in muscle size as a result of resistance training is due to increases in the diameter of existing muscle fibers and not an increase in the number of fibers.
Julius Wolff	1836–1902	Proposed Wolff's law of bone transformation.
Otto Meyerhof	1884–1951	1922 Nobel prize winner for physiology or medicine (shared with A. V. Hill) who studied anaerobic energy transformation.
Erich A. Müller		Conducted pioneering research on various aspects of muscular fatigue (26) and coauthored a popular paper in 1953 with Theodor Hettinger on isometric training and strength gain (27).
H. W. Knipping		Published important papers on respiratory physiology and age changes in maximum oxygen consumption (19, 20).
Wildor Hollmann	1925–	Studied the effect of physical activity on the age trend of loss in aerobic power (17).

Important Scandinavian Exercise Scientists

Name	Date	Contribution
August Krogh	1874–1949	Danish Nobel prize winner in 1920 for physiology or medicine who studied capillary regulation and the effect of nutrition on efficiency of muscle work (23).
Erling Asmussen	1907–1991	Best known for his classic review of research on muscle fatigue (1).

(continued)

TABLE 2.1   Continued

Name	Date	Contribution
Erik Hohwu-Christensen	1904–	Published a classic paper (7) on the effects of exercise and work on heart-rate responses, which was the basis for later tests of physical fitness.
Per-Olaf Astrand	1922–	A student of E. H. Christensen who coauthored a classic textbook with Kaare Rodahl in exercise physiology entitled *Textbook of Work Physiology* (3).

George W. Fitz (1860–1934) earned his M.D. degree at Harvard University in 1891, and it has been suggested that he was influenced by Dudley Sargent, who was at the time the director of the Hemenway Gymnasium, as discussed above (14). He was among the first to deplore the uncritical acceptance of various systems of physical training (Swedish, German, and others) that were in vogue at the time. It was his lifelong contention that the advocacy of various theories and beliefs regarding exercise and its effects on the human organism must be based on solid physiological research. With such beliefs, it is not surprising that he established the first formal research laboratory in physical education in the United States at Harvard University in 1891. Physiological responses to exercise were measured at this site (5). In 1892, the Physiological Laboratory was established as part of the Lawrence Scientific School, a unit of Harvard University. The founding of the laboratory was accompanied by the establishment of the nation's first degree program in physical education, a Bachelor of Science in Anatomy, Physiology, and Physical Training. Each advanced student was required to complete some line of original research and report his results in a thesis. Thus, the emphasis on physiological research, Fitz's special concern, was the hallmark of the Harvard program (14). With these accomplishments in mind, it is not surprising that some have suggested that Fitz was the "father of exercise physiology" (32).

The Harvard Fatigue Laboratory, 1927–1947.   No account of the history of exercise science would be complete without recognition of the outstanding contributions of the *Harvard Fatigue Laboratory,* which became the mecca of exercise research in the late 1920s and until its closure in 1947 and trained many of the U.S. leaders in the field during that time. These leaders in turn trained second- and third-generation leaders, who still reflect this Harvard Fatigue Laboratory influence into the present.

Lawrence J. Henderson (1878–1942), a renowned biochemist, brought together an influential group of people and convinced them to back the formation of this laboratory within the School of Business Administration at Harvard University. *David Bruce Dill* (1891–1986) was the research director from the laboratory's inception until it closed in 1947. Both the name of the laboratory and its location in the business school seem incongruous with the breadth of research conducted and the many world famous exercise scientists who trained in or visited the facility. The laboratory conducted research in both the laboratory and field. Although major emphases were exercise and environmental physiology research, review of the literature reveals classic studies in numerous other areas, such as clinical physiology, gerontology, blood characteristics, nutrition, and physical fitness.

Perhaps most importantly, this laboratory became an example for the development of other important institutions, such as the *Institute for Environmental Stress* headed by Steven Horvath, a student (and son-in-law) of Dill. This institute, at the University of California at Santa Barbara, in turn served as the training ground for many of our contemporary investigators, such as Jack Wilmore, now at the Texas A & M University, and Barbara Drinkwater, who went to the University of Washington but is now in hospital research. Outstanding among the students of Dill was Sid Robinson, who did his doctoral work in a study of aging published in 1938. This study has become a classic source for the effects of aging on heart and lung functions and work capacity in the elderly.

Another famous research institute patterned after the Harvard Fatigue Laboratory was the *Laboratory for Physiological Hygiene* developed by Ancel Keys (1904–   ) at the University of Minnesota. Such renowned and prolific investigators as Ellsworth Buskirk (1925–   ) and Henry Longstreet Taylor (1912–1983) were among the many active researchers in the field of exercise science. Indeed, Buskirk became the director of the Noll Laboratory at Pennsylvania State University, and this might be considered the third generation of research institutes proliferating from the original Harvard Fatigue Laboratory as exemplar.

During the early days of the conception of the Harvard Fatigue Laboratory, Arlie Bock (1888–1984), another Harvard product and already a renowned physiologist, played a key role in its formation as advisor and research collaborator with D. B. Dill. Bock was renowned for analyzing the gas concentrations of venous and arterial blood. He was adept at the painstaking procedures of gas analysis and, in general, a consummate scientist and dedicated physician. He remained close friends with Dill for 59 years before passing on at age 95 (12).

The important papers in exercise science from the Harvard Fatigue Laboratory began to appear in 1928. Over 50 papers on exercise eventually were published during the 20 years of the program's existence. As demonstrated by many of these papers, personnel associated with the laboratory established exceptional technology and developed considerable insight as to the effects of exercise (plus different ambient conditions) on intact human subjects. Among those who worked in the laboratory, most have expressed the presence of a great esprit de corps that developed from working within the Henderson–Dill–Bock–Mayo ambiance (5). The prevailing camaraderie and generous intellectual exchange provided the stage for significant accomplishment and an exemplary laboratory role model for additional generations of exercise scientists (5). It was exceedingly unfortunate that Harvard's president James B. Conant in 1947 decreed the demise of the Fatigue Laboratory, largely because he was doubtful of its postwar value (6, 18).

D. B. Dill later joined Sid Robinson, who had relocated to Indiana University, where he established the Human Physiology Laboratory. In his later years, Dill moved to the new laboratory at the University of Nevada at Las Vegas, where he continued to do important research on exercise and environmental research in the desert and organized high-altitude research at White Mountain, California. The work at Las Vegas and White Mountain continued until his death in 1986.

In summary, it should be pointed out that the influence of D. B. Dill and his colleagues at the Harvard Fatigue Laboratory far exceeded in breadth the important effects on the successor U.S. institutions inspired by their work. Their invited foreign colleagues included such internationally recognized scientists as Erling Asmussen (1907–1991), Erik Hohwu-Christensen (1904–   ), Marius Nielsen (1903–   ), and August Krogh (Nobel Prize winner in 1920; 1874–1949) from Denmark. Rodolpho Margaria (1901–   ) from Italy came to extend his classic work on oxygen debt. Another famous visitor was Peter F. Scholander (1905–1980) from Norway, who developed the very clever respiratory gas analyzer that largely replaced the older Haldane analyzer and that all the older generation of exercise physiologists spent many hours over in the course of their laboratory apprenticeships.

Cooper Institute.   One of the most important figures in bringing about the remarkable increase in running and physical fitness, in general, was *Kenneth H. Cooper,* M.D. (1931–   ), a physician trained at the University of Oklahoma School of Medicine and the Harvard School of Public Health, who has been very persuasive in both his lectures and writing (18). His system, which he called *aerobics,* was well accepted by the U.S. public, who found his aerobics fitness scoring system interesting and simple to use. During the 1970s, jogging became very widely accepted as a desirable form of physical activity for men and women, to a large extent because of the work of Cooper and his wife Mildred. Its rise in popularity is illustrated by the fact that participation in the San Francisco Bay to Breakers run increased from 124 individuals in 1964 to 80,000 in 1985. Cooper also set up a research institute in Dallas, Texas, and he and his colleagues continue to report very important data based on the thousands of clients who participated in the exercise programs at the Cooper Institute.

Contributions of YMCA Leaders to Exercise Science

Scores of outstanding leaders in exercise science have traced their origins to the YMCA. Of these, three deserve mention as major contributors to exercise science.

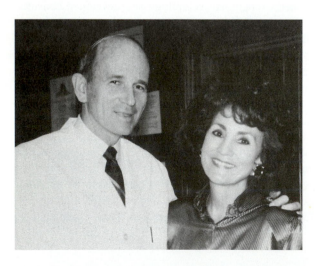

Kenneth H. Cooper, M.D., M.P.H., and Mildred Cooper.

Courtesy of The Cooper Aerobic Center, Dallas, Texas.

Arthur H. Steinhaus (1897–1970) identified himself as a "middle man" between scientists who discover knowledge and consumers who should profit therefrom. Although it is true that he was indeed an interpreter and philosopher of exercise science to the practitioners of health and fitness, he made many original contributions to our knowledge base. He and his students performed research on the tension and resilience of human muscles, components of strength, muscular coordination, and acid–base balance during exercise. Significantly, Steinhaus published two exemplary reviews that had a major impact on exercise physiology in the 1930s and 1940s (5). Indeed, the present author had the great pleasure of knowing this erudite gentleman through a sharing of laboratory interests and methods. Steinhaus felt it to be his good fortune to have been associated with one of the two colleges that were originally founded to train personnel for the YMCA (34). He was the founder in 1923 of the second laboratory devoted to exercise physiology in YMCA-supported schools, in this case at George Williams College in Chicago, where he began training students for laboratory-based research. He authored 165 published articles and was internationally renowned as a guest lecturer. He retired in 1963.

In the early 1900s, physiologic research was begun at Springfield College, another YMCA-supported institution, which was later developed into a true laboratory under the direction of *Peter V. Karpovich* (1896–1975), a Russian immigrant who had been briefly associated with the Harvard Fatigue Laboratory. Some writers have credited him with introducing physiology to physical education in the United States. Karpovich established his own research facility and taught physiology at Springfield College (Massachusetts) from 1927 until his death in 1975. Although he made numerous contributions to physical education and exercise science research, he is best remembered for the outstanding students he advised (35).

Thomas K. Cureton, (1901–1993), who started his career at Springfield College as a swimming coach (while also doing research), moved to the University of Illinois, where he created an exercise physiology laboratory in 1941 that has become famous for its contributions to the understanding of the importance of physical fitness. Probably no single individual deserves more credit for the physical fitness movement since World War II than Cureton. This is so for two reasons: (1) his voluminous writing and motivational seminars (2) the large number of well-trained and highly motivated students who followed him into positions of leadership in university exercise physiology laboratories.

Although there was some awareness in the 1800s of a need for regular physical activity to maintain optimal health, the issue probably seemed unimportant when relatively few could luxuriate in the life of the "couch potato," as is presently possible for many. In any event, Cureton continued his research and lecturing through World War II (when this writer first met and was suitably impressed by both the man and his convictions). Physical fitness programs developed by Cureton and his students, as well as Kenneth Cooper's 1968 book *Aerobics* (8), established a physiological rationale for using exercise to promote a healthy life-style. Cureton continued his research and lecturing until his retirement in 1971.

Important U.S. Leadership by Scientists Trained Abroad

It has been well recognized how much U.S. nuclear science has been aided by German scientists brought to the United States after World War II in the 1940s. Less well recognized is the fact that exercise science and particularly exercise physiology benefited similarly

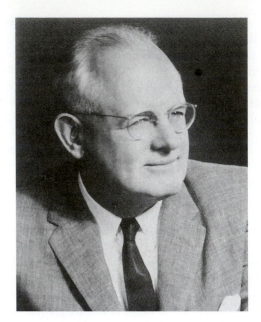

Dr. Thomas K. Cureton.
Courtesy of Dr. Kirk Cureton.

from outstanding scientists who trained in Germany and were induced to move their activity to the United States.

Bruno Balke (1907–1999), M.D., received his training in medicine and physical education in Germany and was invited to this country by *Ulrich Luft* (1910–1991), M.D., in 1950. These two eminent physicians shared an interest in aerospace physiology, and in the 1950s both did research on high-altitude effects and other aerospace research. Luft, who was also trained in Germany, became the director of the Physiology Research Laboratory at the Lovelace Foundation in Albuquerque, New Mexico, where he remained until his death. Although he was mainly recognized for his work in aerospace physiology and respiratory physiology, he was also interested in the physiology of aging and exercise physiology and trained many scientists now active in our field. He also produced many important papers for our field, but he did not achieve the widespread recognition he so richly deserved, because most of the publications from his laboratory appeared in aerospace literature not widely read by exercise scientists.

Balke did research on aerospace questions for the Civil Aeromedical Research Institute and the U.S. Air Force. He also developed one of the most widely used treadmill testing methods for evaluating work capacity, a method that still bears his name.

Balke was an early influence on the American College of Sports Medicine (ACSM), founded in 1954, and he served as its president in 1966. He was a leader in the development of the ACSM program of certification for exercise leaders of fitness and cardiac rehabilitation programs. In 1963, he left government service to start the Biodynamics Laboratory at the University of Wisconsin at Madison. He is reported to have produced 52 Ph.D. graduates from his laboratory (28). Dr. Balke was also a leader in the formation of the ACSM journal entitled *Medicine and Science in Sport* and became its first editor in 1969.

Another German transplant who made important contributions to U.S. exercise science was *Ernst Simonson* (1898–1974), M.D., whose interest in work performance and fatigue dates back to his earlier postdoctoral years and his appointment in 1928 as head of the Division of Industrial Physiology at the University of Frankfurt (Germany). From 1930 to 1937, he was scientific director of the Institute of Labor of the Ukraine (USSR). In 1937, Simonson moved to Prague, Czechoslovakia, to do similar work on the application of physiologic knowledge to the organization of industrial tasks and the conditions of work, but his work there was interrupted by Hitler's invasion of Czechoslovakia in 1939 and Simonson departed for the United States. After a productive period with his sponsor, Norbert Enzer in Milwaukee, he joined the staff of the Laboratory of Physiological Hygiene at the University of Minnesota in 1944, where he spent the rest of his professional life. He published many important papers but, unfortunately, most were in German. However, his greatest contribution, *Physiology of Work Capacity and Fatigue* (33), is in English and represents a compilation of research in exercise physiology (1500 references) from all over the world that only he had the linguistic ability to read and translate.

Another important German (Austrian) scientist who migrated to the United States because of World War II was the cardiologist *Wilhelm Raab* (1895–1970), M.D., who was invited to join the medical faculty at the University of Vermont, where he remained until his death. He spent most of his professional life in an effort to provide a scientific foundation for the need for exercise to aid in the prevention of ischemic heart disease. Two books were seminal in this regard: *Hypokinetic Disease—Diseases Produced by Lack of Exercise* (22) and *Prevention of Ischemic Heart Disease* (29). The first was written jointly with his friend and fellow German expatriate, *Hans Kraus* (1905–1996), M.D., who was also important in calling attention to the poor physical fitness of U.S. schoolchildren (21). Kraus and Raab, in both their many published papers and frequent lectures, pointed out that we in the United States were far behind in the promotion of physical rehabilitation centers such as were well supported in European societies. Table 2.2 illustrates their point. The present author spent 12 weeks visiting the German centers and collaborating in research evaluating the efficacy of the program at the pioneering center at Ohlstadt, headed by the well-known German internist Peter Beckman (9).

Under the impact of rapidly rising cardiac mortality in prosperous postwar Germany and other European countries, several farsighted social insurance organizations and industries initiated in 1955 an organized system of active prophylaxis against ischemic heart disease; they sponsored the development of reconditioning centers for workers who were

TABLE 2.2   Number of Preventive Reconditioning Centers in European Countries Compared to the USA (29)

Soviet Union	2100	Switzerland	4
Czechoslovakia	400	Austria	4
East Germany	400	United States	0
West Germany	20		

showing symptoms of "nervous exhaustion" and early heart disease. Workers were sent for 4 to 6 weeks to locations selected for scenic beauty, usually in mountainous terrain, where they underwent 5 to 6 hours per day of outdoor calisthenics, relaxation training, breathing exercises, and hiking and mountain climbing, complemented by various baths. Such programs were more widespread in the eastern European countries probably because they were largely government supported.

Although Kraus and Raab were successful in bringing about a perception that physical activity was beneficial in reducing the mortality and morbidity of cardiovascular diseases as well as improving the quality of life, the European programs never made their way across the Atlantic. However, in the 1960s the need for exercise and fitness became increasingly recognized by virtue of the work of such leaders as Kraus and Raab, the efforts of the American Alliance for Health, Physical Education, Recreation, and Dance, and the President's Council on Physical Fitness.

Exponential Growth of Leaders in Exercise Science in Contemporary Times

The large number of people who now provide leadership in exercise science prohibits consideration of most contemporary individuals. Fortunately, an outstanding leader in exercise science research, Henry J. Montoye and his colleague, Richard Washburn, at the University of Wisconsin have provided a genealogy of contributors to the *Research Quarterly* (Figure 2.1), which includes most of the leadership in exercise science up to their date of publication, 1980 (25). For the reader interested in pursuing the genealogy of leadership from the allied health professionals, an excellent source is available (24). It must be noted that the effects of any one important research institution are far greater than the work of the leaders themselves because of the multiplicative effect brought about by their students.

History of Exercise Science in Europe

Important British Exercise Scientists

Archibald V. Hill (1886–1977) was awarded the Nobel prize (shared with Otto Meyerhof) in 1922 in the category of physiology or medicine for his findings on energy metabolism. In 1923, he was honored as the Joddrell Professor of Physiology at University College, London. He was also a frequent visitor to the United States as a research collaborator at Cornell University in New York and visited Arlie Bock's Laboratory at Harvard in 1926. Hill was a brilliant scientist whose pioneering work was well received in the United States. Although he could deal with the most complex biochemical processes of his time, he was also able to focus his keen mind on the problems of muscle physiology of interest to athletes and runners in particular. His development of the inertia wheel for studying accelerated muscular contraction in the human body is a case in point. His publications are too numerous for description here, but two of his most important books deserve a place in every exercise scientist's library: *Muscular Movement in Man* (15) and *Living Machinery* (16). He was truly one of the greatest philosophers in the field of exercise physiology.

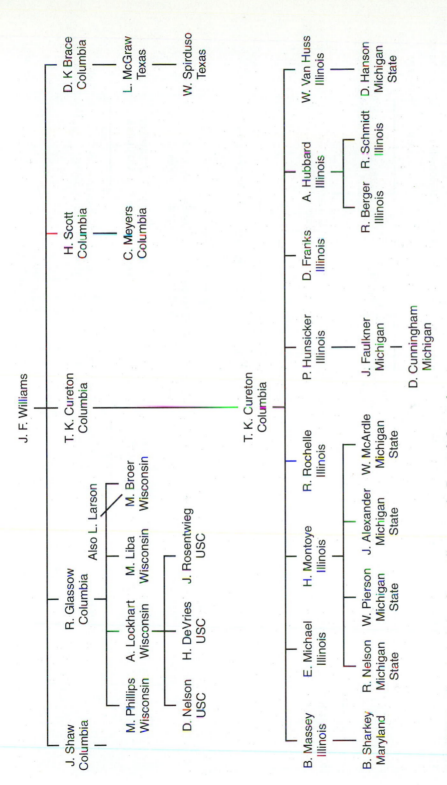

FIGURE 2.1 Genealogical chart for contributors to the *Research Quarterly*.

(*continued*)

FIGURE 2.1 *Continued*

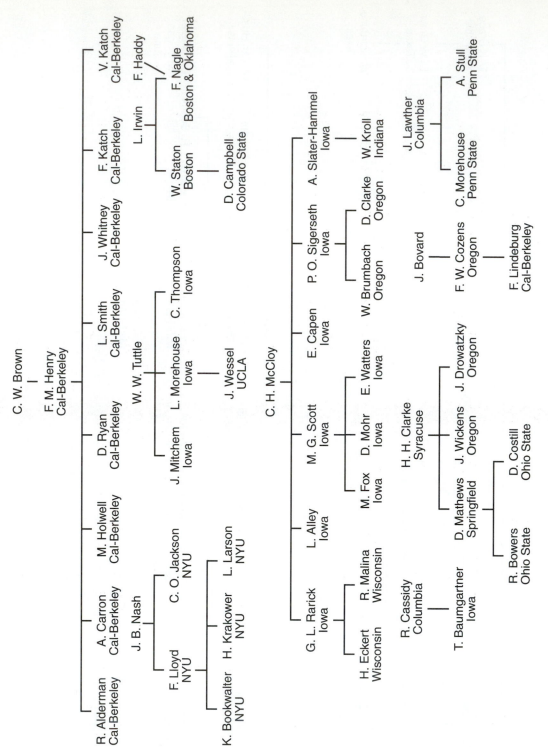

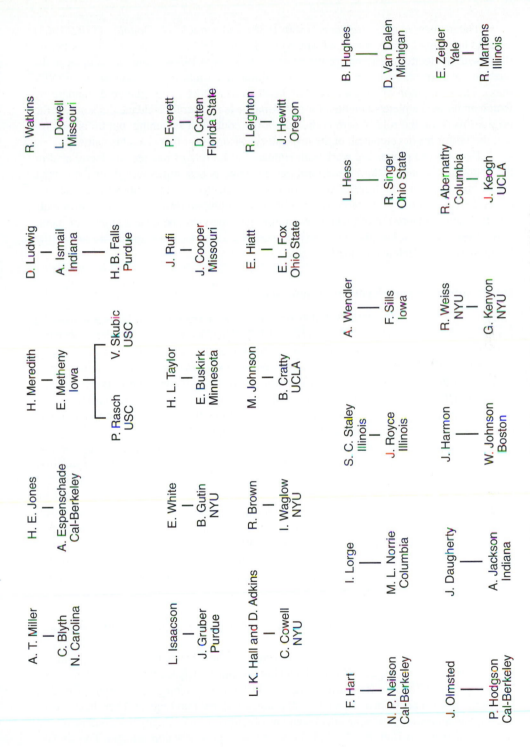

Reprinted with permission from *Research Quarterly for Exercise and Sport*, Vol. 51, No. 1, pp. 261–266, © 1980 by the American Alliance for Health, Physical Education, Recreation and Dance, 1900 Association Drive, Reston, VA 20191.

The names *John S. Haldane* (1860–1936) and *Claude G. Douglas* (1882–1963) became household words among all who worked in the field of exercise physiology before the advent of electronic gas analyzers and computers (circa 1950s) made life simpler in the analyses of respiratory gases necessary to estimate maximal oxygen consumption (VO_2 max). The estimation of VO_2 max was and still is, to a large extent, the gold standard by which endurance athlete's potential for performance is measured. Haldane did some of the original work on the role of carbon dioxide in the control of breathing, but he is best remembered for his development of the respiratory gas analyzer that bears his name.

Douglas did pioneering work with Haldane in the role of oxygen and lactic acid in the control of breathing during exercise, but his name is best remembered for the canvas and rubber bags in which respiratory gases were collected while a subject exercised on either a treadmill or cycle ergometer. We now have computerized electronic instruments that take the drudgery out of making respiratory gas analyses and measurements of metabolic rates and capacities, but none has yet surpassed the accuracy and reliability of the Douglas Bag and Haldane method.

Important German Exercise Scientists

Among the earliest experimental studies of human gait were those by *Christian Wilhelm Braune* (1831–1892) and *Otto Fischer* (1861–1917). Their work is still considered of major importance as the foundation for studies involving biomechanical aspects of walking (30).

Werner W. Siebert was the first to demonstrate experimentally that muscular hypertrophy develops only after a muscle is forced to work intensively: the forerunner to what we now call the *overload principle.* Siebert and his colleagues showed that increased strength and hypertrophy are a result of an increase in the diameter of the individual fibers of a muscle and not of an increase in the numbers of fibers (34).

In 1892, *Julius Wolff* (1836–1902) expressed the classic concept regarding the formation of bony tissue: Every change in the form and function of a bone or, of their function alone, is followed by certain definite changes in their internal architecture and equally definite secondary alteration in their external conformation in accordance with mathematical laws. However, Wolff's law of bone transformation is thought to be an overstatement. Bone forms in response to many factors, including hereditary tendencies, nutrition, disease, and hormonal and biochemical influences (30).

Otto Meyerhof (1884–1951) was one of the earliest investigators to shed light on the energy transformations involved in anaerobic metabolism. In 1922, he shared the Nobel prize for physiology or medicine with A. V. Hill for their work on the metabolism of lactic acid in muscle.

Erich A. Müller is best known for his work on questions relating to work, endurance, and fatigue and the related questions of interest in industrial physiology (*arbeitsphysiologie*). Müller did some of the pioneering work concerning the relationships between load and endurance (26). The only aspect of his work that has become widely known in the United States is his paper with Theodor Hettinger on the use of isometric training for strength gain (27), one of the few papers from his laboratory that was translated into English. Their findings indicated that a maximum training effect could be obtained from one daily 6-second isometric contraction against two-thirds of an individual's maximum contraction strength. This finding has been widely reported in the exercise science literature and in the popular press, but much of Müller's other work has been of greater scientific importance.

H. W. Knipping contributed to the literature on respiratory physiology (19) and also important data on the age changes in maximum oxygen consumption (20).

Wildor Hollmann (1925–) provided the most convincing demonstration of the delay of the age trend of losses in aerobic power by physical training. Maximal oxygen consumption was measured from 1949 to 1952 and again in 1964. The maximal oxygen consumption of the sedentary group decreased to 69% of the initial value, whereas the physically active group only declined to 90% of the original value (17). Later work in the United States substantiated these data.

Important Scandinavian Exercise Scientists

We are indeed fortunate that so much of the important work by the exercise scientists of Scandinavia has been published in English. Since this is not true to the same extent for the scientific papers of France and Germany, it is not surprising that we have probably been influenced to a greater degree by the Scandinavians. Also, it has been pointed out that early contacts between D. B. Dill and *August Krogh* (1874–1949), a Danish Nobel prize winner in 1920 for physiology or medicine, led to the coming of three outstanding Danish physiologists to the Harvard Fatigue Laboratory in the 1930s. Krogh encouraged E. H. Christensen, E. Asmussen, and M. Nielsen to spend time at Harvard studying the effects of heat and high altitude on exercise (35). Krogh himself made many contributions to exercise science; one of the earlier studies of the effect of nutrition upon efficiency of muscle work was published with J. Lindhard in 1920 (23); they compared the relative values of fat and carbohydrate as sources of muscular energy. Their work has long been used to support the concept of greater mechanical efficiency of work done using carbohydrate rather than fat, although the difference is small (circa 5%). After visiting scientist stints at the Harvard Fatigue Laboratory, Christensen moved to Stockholm, Sweden, to become the first physiology professor at the College of Physical Education at Gynastik och Idrottshogkolan, while Asmussen and Nielsen became professors at the University of Copenhagen in Denmark.

The work of *Erling Asmussen* (1907–1991) contributed to many areas of physiology, but the greatest number of papers dealt with problems of exercise physiology, usually with direct application to physical education and sports. Thus, some of his more important papers covered (1) the importance of warm-up, (2) a comparison of oxygen consumption in positive versus negative work, (3) causes of muscle soreness, (4) uses of electromyography, and possibly his most important and best known work, (5) a summary of research on muscle fatigue (1).

In 1931, *Erik Hohwu-Christensen* (1904–) provided a classic study regarding the effects of exercise and work on heart-rate responses. This study formed the basis for much further research and for many of our later tests of physical fitness based on heart-rate response (7).

Christensen teamed with Ole Hansen in the late 1930s to publish a series of five studies of carbohydrate and fat metabolism during exercise. These studies are still cited frequently and are considered to be among the first and most important sport nutrition studies. In 1939, Christensen and Hansen provided the basis for the use of sugar in endurance athletics or in hard work, and their work suggested that the beneficial effect was in raising the blood sugar level for the central nervous system.

While Christensen's own studies became classic worldwide in their effects on the physiology of exercise, possibly an even greater effect on U.S. exercise science was indirect through his mentoring of Per-Olaf Astrand.

Per-Olaf Astrand (1922–   ) credits E. H. Christensen for having introduced him to the field of work physiology at the College of Physical Education at Gymnastik och Idrott-shogskolan (G. I. H.) in Stockholm, where he spent most of his academic career (3). In a visit to their laboratory in 1965, the present writer acquired a publication list in which Astrand had credit for 62 publications starting in 1952. Fortunately, most of his publications are available in English and thus have been of great interest to U.S. exercise science students. This level of production has not slowed down since 1965, and one must assume that he and his colleagues (including his wife I. Astrand) have probably published close to 500 meaningful contributions to our knowledge of exercise physiology. One of his important works is *Textbook of Work Physiology* (3), written with his colleague Kaare Rodahl and first published in 1970. Among exercise scientists, he is best known for the test of physical fitness based on heart-rate response to a measured power output on a cycle ergometer. This test is based on the Astrand–Ryhming Nomogram (2) and is usually referred to simply as the Astrand test, since I. Ryhming became P. O. Astrand's wife. Both Astrands have had a long-term interest in the physiology of aging and have contributed important papers on this subject.

Present and Future Trends in Exercise Science

It is presently very difficult for most university departments of physical education to serve the needs of both teacher preparation and the next generation of exercise scientists. To begin with, even the high school background in sciences required for successful progress as undergraduate students is very different between those heading into teaching jobs and those whose destination lies in exercise science. In this writer's experience, we have required very little science background for matriculation as physical education students. On the other hand, students heading toward careers in exercise science must be required to present with a solid high school background in at least biology, physics, chemistry, and mathematics, including introduction to calculus. Whether such a science background for those going into teaching physical education or coaching is necessary or even desirable is debatable. However, students going into exercise science must be so prepared in order that they will have the prerequisite knowledge and skills to handle university undergraduate courses such as physiology, biochemistry, kinesiology, and biomechanics in depth. The undergraduate courses must be in depth in order to allow successful participation in professional schools of medicine or physical therapy and in graduate work, which will probably be focused evermore on molecular biology, advanced biochemistry, and biophysics.

Thus, we are on the horns of a dilemma if a (usually) small faculty of physical education (usually) poorly supported by research funds is to be expected to produce both physical education teacher–coaches and also scholar–practitioners to attack the increasingly complex problems of exercise science research. To exacerbate this problem, it must also be recognized that very seldom can we find faculty members who are capable of leadership in both domains, even if there were enough hours in the day.

Many university programs have already recognized these problems, and the solution seems to lie in the division of what has in the past been simply physical education into what has become two departments: (1) a department directed toward pedagogy (now usually called Physical Education) and (2) a department directed toward the development of the scholar, which currently often assumes the name Exercise Science or Kinesiology.

In this writer's opinion, this trend will continue and will probably accelerate for many reasons: (1) an increasing level of sophistication in exercise science, (2) an ever increasing cost of instrumentation, (3) a movement from systems-oriented physiology of exercise toward molecular biology, (4) an ever increasing competition for limited research grants, (5) student interest in nonteaching options related to exercise and physical fitness, and (6) the science-based entrance requirements for professional schools.

This writer is optimistic that the enhanced preparation of exercise scientists may result in an interesting and rewarding future in which the new problems of health care and delivery can only help to open up the job market, as more and more of the general public continue to be interested in the effects of exercise as a preventive and therapeutic modality.

Summary

Many of the pioneers in exercise science were medical doctors who recognized the need for science-based principles to guide the development of exercise programs for athletes and nonathletes. There were a number of important individuals who contributed to the development of exercise science and many were in some way associated with the Harvard Fatigue Laboratory (1927–1947). Still today, the lineage of prominent exercise scientists can be traced to the Harvard Fatigue Laboratory. In addition, scores of outstanding leaders in exercise science from the United States were associated with the YMCA through George Williams College and Springfield College. Furthermore, many well-recognized exercise scientists were trained abroad, particularly in Germany, England, and Scandinavia.

Critical to the evolution of exercise science in the United States was the establishment of the American College of Sports Medicine in 1954. The ACSM is widely recognized throughout the world as the preeminent professional association for exercise scientists.

S T U D Y   Q U E S T I O N S

1. Discuss the role of the American College of Sports Medicine in the evolution of exercise science.

2. Name two important figures associated with the Harvard Fatigue Laboratory and describe their contributions to exercise science.

3. Briefly discuss the contributions of the Cooper Institute and its founder Kenneth Cooper to the physical fitness movement.

4. Discuss the implication of the end of World War II to the development of exercise science in the United States.

5. Describe and defend your opinion of the future of exercise science based on the current trends in the field.

GLOSSARY

ACSM   American College of Sports Medicine.

Aerobics   Any physical exercise that requires additional effort by the heart and lungs to meet the increased demand by the skeletal muscles for oxygen.

Anatomy   The study of the parts of an organism and their relationship to each other.

Athletes heart   Enlarged heart of a trained endurance athlete.

Fatigue   A state of exhaustion or a loss of strength or endurance, as may follow strenuous physical activity.

Hypokinetic disease   A disease associated with a lack of physical activity.

Ischemic heart disease   A pathologic condition of the myocardium caused by lack of oxygen reaching the tissue cells.

Kinesiology   The study of human motion.

Physical fitness   The ability to perform daily tasks with vigor and without undue fatigue.

Physiology   The study of the processes and function of the human body.

YMCA   Young Men's Christian Association.

SUGGESTED READING

Berryman, J. W. *Out of Many, One.* Champaign IL: Human Kinetics, 1995.

REFERENCES

1. Asmussen, E. Muscle fatigue. *Med. Sci. Sports* 11:313–321, 1979.

2. Astrand, P. O., and I. Ryhming. A nomogram for calculation of aerobic capacity (physical fitness) from pulse rate during submaximal work. *J. Appl. Physiol.* 7:218–21, 1954.

3. Astrand, P. O., and K. Rodahl. *Textbook of Work Physiology.* New York: McGraw-Hill Book Company, 1970.

4. Belloc, N. B., and L. Breslow. Relationship of physical health status and health practices. *Prevent. Med.* 1:409–421, 1972.

5. Buskirk, E. R., and C. M. Tipton. Exercise physiology. In: *The History of Exercise and Sport Science,* J. D. Massengale and R. A. Swanson (Eds.). Champaign, IL: Human Kinetics, 1997, pp. 367–438.

6. Chapman, C. B. The long reach of Harvard's Fatigue Laboratory, 1927–1947. *Perspect. Biol. Med.* 34:17–33, 1990.

7. Christensen, E. H. Beitrage zur physiologie schwerer körperlicher arbeit. *Arbeitsphysiologie* 4:453–469, 1931.

8. Cooper, K. H. *Aerobics.* New York: Bantam Books, 1968.

9. deVries, H. A., P. Beckman, H. Huber, and H. Dieckmeier. Physiological effects of sauna on the neuromuscular system. *J. Sports Med. Phys. Fitness* 8:16–19, 1968.

10. deVries, H. A. Physiological effects of an exercise training regimen upon men aged 52–88. *J. Gerontol.* 25:325–336, 1970.

11. deVries, H. A., and T. J. Housh. *Physiology of Exercise,* 5th ed. Madison, WI: Brown and Benchmark, 1994.

12. Dill, D. B. Arlie V. Bock, Pioneer in sports medicine, Dec. 30, 1888–Aug. 11, 1984. *Med. Sci. Sports Exerc.* 17:401–404, 1985.

13. Fiatarone, M. A., E. C. Marks, N. D. Ryan, C. N. Meredith, L. A. Lipsitz, and W. J. Evans. High intensity strength training in nonagenarians. *J. A. M. A.* 263:3029–3034, 1990.

14. Gerber, E. W. *Innovators and Institutions in Physical Education.* Philadelphia: Lea and Febiger, 1971, pp. 292–297.

15. Hill, A. V. *Muscular Movement in Man.* New York: McGraw-Hill Book Company, 1927.

16. Hill, A. V., *Living Machinery.* New York: Harcourt Brace Jovanovich, 1927.

17. Hollman, W. *Körperliches Training als Prävent von Herz-Kreislaufkrankheiten.* Stuttgart: Hippocrates-Verlag, 1965.

18. Horvath, S. M., and E. C. Horvath. *The Harvard Fatigue Laboratory: Its History and Contributions.* Englewood Cliffs, NJ: Prentice Hall, 1973.

19. Knipping, H. W. Uber die respiratorische insuffizienz. *Klin. Wschr.* 14:406, 1935.

20. Knipping, H. W., W. Bolt, H. Valentin, and H. Venrath, *Untersuchung und Beurteilung des Herzkranken.* Stuttgart: Enke-Verlag, 1960.

21. Kraus, H., and R. Hirschland. Minimum muscular fitness tests in school children. *Res. Q.* 25:178–185, 1954.

22. Kraus, H., and W. Raab. Hypokinetic Disease—Diseases Produced by Lack of Exercise. Springfield, IL: Charles C Thomas, 1961.

23. Krogh, A., and J. Lindhard. The relative value of fat and carbohydrate as sources of muscular energy with appendices on the correlation between standard metabolism and the respiratory quotient during rest and work. *Biochem. J.* 14:290, 1920.

24. Massengale, J. D., and R. A. Swanson (Eds.). *The History of Exercise and Sport Science.* Champaign, IL: Human Kinetics, 1997.

25. Montoye, H. J., and R. Washburn. *Research Quarterly* contributors: An academic genealogy. *Res. Q.* 51:261–266, 1980.

26. Müller, E. A. Das arbeitsmaximum bei statischer haltearbeit. *Arbeitsphysiologie* 5:605, 1932.

27. Müller, E. A., and T. Hettinger. Muskelleistung und muskel-training. *Arbeitsphysiologie* 15:111, 1953.

28. Powers, S. K., and E. T. Howley. *Exercise Physiology,* 2nd ed. Madison, WI: Brown and Benchmark, 1990.

29. Raab, W. *Prevention of Ischemic Heart Disease.* Springfield, IL: Charles C Thomas, 1966.

30. Rasch, P. J., and R. K. Burke. *Kinesiology and Applied Anatomy.* Philadelphia: Lea and Febiger, 1974.

31. Robinson, S. Experimental studies of physical fitness in relation to age. *Arbeitsphysiologie* 10:251–323, 1938.

32. Siedentop, D. *Introduction to Physical Education, Fitness and Sport.* Mountain View, CA: Mayfield Publishing Company, 1994.

33. Simonson, E. *Physiology of Work Capacity and Fatigue.* Springfield, IL: Charles C Thomas, 1971.

34. Steinhaus, A. H. *Toward an Understanding of Health and Physical Education.* Dubuque, IA: William C. Brown Company, 1963.

35. Wilmore, J. H., and D. L. Costill. *Physiology of Sport and Exercise.* Champaign, IL: Human Kinetics, 1994.

CHAPTER

3

Anatomy

GLEN O. JOHNSON

Definition of Anatomy

Anatomy and Exercise Science
Why Study Anatomy in Exercise Science?

History of Anatomy
Prescientific Period
Scientific Period
The Middle Ages
The Renaissance
Seventeenth through Twentieth Centuries

**Present-day Anatomy: Instrumentation
and Techniques**
Electron Microscope and Scanning
Electron Microscope
X-rays
Computerized Tomography

Positron Emission Tomography
Magnetic Resonance Imaging
Dual Energy X-ray Absorptiometry
Ultrasound Imagery Sonography

Employment Opportunities in Anatomy

Professional Associations

Prominent Journals

Concluding Remarks and Future Trends

Summary

Study Questions

Glossary

Suggested Readings

References

An old joke in departments of anatomy concerns a professor of anatomy being asked, "What do anatomists do?" The typical reply is "They do anatomy!" The response, although correct, tells us nothing about what anatomy is or what anatomists do. This chapter will describe what anatomy is and what anatomists do, present a brief history of anatomy, and describe how the study of anatomy is important and useful to the student in exercise science.

Definition of Anatomy

The word *anatomy* is from Greek origins and means "to cut" or "to cut up"(4). Today we refer to "cut up" as dissection. *Dissection* is the careful cutting up of cadavers (human bodies) to study body structures such as muscles, nerves, and vessels.

Modern textbooks of anatomy, however, define *anatomy* as follows: The study of the parts of the body and their relationship to each other. Anatomy can be broken down into different types of anatomical study or what are often called the subspecialties of anatomy. The major subspecialties of anatomy include the following:

Gross anatomy. The study of those body structures that one can see without the aid of a microscope. The beginning exercise science student will be particularly concerned with the study of gross human anatomy.

Histology (microscopic anatomy). The study of structures with the aid of a microscope. For example, the study of different types of cells and the structures within the cells.

Comparative anatomy. The comparison of anatomical structures of different animals, both the similarities and differences. For example, how does the wing of a bird compare to the arm and forearm of a human.

Embryology. The study of the anatomical changes that occur from conception to birth.

Developmental anatomy. The study of embryology as well as the anatomical changes that occur from birth to death. This type of anatomy is used in exercise science studies when studying the effect of exercise on growth and development.

Pathological anatomy. The study of the anatomical changes that occur in structures as a result of disease (1, 4, 9).

A student's first exposure to anatomy is likely to be a course in gross human anatomy. The method by which gross anatomy is presented or studied can vary. Most beginning courses in human anatomy use the *systemic* method of study. Systemic anatomy means that each of the systems of the body is studied independently before moving on to the next system. Typically, the skeletal system is studied first, then the muscular system, nervous system, circulatory system, and the rest of the 11 body systems in various order. The other method of study is *regional anatomy,* which means that everything about a specific region of the body is studied together. In this method, all the bones, muscles, nerves and vessels of the upper limb are learned at the same time before moving on to another body area. Beginning courses in anatomy typically use the systemic method, whereas advanced courses, such as those offered in medical schools, usually use the regional method of study. Gross human anatomy is best studied using dissected human cadavers. When cadavers are not available, reasonable knowledge can be obtained by studying animal bodies, such as cats or fetal pigs. Computer simulations of dissection and models are also helpful learning aids when used in conjunction with cadavers.

Anatomy and Exercise Science

Exercise science draws on many fields of science to accomplish its goals. Anatomy is one of the important specialty sciences used in exercise science.

Many of us began to study anatomy shortly after we learned our first words. What child has not been asked, "Where is your nose?" or "Where is your ear?" The child then points to the appropriate structure. This is the individual's first lesson in anatomy, learning the names of structures. It must, however, be emphasized that the study of anatomy involves more than just learning the Greek and Latin names of structures, although this is, in the author's opinion, certainly necessary. Where structures are located, their relationship to other structures, their growth, and their basic function are also critically important to the student of anatomy.

Why Study Anatomy in Exercise Science?

Anatomy is an essential science for many professions, including medicine, dentistry, physical and occupational therapy, nursing, physical education, and, of course, exercise science. The beginning exercise science student has several career options where a sound background in anatomy will be useful. Some will become certified exercise specialists designing exercises and leading exercise groups and/or coaching athletes. Others may move on to teaching and research positions at universities or pursue professional degrees in the medical or paramedical fields. In all situations, a firm grasp of basic anatomical concepts is essential.

For the exercise specialist and coach, an understanding of bone growth and its reaction to stress, the structure and function of joints and muscles, as well as vessel and nerve pathways, will aid them in designing appropriate exercises, eliminating commonly used but harmful exercises, and understanding injury and the repair of tissues.

The exercise science researcher must possess the above knowledge, as well as more in-depth insights regarding the structure of cells and tissues and the response of these to different types of exercise stress. For example, we are daily exposed by television and other media to a plethora of exercise devices and/or exercise systems, which more or less guarantee that we will lose weight, gain muscle, or attain super abdominals in "just a few minutes a day." Exercise scientists, by way of their training in anatomy and other sciences, must be credible sources about which claims are true and which have no realistic scientific validity. In addition, the relationship of exercise to growth and development, body composition, and the design and improvement of athletic equipment involves a knowledge of anatomy.

Children's sports participation and the appropriate amounts and types of exercise for schools are also important issues for exercise scientists, using their knowledge of anatomy. Children are not just small adults. Exercise and training programs must therefore be designed for them based on an intimate knowledge of a child's anatomy and the variation in growth at different ages. Body composition (basically the relationship of the amount of fat to the amount of lean tissue in the body) and its change during growth and training are other frequently studied areas in exercise science and are important with regard to sports performance and health. Anatomy provides the basis for the study and understanding of these areas. The study of biomechanics, described in Chapter 5, demands a thorough knowledge of anatomy with regard to boney levers, muscle attachments, and the types of movements of which different joints are capable. These few examples, however, merely scratch the surface about the importance of anatomy and how anatomy is used in exercise science. Figure 3.1 presents an abstract of a body composition research study.

FIGURE 3.1   **Abstract of a body composition study.**

Housh, T. J., G. O. Johnson, J. Stout, and D. J. Housh.
Anthropometric growth patterns of high school wrestlers.
Med. Sci. Sports Exerc., Vol. 25, No. 10, pp. 1141–1150, 1993.

The purpose of this investigation was to examine the anthropometric growth patterns of high school wrestlers; 477 high school wrestlers volunteered as subjects for this study. The total sample was divided into four independent age groups: Age group 1 (AG1) = 14.00–14.99 yr (N = 38); AG2 = 15.00–15.99 yr (N = 130); AG3 = 16.00–16.99 yr (N = 163); and AG4 = 17.00 – 17.99 yr (N = 146). Thirteen anthropometric dimensions (seven diameters and six circumferences) were taken on each subject. To examine normal growth patterns, the anthropometric data were compared with values from a national representative sample of adolescent males. The results indicated that there were few differences between the wrestlers and the national sample for yearly changes in the anthropometric dimensions. These findings suggest that participation in high school wrestling, which typically includes repeated bouts of weight cycling, does not adversely affect normal growth patterns.

Source: T. J. Housh et al., *Medicine and Science in Sports and Exercise* 25(10): 1141, 1993. Reprinted with permission.

History of Anatomy

As scientists, we must always be ready to ask the most basic, and to some infuriating, questions. In this case, I can already hear the groans of the students that might be assigned to read this chapter and I can hear their silent question. Why? Why study the history of anatomy, or any science, or any subject at all? One logical response is that if we do not study history we have no measure of the progress of human beings. In fact, the essence of human progress is increased knowledge. The following quote was written in 1930:

> Indeed the history of mankind is essentially the history of a gigantic struggle between light and darkness, between knowledge and ignorance. As the light gradually conquers the surrounding gloom, as science gradually destroys superstition, as rationality gradually replaces irrationality, and order, chaos, so—and not otherwise—does civilization increase. (10)

In today's tumultuous world we would do well to remember these words of wisdom and take some time to study how these beneficial changes came about.

Prescientific Period

Anatomy is one of the basic sciences and can be accurately considered one of the oldest branches of medicine (7). To the Paleolithic (cultural period from 750,000 to 15,000 years ago) hunter, some knowledge of anatomy must have been essential for survival. Drawings on the walls of caves of prehistoric peoples in Spain and France accurately show the location of the heart and other vital organs of mammoths and bison (Figure 3.2). Carvings

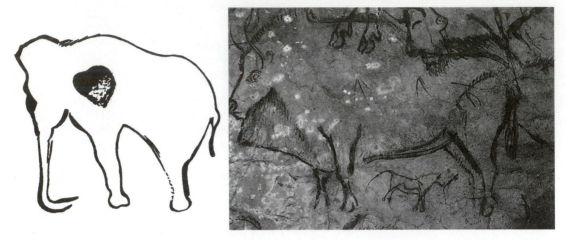

FIGURE 3.2   Paleolithic cave drawings from Spain and France showing elephant heart and bison with arrows in their hearts.

12,000 years old made from reindeer horns found in these caves demonstrate the dissected skull of a horse's head, as well as the shape of some of the surface muscles of the horse's head (7, 12, 15).

Paintings of human hands, estimated to be 30,000 years old, have also been found in a cave in France (12). We can only speculate what the paintings mean, but a good guess would be that the ancient humans were intrigued by the structure of the hand, either as a form of art or from a structural and functional perspective. Without question, the butchering of animals for meat and other tissues provided these hunters with practical knowledge about the structure and function of some organs. Knowing the location of the heart and the fact that piercing it was an efficient method of killing an animal would most certainly be important for these hunters' survival.

Prehistoric hunter and forager people were also probably knowledgeable about some aspects of their own bodies. They surely recognized that severely broken limb bones or torn muscles healed, but could lead to loss of motion or ineffective movement. They would know which wounds most likely meant death and which would heal well, and they likely had methods of hastening the healing of some injuries, perhaps by cauterization (burning of wounds) or the use of certain healing plants. Differences between the genders would have been apparent, but these people would probably not have understood reproductive functions (8, 16). There is evidence that 100,000 years ago humans used sharp flint stones to cut out round sections of living human skulls to expose the brain, a process called trephining (also trepanation: see Figure 3.3). The reasons for trephining are probably varied. One would be medical, that is, relief of head pain or repair of skull wounds. Another may have to do with superstition, perhaps to satisfy mystical gods or spirits (5, 8). However, we can only speculate about their knowledge about themselves and the world around them, although in this author's opinion they were likely far more attuned to their immediate envi-

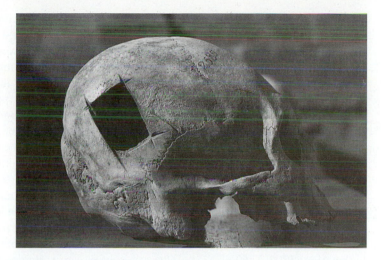

FIGURE 3.3   A prehistoric skull showing trephination.
Copyright © 1982 Daniele Pelleguni/Photo Researchers, Inc.

ronment than are many people today. Because there are no written records of these times, the era is referred to as the prescientific era.

Scientific Period

It is not realistic to present a complete, comprehensive review of the written history of anatomy in this chapter. An attempt will be made to cite some of the major contributors and events in the early development and advancement of anatomical study, recognizing that some individuals and some geographical areas will receive reduced coverage or not be mentioned. The interested student is encouraged to use the references at the end of this chapter for more detailed information.

It is also important that the student comprehend that, although dates of events or peoples' lives will be cited, the history of any subject is not just a series of dates. Ideas, concepts, and practices develop over periods of time (often many years), and these new ideas, even when correct, are often not readily accepted by the scholars and political and religious leaders of any historical period, including new discoveries or ideas that occur in today's world. Sometimes this nonacceptance of a new idea is a good thing when its reason is healthy scientific skepticism. At other times, nonacceptance is unhealthy when it is done to preserve questionable political, social, and/or religious power for the few to the detriment of peoples' lives. Dates are presented only to emphasize the approximate era when certain advances occurred. The development of anatomical knowledge closely paralleled advances in medicine; hence many important historical figures in anatomy were also famous physicians, or vice versa.

Traditional Western thought places the beginning of the scientific period, at least regarding anatomy, with the Greeks around 500 B.C. (1, 12, 15), although Homer describes the anatomy of wounds in the *Iliad* in 800 B.C.) (8, 16).

The Greeks, however, undoubtedly obtained some of their concepts regarding the human body from earlier Mesopotamian and Egyptian civilizations. The present country of Iraq contains the Tigris and Euphrates rivers. The fertile land between the two rivers was called Mesopotamia and is often referred to as the cradle of civilization (2, 8, 15, 16). Clay models of sheep's liver have been found (dated around 2000 B.C.) in Mesopotamia. Writings on them indicate that they were used more for religious purposes than anatomical study, but they were also important in medicine. For example, in Babylon (an ancient city on the Euphrates River) the liver was considered the seat of life (or guardian of the soul) and was much used in diagnosis. Sick people would breathe into the nose of a sheep, after which the sheep was killed and its liver removed. The medical diagnosis was made by comparing the sheep's liver to a clay model of a sheep's liver (5, 16). Obviously, such diagnoses were based on superstition and religious beliefs but the connection of illnesses to specific body organs was an important concept. A few records from Mesopotamia also describe surgeries that reflect a knowledge of anatomy. Some of these medical procedures are described in the Code of Hammurabi, which was mandated by *Hammurabi,* a great Babylonian king (1792–1750 or 1738–1686 B.C.; sources vary). Hammurabi may have begun building the Tower of Babel mentioned in the Christian Bible (Genesis 11:4)(2). The Code of Hammurabi was a generally wise set of rules for society. Some punishments, however, were severe. For example, if a physician operated on an eye and the patient was blinded, the physician's hands were cut off. The carrying out of these punishments was probably not always strictly enforced, because, if they had been, no one would have dared practice medicine (2, 8). Perhaps today's physicians should be more tolerant of their high malpractice insurance.

Egypt.   Some ancient Egyptian (Egypt is west of the Mesopotamian area) papyruses (documents written on a material from the papyrus plant), thought to be written around 3000–2000 B.C., described such maladies as tumors, ulcers, and fractures and treatments such as splinting techniques, suturing, and cauterizing wounds. They also contained the first known mention of the word *brain,* along with a description of the meninges (membranes around the brain) and the gyri (ridges on the surface of the brain). Another papyrus of that period (around 3000 B.C.) describes the heart and vessels from it to various parts of the body (5, 8, 12). Although anatomically inaccurate with regard to present knowledge, these records indicate a rudimentary understanding of the heart's function.

The Egyptians also practiced embalming and mummification of the body with great skill. Mummification, which began around 4,000 B.C., was more of religious than medical or anatomical significance, but the process involved intimate knowledge about the body. It is known that they removed most of the brain by inserting a hook through the nostrils. They also removed internal organs such as the liver, lungs, and intestines and stored them in special clay pots. The lids of the pots represented the particular god who was a protector of that particular body part. The concept of body parts being related to a specific deity or cosmic affiliation continued, as we shall see, long into the Middle Ages. Herodotus, a Greek historian, visited Egypt in the fifth century B.C. and presented a vivid description of the mummification process (8, 12).

China, Japan, and India.   China has one of the oldest known civilizations, but due to geographic and cultural isolation, Chinese knowledge in the area of science and medicine has not had great influence on Western cultures, although some information exchange did occur between China, India, and the Mediterranean area during ancient times. Chinese religious beliefs (mainly Confucianism) forbade defiling the body; thus, dissection was forbidden and knowledge of organs was obtained only from wounds (12, 16). However, an ancient Chinese book on anatomy indicates that condemned criminals may have been dissected around 1000 B.C. (7). For the most part, however, Chinese physicians were taught only about the surface of the body from models and diagrams (8, 12).

The Chinese believed in two basic forces or principles, the yin and the yang, which governed everything from the universe to the human body. With regard to the body, it was believed that balance between these forces was essential for good health (3, 7, 8, 12). These beliefs thwarted, to some degree, studying the structures of the body, because the major concern was identifying these forces and keeping them in balance. Belief in yin and yang did not foster a spirit of exploration of the internal body. However, certain aspects of the yin and yang were related to specific body structures and, as a result, acupuncture was developed by the ancient Chinese to attain balance between the forces of yin and yang. Acupuncture involved 365 vital points and thus demanded a detailed anatomical knowledge of the body's surface. This technique is still much used in China, as well as in some medical facilities throughout the world, to relieve pain or perform surgeries. Why acupuncture works with some people is still not known (3, 8, 16). Some ancient Chinese, however, knew more than just surface anatomy. In 2600 B.C., Huang Ti, who is considered the father of Chinese medicine, stated that "all the blood of the body is under control of the heart. The heart is in accord with the pulse. The pulse regulates all the blood and the blood current flows in a continuous circle and never stops" (12). This astounding concept was not confirmed in the Western World until described by William Harvey in 1628, 4200 years later. This emphasizes the importance of communication. If the ancient scientists had the communication systems of today, advances in anatomy and medicine and all other areas would have occurred at a much accelerated pace, and the credit for specific discoveries would be much different from what we recognize today.

The development of anatomy in Japan mirrored that of China, largely because Japan sent Buddhist monks (in the sixth Century) to study anatomy in China. The Japanese adopted these teachings because their cultural tradition, as with many cultures of that era, was not a questioning one, so they readily accepted the information from the Chinese (3, 8). Later, after some initial association with a few European powers, the Japanese government banned all contact with Western countries in 1603. However, some medical texts (mainly Dutch) with anatomical drawings had already circulated among Japanese physicians, and they contradicted the traditional Chinese models of anatomy that had been used for centuries. Finally, in 1771, a Japanese physician, Genpaku Sugito, was able to observe a dissection and compare the Dutch model with the Chinese concepts then in use. He was disturbed because the dissection proved the errors in the Chinese model. In 1774, Sugito and his colleagues published an anatomy book based on the more correct Dutch anatomical work. Interestingly, they used exact copies of the Dutch anatomical drawings of the body, but they drew Japanese heads and eyes onto the more rotund Dutch bodies, probably to make them more acceptable to Japanese scientists and physicians (3, 12, 16).

Writings from ancient India indicate that Indians were also contributing to the advance of anatomical and medical knowledge (8, 12). Susruta was a well-known Hindu physician, who is thought to have lived in the sixth century B.C. Susruta stated that "the surgeon, who wishes to possess the exact knowledge of the science of surgery, should thoroughly examine all parts of the dead body after its proper preparation" (12). Hindu religious laws, however, banned touching the deceased or using a knife for dissection. Thus, bodies were placed in water until they were soft enough to scrape off skin and other tissues with a broom or scraper to view deeper structures (7, 12). Because the penalty for adultery in ancient India was to cut off the offender's nose, other writings describe detailed plastic surgery techniques to repair the nose (called rhinoplasty), as well as other fairly sophisticated surgeries (8, 12).

The Greeks.   The Greeks laid the foundations for the study of science, medicine, and anatomy, as well as other disciplines. The focus of Greek children was on physical training and development of the body up to age 18, at which time they began to study science and philosophy, which naturally led to considerable advances in these areas (7, 16).

The first systematic writings about anatomy were by *Alcmaeon* of Crotona around 500 B.C. (Crotona was a Greek colony in southern Italy). From animal dissections, he described the optic nerves and the auditory tube (the auditory tube connects the ear to the throat) (1, 8, 12, 15). He also asserted, in contrast to some others of that time, that the brain, not the heart, was where human intelligence was located (12). Although Alcmaeon may have dissected a human, it is not likely that most of the great Greek scientists/philosophers had, although considerable animal dissection was accomplished (1, 12). [Another historically famous person from Crotona is the athlete Milo of Crotona. Legend says he could carry a four-year-old bull because he had done so every day since the bull was born. In a modern replication of Milo's feat, a 17-year-old who weighed 149 pounds began lifting a calf daily. At the start the calf weighed 75 pounds. The boy lifted the calf every day for 201 days, at which time the calf weighed 290 pounds and the boy weighed 152 pounds (6).]

Empedocles (493–433 B.C.) was from a Greek colony in Sicily (the southern tip of Italy) and lived about the same time as Alcmaeon. He is important because some of his anatomical theories affected anatomical, medical, and scientific thinking for several thousand years. Empedocles taught that the heart was the center of the vascular system (correct), but also that it was the site of and/or distributor of "pneuma" (incorrect). Pneuma was considered to be the "life and soul" of the body. It was thought to be the steamlike substance that could be seen rising from the blood of people or animals slain in the open air. Unfortunately, Empedocle's concept of pneuma and other body functions remained a standard belief for thousands of years (5, 7, 12, 15). It is necessary to remember, however, that even though the early anatomists and/or scientists were not always correct, their ideas were important for the next generation of developing scientists and the advances that came after them.

Hippocrates (460–377 B.C.), the Father of Western Medicine, was a Greek physician whose Hippocratic oath (the oath basically describes a physician's obligations to their patients) is still recited at some medical schools (1, 8, 16). A collection of medical and philosophical writings called the Hippocratic Collection has been attributed to Hippocrates, but evidence indicates he wrote very few of the papers. Most were written by other physicians of his time and were put together 100 or so years later by Alexandrian scholars (7, 8, 12). Hippocrates stated that "anatomy is the foundation of medicine" (12), but he never dissected a human body and had little knowledge of internal organs. He described tendons as nerves and thought the brain to do nothing more than secrete mucus, although in the Hippocratic writings the human brain is correctly described as having two identical halves separated by a membrane (6, 10, 13, 14). Hippocrates believed that the mucus secreted by the brain cooled the heart and that the arteries contained nothing but air. In fact, the word *artery* is of Latin and Greek origin and means "to keep air" or an "air duct." Many ancient scientists and physicians held this concept (1, 7).

Medicine was kept in the family because Hippocrates' son-in-law, Polybus (390 B.C.), devoted studies to the human body, although his anatomical descriptions were largely inaccurate and very crude. Both Hippocrates and Polybus promoted the humoral theory of the body. According to this theory, there were four body humors and each was associated with a particular organ. The four humors were blood (with the liver), phlegm (with the lungs), yellow bile (with the gallbladder), and black bile (with the spleen). Hippocrates, Polybus, and others maintained that these four humors must be in balance for a person to be in good health, to some degree a concept somewhat similar to the Chinese yin and yang (11, 12, 15, 16).

Unfortunately, the erroneous humoral theory remained a strong force in medicine for some 2000 years (8, 16). While certain of Hippocrates anatomical concepts were erroneous, he contributed greatly to anatomy and medicine because he believed that diseases are the result of natural causes and not due to the whim of the gods (1, 16), a considerable advance, although during the Middle Ages in Western Europe and England most still believed that diseases were the result of sin or punishment by God. Relative to exercise science, Hippocrates stated that "diseases caused by overeating are cured by fasting…diseases caused by indolence are cured by exertion…and tenseness by relaxation" (15). One might argue that the Father of Western Medicine was also an exercise scientist.

Although some of the anatomical concepts provided by the Greek scientists, physicians, and anatomists may seem ludicrous and humorous today, their contribution to the advance of knowledge is invaluable. They developed systematic methods of inquiry, were careful observers, and dissected animals. These were the beginnings of the scientific method (7, 15). For example, a part of the Hippocratic Collection titled "On the heart" (circa 340 B.C.) describes how air enters the heart and that the heart is where intelligence is located, which is totally erroneous. However, the writing also accurately describes the atrioventricular valves (AV valves; valves between the atria and ventricles), the chordae tendinae ("heart strings," which prevent inversion or prolapse of the AV valves), and the semilunar valves (valves guarding the pulmonary and aortic exits out of the right and left ventricles, respectively) (15).

Aristotle (384–322 B.C.), one of the most well known of the ancient Greeks was a scientist and philosopher. He was the son of the physician to King Philip of Macedonia (a region on the Balkan peninsula, an area around the Black, Aegean, and Mediterranean seas) and a student of Plato. He became the tutor for King Philip's son, who is well-known historically as Alexander the Great (8, 15, 16). Aristotle never dissected a human body, but he dissected many animals and thus his comments about human anatomy were based on these dissections (7). Due to his excellent biological descriptions of animals, Aristotle is considered the founder of comparative anatomy, and he also developed ideas concerning organic evolution later praised by Charles Darwin (7, 12, 15).

Aristotle was the first to use the term *aorta* (the large artery leaving the left ventricle of the heart), presented a fairly accurate description of the pathway of the esophagus, and had many other significant insights (7, 15). However, his works also contained considerable anatomical errors due in part to the lack of human dissection and in part to the fact that Aristotle was more a natural philosopher than anatomist. Whereas his teacher, Plato, believed the brain to be the seat of intelligence, Aristotle placed intelligence in the heart. He considered the brain to function only to cool the heart. He also believed that arteries sometimes carried only air and sometimes only blood (1, 7, 12, 15, 16). Despite such errors, Aristotle is considered one of the greatest contributors to anatomy and medicine.

Interestingly, it was Aristotle's philosophy, more than his scientific logic, which influenced biological and anatomical thought for 2000 years (7, 15). In many instances however, his thinking was incorrectly interpreted or misused. Appropriate discussion of Aristotle's influence is beyond the scope of this chapter so a small example about why his thoughts were so long accepted will have to suffice. One of Aristotle's fascinations was with reproduction, and he believed that the female provided the material substance of the embryo (the soil in which the life grows), but only the male contributed the *psyche* or actual life to the organism. Because this psyche is not a material thing, he thus believed that no substance needed to pass from the male to the female. This view of reproduction (in this case human reproduction), is called parthenogenesis (virgin birth). In fact, a number of Greek mythologies contained stories about virgin births. This concept was accepted by many scientists up to the nineteenth century. Virgin birth is a major belief of Christianity, and thus many of Aristotle's views were readily accepted by the early Christian Church, whereas many other ancient ideas and writings, although correct, were considered pagan beliefs, not accepted, and thereby often destroyed by the churchmen (7, 12, 15).

When the Greek cultures of the mainland began to decline, the center of knowledge passed to Alexandria (around 300–250 B.C.), a city on the coastline of Egypt. Alexandria was founded by Alexander the Great (Aristotle's pupil) and became the center of intellectual pursuits for several centuries (1, 12). A library in Alexandria contained 700,000 written works, virtually all the written knowledge of the Western civilized world at that time (12). (Alexandrian scholars put together the previously mentioned Hippocratic Collection.) Anatomical study advanced in the Alexandrian School of Medicine due primarily to the work of two Greek scholars, *Herophilus* and *Erasistratus* (1, 12, 15). Alexandria attracted many famous scholars of the time, including the mathematicians Euclid and Archimedes. Archimedes calculated the value of pi, but is more famous for his principles of buoyancy, which are used in exercise science studies of body composition with underwater weighing (2, 8).

Advances in anatomy were particularly enhanced by the acceptance in Alexandria of human dissection. Although some human dissection had been accomplished in earlier civilizations, the dissections of Herophilus and Erasistratus were probably the first public dissections (that is, viewed by other scholars) (1, 8, 12, 15). Herophilus was born around 335–300 B.C. (sources vary) and is referred to as the Father of Anatomy (12, 15). He is credited with dissecting up to 600 human bodies, which gave him anatomical insights none before him could have obtained. Unfortunately, his manuscripts were destroyed, but some later scholars, such as Galen, described his work. Among other things, Herophilus made the first distinctions between motor and sensory nerves, described the difference between the cerebrum and cerebellum of the brain, and gave detailed descriptions of the liver and uterus. Unlike Aristotle, he correctly maintained that intelligence was located in the brain. His many human dissections probably included some vivisections (dissecting a living person, usually a criminal), but scholars are unclear about this. Herophilus was a noted teacher and is thought to be one of the first teachers of anatomy and medicine to have female students (1, 7, 12, 15).

Erasistratus (310 to 250 B.C.) was a slightly younger contemporary of Herophilus and is referred to as the Father of Physiology, although he was a superb anatomist for his time. He noted that the human brain had greater convolutions than animal brains and believed that it was the reason for their greater intelligence. He studied the heart and described many vessels such as the renal arteries and the vena cavas (the large veins bringing blood back to the heart), but thought that tendons and nerves were the same thing, as did most of the Greek physicians and anatomists.

Erasistratus made significant contributions to knowledge about the heart and circulatory system, but believed that only veins carried blood and that arteries carried the airlike "vital spirit," much as Empedocles and Hippocrates had thought. When he saw people with bleeding arteries, he argued that the injury caused a vacuum and that blood was "sucked into the arteries from veins through very fine intercommunications between the two types of vessels" (15). Far before their discovery, and without knowing it, Erasistratus had perceived the capillary system.

Eventually, Alexandria and its scholarly atmosphere began to decline, and unfortunately many of the written works stored in the great libraries were destroyed by fanatical Christians or stolen and sometimes lost by the later invading Arabian forces (7). However, although the Arabian armies often destroyed the buildings, they took many of the libraries written works with them. Thus, they preserved many of the anatomical papers, particularly those of the Greeks, that would otherwise never have survived. These important records, which were translated from Greek to Arabic, were later returned to European countries and then retranslated from Arabic to Latin (7, 15). The Arabs had a long-standing interest in studying the works of the Greeks and translating them into Arabic. The Arabs also established centers of learning similar to Alexandria in the Persian (now Iraq) city of Bagdad and in Cordova or Cordoba in Spain (10)].

The preservation of these writings was a critically important event because, during the Middle Ages, the church forbade studying the human body, as well as any writings concerned with anatomy or the body, and even destroyed any materials it found. If the Arabian invaders had not saved these works, they would have been forever lost. Fortunately, these anatomical papers began to appear in Europe during the thirteenth century, where they helped stimulate a rebirth of anatomical and medical study (3, 15, 16). The Arabs likewise benefited, because their religion strictly forbade dissection and did not even allow pictures of the human body. There were no courses on anatomy in Arabian medical schools at that time. Thus, Arab physicians and scientists, probably at great personal risk, studied and preserved the anatomical works of the Greeks and others (3, 10).

The slow but steady decline of Alexandria as an intellectual center continued with the advance of the Romans, and the city became part of the Roman empire in about A.D. 30. With the decline of Alexandria and the advent of the Roman Empire, anatomical and medical knowledge suffered a decline or, at best, made few advances. Dissection was either forbidden or not encouraged. The inquisitiveness, promotion of philosophical theories, and questioning mind-set of the Greeks were no longer prominent, if not discouraged in the Roman Empire. The Romans were practical; that is, they wanted what was immediately useful and believed the theoretical pursuits of the Greeks to be relatively unimportant (7, 12, 15).

Even at the height of the Roman Empire, most of the physicians were Greek, because the Romans felt that medicine was a lowly profession "fit only for slaves and immigrants" (7). A medical school was started in Rome in 60 B.C. by Asclepiades (120 to 70 B.C.) called the Asclepiadic sect in physic (7, 8, 12, 15, 16). (The name Asclepiades likely was derived from Aescalapias, who was the Greek god of medicine and a son of Apollo.) The Asclepiades school recommended exercise-science-like prescriptions such as diet, exercise, massage, and even listening to music. It also used drugs such as opium and wine to treat patients. Asclepiades also rejected Hippocrates concept of the four humors. However, virtually no advances in anatomy or understanding of the human body were made by Asclepiades or the medical school and, unfortunately, the humoral theory remained prominent (8).

Little advance in anatomy and medicine occurred because both the Romans and the beginning of the Christian era forbade dissection. The antidissection attitude and overall progress of medicine (and other areas) continued for over a thousand years, an era known as the Early Middle Ages (15, 16).

Two notable individuals from the Roman era had considerable influence on anatomy and medicine, Aulus Celsus, a Roman, and Claudius Galen, a Greek scholar and physician. Celsus (circa 30 B.C.–A.D.45) was not a physician, but a very educated person who wrote on many subjects. Many of his books were lost, but eight of them on medicine, called *De Re Medicina,* were found in the fourteenth century. It is suspected that many of his anatomical and medical writings came from the Hippocratic Collection and other Greek sources, but his writings in Latin on these subjects are considered exceptional. Celsus described the trachea (windpipe), esophagus, diaphragm, lungs, liver, spleen, and kidneys. His descriptions of surgeries were particularly detailed regarding the skeleton of the extremities. The latter knowledge was likely gained from battlefield physicians. He approved of human dissection but probably never experienced one himself (6, 7, 12, 15).

Claudius Galen (129–A.D. 199), along with Hippocrates, is considered to be the greatest of the early physicians. His influence on medicine was so dominant that during the Middle Ages (some 1300 years later) he was called the Prince of Physicians (7, 15). His writings on medicine and anatomy were considered virtually infallible for 1500 years in Western medicine. Galen also wrote about other subjects, such as mathematics, philosophy and religion. His religious writings (which were sometimes misinterpreted) in particular helped preserve his medical and anatomical views because they were supported for many years by Canon Law (5). (Canon Laws are the official rules of faith and practice of the Catholic church.) Because the Catholic church did not allow Galen's anatomical concepts to be criticized, the incorrect ideas persisted and stifled the progress in anatomical study from his death in A.D. 201 until the Renaissance period of the late Middle Ages. His influence was so dominant that in the 1550s the Royal College of Physicians of London demanded that one of their members retract a statement that described some errors in Galen's work. The accused physician quickly did so (1, 7, 12, 15). The French anatomist Jacobus Sylvius (1478–1555), when faced by dissection with obvious errors in some of Galen's writings, stated that "man must have changed his structure in the course of time, for the teaching of Galen cannot err" (12).

Galen never dissected a human body, but did considerable dissection work on many animals, including apes, pigs, and bears, and often attributed structures in them to be the same in humans. For a time he served as physician to the gladiators, whose severe wounds allowed him to observe considerable human anatomical structures. Even though Galen's views were erroneous in some areas, in others he presented very accurate anatomical descriptions. He was particularly accurate in his descriptions of the skull and vertebral column and the bones of the extremities. He described the difference between arteries and veins and proved that arteries contain blood instead of air, as had been believed since the time of Aristotle (7, 8, 11, 12).

Galen's dominance for so many centuries was due in part to his brilliance, his forceful personality, and his voluminous writing, as well as the political–religious atmosphere of the time (5, 7, 8, 11, 12, 15). It is unlikely that any future scientist will dominate any field to the degree of Galen, and we are indebted to him for preserving and describing anatomical and medical knowledge from a time in history that would have otherwise been lost (12).

The Middle Ages

The Middle Ages is generally accepted to have occurred from the fourth or fifth century A.D. to the middle of the fifteenth century. This would roughly be from the fall of Rome in 476 A.D. to the end of the Byzantine Empire in 1453 when the Turks captured Constantinople (now Istanbul) (8, 12, 16).

The fall of the Roman Empire, the death of Galen, and the rise of a powerful, tyrannical church caused a considerable decline in the advance of anatomy and other scholarly pursuits. The Early Middle Ages (circa A.D. 450–750) is sometimes called the Dark Ages due, in part, to the lack of advance in learning during this period. However, a few centers of learning survived, which helped at least to preserve existing anatomical knowledge. The most well-known were the universities at Salerno and Bologna and a Benedictine monastery in Monte Cassino, Italy. At Salerno and/or Monte Cassino, a much-traveled Benedictine monk, Constantinus Africanus (Constantine the African, 1020–1087), translated the works of Hippocrates and Galen (which had been rescued by Arabian invaders) from Greek and Arabic into Latin. He also included some new insights in anatomy provided by Arabian physicians because, while western Europe stagnated in the Early Middle Ages, Arabian physicians studied the ancient Greek works and developed some new anatomical descriptions during the seventh to tenth centuries. The Arabian physician Avicenna (980–1087), for example, presented an accurate description of the six muscles that move the eyeball. Another, Haly (Ali) Abbas (circa 994), gave a very accurate description of the heart and circulation, including the heart valves and the fact that the left and right ventricles contracted simultaneously (7, 8, 12). Thus, some progress, however minimal, was being made.

For the most part, Western European countries stagnated from the fourth and fifth centuries up to the eleventh century. Anatomy and medical advances were minimal at best. The powerful and political church forbade dissection; in fact, none had occurred since the Alexandrian period. The prevailing attitude was one of greater concern for what occurred after death, rather than while living. Scholars sought "truth" using philosophical or religious concepts, rather than by experimentation or observation. The foundation of knowledge was faith instead of reason (5, 7, 10, 12). With little progress in technology combined with the dominant belief that life on Earth was unimportant except for its preparation for the rewards of an afterlife, little overall progress occurred.

An interest in astrology developed, and a figure called the zodiacal man became popular (Figure 3.4). Different parts of the zodiacal man were related to specific constellations in an attempt to relate body functions and illnesses to the movements of planets, a concept somewhat similar to that of the ancient Egyptians (3, 7, 8, 12). The carry-over regarding astrological predictions about a person's daily life persist and remain a popular (and believable to many) part of today's daily newspapers.

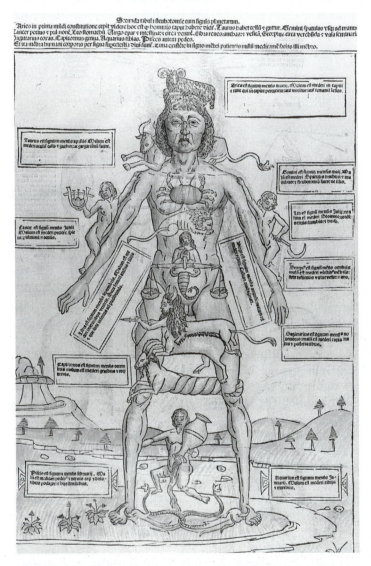

FIGURE 3.4   The zodiacal man from the Middle Ages. Different body parts are related to the stars that were thought to influence a person's health.
Yale University, Harvey Cushing/John Jay Whitney Medical Library.

Eventually, society began to slowly change, and during the twelfth and thirteenth centuries new universities emerged in Italy, France, Germany, and England. A renewed interest in anatomy and the study of the body began in these universities. Between 1200 and 1350, fifteen universities in Italy alone were formed. The most important of these with regard to anatomy was the previously mentioned University of Bologna (3, 12). The first medical faculty in Europe was established at Bologna about 1156 (7). Human dissection began to occur, and the first detailed descriptions were given by William of Saliceto (1215–1280). The reasons for these dissections, however, were not for learning or the advance of knowledge about the human body. The dissections were done for legal purposes, because the law schools wanted information about how the person died, that is, legal evidence, as in cases of poisoning or knifing. Thus, the physicians recorded, to the best of their ability, the potential causes of death, but the major emphasis was on "how to dissect." In other words, the method of dissection was far more important than the study of structures to determine function (3, 7, 15)

The church's ban on dissection at this time was due to a Papal Bull issued by Pope Boniface VIII in 1300. It prohibited cutting up the dead, but the actual reason for the Bull was misinterpreted by many priests. The reason for the Bull was to stop the common practice of the Crusaders from stripping the flesh of their dead soldiers and boiling the remaining flesh from the bones. The bones could then be easily carried home to avoid being buried in what was considered heathen soil. The ban on this practice was interpreted as a ban on any type of dissection (7).

Church authorities did not protest anatomical demonstrations at Bologna in the early 1400s, and in 1482 Pope Sixtus IV issued a Papal Bull allowing dissection if the local clergy granted permission. We can wonder if there is any significance to the fact that Sixtus IV had been a university student at Bologna (11). The student must understand that in the medical schools of the Middle Ages, medicine (that is, physicians) and surgeons were quite different. Medical schools taught medicine to physicians, and most physicians considered surgery beneath their dignity and felt that a detailed knowledge of anatomy was unnecessary. Knowing the position of internal organs was good enough for them. Surgery was done by barbers, bathhouse keepers and sometimes even executioners (10). With time, surgery became a part of the training for medical doctors and is one of many medical specialties today.

The Renaissance

With the rise of the universities, the Middle Ages moved into the Renaissance, a period ranging from the early fourteenth to the late sixteenth or early seventeenth century. During this time, major advancements in literature and art and a virtual revolution in science occurred (2). The invention of the printing press in the 1450s was particularly important because this allowed the anatomical knowledge or theories of a particular scholar or university to more easily spread to anatomists in other countries. The most well known early anatomy text was written by Mondino de' Luzzi (1276–1326). The book, entitled the *Anathomia,* was first published in 1316 but not printed until 1487. It was not a particularly accurate book regarding anatomical structure and generally was mostly a reproduction of Galen's descriptions. It contained no illustrations, but it was the best available at the time, became required reading in European medical schools for hundreds of years, and underwent many revisions. Mondino had supervised dissections of executed criminals and accurately described some vessels and heart structures, but he could not bring himself to question Galen's materials; thus the book continued the attitude that Galen could not be wrong. However, Mondino made detailed descriptions of the dissection process that were useful at the time. As a result, Mondino is called the Restorer of Anatomy (3, 5, 7, 12, 15).

The increased emphasis on dissection during the Renaissance created a shortage of cadavers. Due to the lack of embalming techniques, with the resulting decay of tissues, dissection had to be completed quickly. Dissections would often continue nonstop, day and night, for several days. Grave robbing to obtain cadavers became a problem, and some medical students were convicted for it. The main source of bodies for dissection was executed criminals. Because most of these were males, there was little opportunity for dissection and observation of female anatomy, so knowledge about female reproductive organs was scarce (7, 11).

There were many who contributed much to anatomy during the Renaissance, but two individuals are particularly noteworthy, one an artist and the other a physician. The artist was Leonardo da Vinci (1452–1519), better known by most as the painter of the Mona Lisa and the Last Supper (2). Da Vinci, one of the great geniuses of all time, was also a scientist, inventor, mathematician, astronomer, and philosopher. He dissected many human bodies and produced exquisitely detailed anatomical drawings. He also made many anatomical discoveries and developed technical procedures that enhanced anatomical study. He was the first person to demonstrate the shape of the ventricles (fluid-filled cavities) in the brain by pouring melted wax into them through a hole he had drilled into the brain of an ox. He did this with other body cavities as well. He described *arteriosclerosis* (hardening of the arteries) by comparing the dissected arteries of an old man to those of a young man, along with many other functional anatomical observations. He had intended to publish his drawings and interpretations with a professor (Marcantonio della Torre), but the professor died at an early age, which halted the project. Had they been published at that time they would have advanced knowledge about anatomy and physiology by several hundred years. However, da Vinci's progressive thinking and discoveries in anatomy had little effect at the time, but his advances are well worth mention in any history of anatomy. Unfortunately, his drawings were lost and not found again until the twentieth century (3, 5, 7, 10, 12, 14).

Figure 3.5 presents da Vinci's sketches of the arm and forearm. Many artistic contemporaries of da Vinci also used dissection and drawings of dissection in order to more accurately depict the human form. Among these are Michelangelo and Raphael. Few representations of the beauty of the human body can equal Michelangelo's 17-foot sculpture entitled David (Figure 3.6), which was carved from a single block of white marble (10, 16).

A physician, *Andreas Vesalius* (1514–1564), provided the foundation for modern medicine and revolutionized the study of anatomy. Vesalius was the greatest anatomist of his time and is called the Reformer of Anatomy because he initiated, at that time, a unique change in the teaching of anatomy. When anatomy and dissection were finally approved as a university course, the professors of anatomy became elitist. They disdained touching the body and sat in elevated high-backed wooden chairs (the origin of chairs in today's university) and pointed with a long pole at what they wished their helpers (often local butchers) to cut (the origin of the statement "I wouldn't touch that with a 10-foot pole"). The main

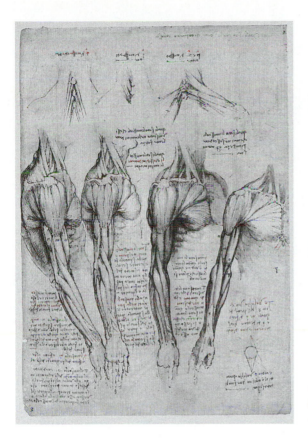

FIGURE 3.5   Drawings of the arm and fore-arm by Leonardo da Vinci.

The New York Academy of Medicine

intent of these professors was to demonstrate the proper dissecting technique and substantiate what Galen had described.

Vesalius, who had been trained in this method, came down from the chair, dismissed the helpers, and did the dissecting himself, all the while lecturing to the students and surrounding audience in a stimulating, challenging manner (3, 11, 12, 14–16). His participation in the dissection, his challenge of previously held beliefs about structure, and his stimulating narrative particularly delighted the students (11, 14). Like today's students, Vesalius's students probably enjoyed seeing some of the more stuffy professors' stodgy thinking challenged by the intelligent, logical, and charismatic Vesalius. In 1543, at the age of 28, Vesalius published *De Humani Corporis Fabrica* (*On the Fabric of the Human Body*), often referred to simply as the *Fabrica*. It challenged the long-held beliefs of Galen, as well as being the first accurately illustrated text on human anatomy that also described specific dissection techniques (11, 12, 14, 15). As with most new concepts, Vesalius's teaching methods and the *Fabrica* were not readily accepted by many of the traditional scholars at the time, but both certainly certify Vesalius's label as the Reformer of Anatomy.

A number of other anatomists of that time also made important contributions, but none had the overall impact of Vesalius. His teaching method of dissection or demonstration while

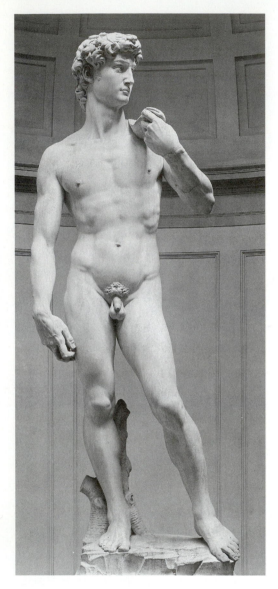

**FIGURE 3.6   Michelangelo's David, which was
sculpted from a single block of white marble.**

Archivi Alinari/Art Resource, NY

lecturing to students still remains a favored method in anatomy laboratories today. Unfortunately, criticism of new ideas then as now can be harsh. Vesalius became so disturbed by the
abuse that he allegedly took all his unpublished papers and burned them. Others argue, however, that the reason Vesalius burned his papers was strictly symbolic. It marked the end of
his academic career as a researcher in anatomy to begin a more financially secure career as a
court physician. Not only was the new career more lucrative with regard to monetary rewards, but Vesalius considered himself a physician first, and his pursuit of increased anatom-

ical knowledge was merely a process of making himself a better physician (11). Whatever the reason, he later regretted burning the papers (12). Figure 3.7 shows a drawing of muscles from the *Fabrica* by Vesalius.

Seventeenth through Twentieth Centuries

Following the Renaissance, science in general and anatomy made many advances. Anatomy even became a form of entertainment; amphitheaters were built throughout Europe and high-priced tickets sold to the wealthy, who were then allowed to witness dissections performed by anatomists in decorative scholarly gowns. Most of these dissections were done during cold weather primarily due to the lack of embalming techniques (3, 7, 16).

The two major advances that occurred during the seventeenth century were an explanation of how the blood circulates and the development of the microscope (7, 8, 11, 16). In

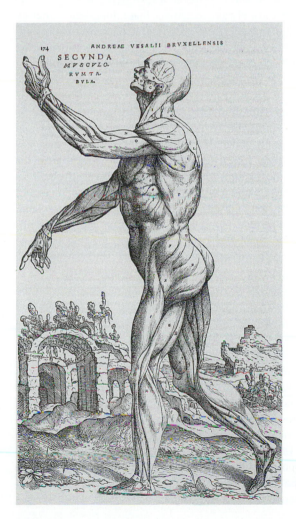

FIGURE 3.7   Diagram of surface muscles from the *Fabrica* by Andreas Vesalius.

The New York Academy of Medicine

1628, *William Harvey* (1578–1657), an English anatomist, published a book entitled *Anatomical Studies on the Motion of the Heart and Blood in Animals* in which he described his solution about how the blood travels in a circle. Some believe this description to be the greatest anatomical–medical–physiological development of the seventeenth century (7, 8, 11). Some earlier anatomists had alluded to this fact, but it was Harvey who proved it by experimentation and, due to the availability of printing, was able to publish it and have it distributed.

Harvey's major problem was that he had no way of explaining how blood passed from the smallest arteries to the veins because he had no microscope. Harvey hypothesized that tiny "pores" must exist to connect the arterial–venous system. Thus, he correctly predicted the existence of the capillaries, although he did not perceive their structure as we know them (8, 11, 15). Today, the basic workings of the heart and circulation and the benefits of exercise to this system are taught to elementary schoolchildren.

We may be astounded, even amused, as to why it took so long for the circulatory system to be described and why this concept was considered a revolution in anatomy and physiology at the time. As scientists, we must always remember that a long-held belief by a society is difficult to change, even when that society is presented with overwhelming evidence refuting previous beliefs. It was even more difficult when effective communication was lacking. We must also remain cognizant of the fact that small, seemingly insignificant discoveries may eventually lead to a giant leap forward in the understanding of how the human body works.

With the increased emphasis on dissection relating structure to function started by Vesalius and Harvey's description of the circulation of the blood, advances in anatomy (and medicine) occurred rapidly in the seventeenth and eighteenth centuries. A major factor was the development of the microscope. Crude lenses for eyeglasses were available in the Middle Ages, and some early microscopes achieved a magnification power of about 10 times. In 1665, Robert Hooke (1635–1703), using a primitive microscope, coined the word *cells* to describe the honeycombed appearance of dried cork. Later, a Dutch cloth merchant, Antony van Leeuwenhoek (1632–1723) ground lenses in his spare time and greatly improved the magnification power of microscopes. Van Leeuwenhoek was the first person to describe and measure red blood cells and the striated appearance of skeletal muscle (7, 8, 11, 16). [Van Leeuwenhoek once ground a tiny lens from one grain of sand (7).]

An Italian, Marcello Malpighi (1629–1694), developed techniques for preparing tissues for microscopic study and confirmed the existence of capillaries, which Harvey had hypothesized (3, 7). Considering that 1 cubic millimeter of blood (the size of a large grain of sand) contains 4 to 6 million red blood cells, the discovery of such small entities was an amazing achievement and advancement. [Van Leewenhoek's measurements of one red blood cell were quite close to their actual size compared to today's sophisticated measures. One red blood cell is about 8.1 micrometers or 3/10,000 inch in diameter. A row of five red blood cells would about equal the diameter of one period at the end of a sentence (1, 3, 7).]

Many other anatomical structures were described during the seventeenth and eighteenth centuries by anatomists whose names were subsequently given to the structures that they described, an *eponym*. The most well known eponym in the human body is the Achilles tendon (3). Eponyms are not supposed to be used in present-day anatomy, but some (such as Achilles tendon) will likely remain indefinitely. Table 3.1 presents some still commonly used eponyms along with the modern anatomical name.

TABLE 3.1   Some Commonly Used Eponyms and the Appropriate Modern Anatomical Name

Eponym	Named for:	Appropriate Term
Achilles tendon	Greek Warrior in the Iliad whose only vulnerable spot was this tendon.	Calcaneal tendon
Adam's apple	Adam in Christian Bible. Legend states he tried to cough up the "forbidden fruit" and it was trapped in his throat, making it protrude more in men than women. (Actually, men have a larger and differently shaped thyroid cartilage and less fat over it.)	Laryngeal prominence of the thyroid cartilage
Circle of willis	Thomas Willis (1621–1675). Described the arteries that encircle the base of the brain.	Arterial circle
Eustachian tube	Bartolomeo Eustachio (1524–1574). The tube connecting the middle ear with the throat.	Auditory tube
Fallopian tube	Gabriele Fallopius (1532–1562). Tubes that carry ovums (eggs) from the ovaries to the uterus.	Uterine tubes
Graafian follicle	Regnier de Graaf (1641–1673). Structure in the ovary containing the developing egg.	Ovarian follicle
Haversion system and Haversion canal	Clopton Havers (1650–1701). System of canals in bone that carry capillaries and nerves.	Osteon and central canal
Schwann cell	Theodor Schwann (1810–1882). Cell that forms the fatty sheath (myelin) around nerve fibers.	Neurolemmocyte
Wormian bones	Olaus Worm (1588–1654). Extra sutures in some skulls that create islands of bones in the skull; they are not detrimental.	Sutural bones

During the nineteenth century, progress in anatomy and the understanding of the human body was rapid due to improvements in the microscope. A major development was the cell theory developed by two Germans, M. J. Schleiden and Theodor Schwann in 1838. Schwann (with credit to Schleiden) stated that "cells are organisms and entire animals and plants are aggregates of these organisms arranged according to definite laws" (5, 7, 11). However, Schleiden and Schwann did not know where cells came from. One thought that they proposed was that the cells came from "spontaneous generation" (that is, they simply develop), which goes back to the time of Aristotle. In 1858, another German, Rudolf Virchow, published a book called *Cell Pathology* in which he correctly described that cells came from other cells (7, 11). Again, we see that what seems so simple today was a revolutionary concept at the time.

In 1858, Henry Gray published the famous *Gray's Anatomy*. This book, which is still in print and contains some of the original illustrations, is probably the most used gross anatomy text of all time and likely remains on the shelf of virtually all anatomists. For many years it was the equivalent of the anatomical bible to physician training, although it is minimally used in most present-day anatomy courses due to improvements in atlases and other medical anatomy texts (1, 16).

Anatomical study during the twentieth century has become very specialized, and research about structures is relegated to the cellular and subcellular level. One helpful development in gross anatomy that began in the late nineteenth century and continues today is the standardization of anatomical nomenclature such that eponyms (Table 3.1) and/or different terms for the same structure are changed to one name used worldwide. The organization that monitors these and other anatomical interests is called the International Congress of Anatomists (16). Table 3.2 presents a brief review of some major contributors to anatomy.

Present-Day Anatomy: Instrumentation and Techniques

Electron Microscope and Scanning Electron Microscope

The electron microscope and scanning electron microscope revolutionized our understanding of the cell. These instruments showed that the cells of each tissue were far more complex than imagined by the simple light microscope. Whereas the light microscope can magnify an object about 1400 times, electron microscopy can magnify beyond 150,000 times normal. These instruments resulted in the discovery of new cell structures and aided in the understanding of their function, which led to a better understanding of injury and disease and thus new treatments.

The light microscope, as its name implies, uses a beam of light to reveal body tissues. Electron microscopy uses a beam of electrons. Other differences between light and electron microscopy involve the type of stains used on the tissues. For example, tissues prepared for light microscopy use various colored dyes to stain the tissues, whereas electron microscopy must use heavy-metal salts. Because of this, micrographs (pictures from an electron microscope) are grayish in color because only light waves have the property of color; electron waves do not. (Crudely, this is somewhat like black and white photographs versus color photographs.) The scanning electron microscope offers further advantages because it can produce three-dimensional images.

In addition to microscopy, advances in radiology or medical imaging techniques have also been useful in anatomy. Imaging techniques are important tools in clinical diagnosis, research, and teaching, and their interpretation requires a sound knowledge of anatomy. Following are brief descriptions of medical imaging techniques, all of which are or may be used in exercise science research.

X-rays

X-rays were discovered in 1895 by *Wilhelm Roentgen* (1845–1923). Originally called Roentgen rays, X-rays are a short electromagnetic wave. Roentgen called them x-rays because he didn't understand where they came from.

When a part of the body is x-rayed, some of the waves are absorbed by tissues. The amount of absorption depends on the density of the tissue; the more dense the tissue, the

TABLE 3.2 Major Contributors or Events to Human Anatomy up to the Nineteenth Century

Event or Person	Civilization or Country	Date	Major Contribution
Papyruses	Egypt	Ca. 3000–2000 B.C.	Described treatments of wounds and described some brain structures.
Huang Ti	China	Ca. 2600 B.C.	Stated that blood traveled in a circle; Father of Chinese medicine.
Hammurabi	Babylon	Ca. 1750 B.C.	Code of Hammurabi; contained rules for physicians.
Susruta	India	Ca. 600 B.C.	Recommended that surgeons study the dead body.
Alcmaeon	Ancient Greece	Ca. 500 B.C.	First systematic writings about anatomy.
Empedocles	Ancient Greece (Italy)	493–453 B.C.	Taught that the heart was the source of pneuma or "life and soul" of the body.
Hippocrates	Ancient Greece	460–377 B.C.	Father of Western Medicine. Developed Hippocratic Oath.
Aristotle	Ancient Greece	384–322 B.C.	Father of Comparative Anatomy; first to use term *aorta*.
Herophilus	Alexandria (Egypt)	335–300 B.C.	First distinction between motor and sensory nerves and the difference between the cerebrum and cerebellum. Considered the Father of Anatomy.
Erasistratus	Alexandria (Egypt)	310–250 B.C.	Father of Physiology.
Asclepiades	Roman	120–79 B.C.	Founded medical school in Rome that recommended exercise, diet, and massage.
Aulus Celsus	Roman	30 B.C.–45 A.D.	Wrote *De Re Medicina* describing internal organs and surgeries.
Claudius Galen	Roman	129–199	Prince of Physicians; writings on anatomy and medicine influenced Western medicine for over 1000 years.
Constantinus Africanus	Carthage Africa	Ca. 1020–1087	Translated Arabic and Greek anatomy papers into Latin at Monte Cassino in Italy.
Avenzoar Avicenna	Arabian	980–1037	Described the muscles that move the eyeball
Ali Abbas	Arabian	Ca. 994	Described heart structures, including heart valves.

(continued)

59

TABLE 3.2 Continued

Event or Person	Civilization or Country	Date	Major Contribution
University of Bologna	Italy	1156	First European medical facility established. Human dissection approved in 1405.
William of Saliceto	Italy	1215–1280	Detailed descriptions of human dissection.
Pope Sixtus IV	Italy	1482	Issued Papal Bull allowing human dissection if approved by local clergy.
Mondino de Luzzi	Italy	1276–1326	Published the *Anathomia*, an anatomy text; known as the Restorer of Anatomy.
Leonardo da Vinci	Italy	1422–1519	First to demonstrate ventricles in the brain. Detailed anatomical drawings.
Andreas Vesalius	Belgium	1514–1564	Reformer of Anatomy; published *Fabrica* with accurate anatomical illustrations.
William Harvey	England	1478–1657	Proved by experimentation how blood flows throughout the body.
Robert Hook	English	1635–1703	Coined the word *cells* from studying dried cork with a microscope.
Antony van Leeuwenhoek	Dutch	1632–1723	Greatly improved microscopic lenses; described and measured red blood cells.
Marcello Malpighi	Italy	1629–1694	Developed techniques of preparing microscopic tissues.
Theodor Schwann and M. J. Schleiden	German	1838	Developed cell theory.
Rudolph Virchow	German	1858	Described how cells came from other cells.
Henry Gray	English	1858	Published *Gray's Anatomy*.
Wilhelm Roentgen	German	1845–1923	Discovered x-ray in 1895.

more x-rays that are absorbed, causing different exposures on film. X-rays are particularly useful for detecting fractures and locating tumors. Sometimes the patient will swallow or be injected with a contrast medium such as barium before the x-ray is taken. These are called contrast x-rays. For example, in coronary angiography, a dye is injected into the arteries that supply the heart and an x-ray is taken. Problems in blood flow to heart muscle may then be detected on the film (1, 2, 4, 8, 9, 16).

Computerized Tomography (CT scan or CAT scan)

The *CAT scan* utilizes x-rays with computers to obtain three-dimensional transverse (cross) sections of a body part, such as the abdominal cavity. A clinician can obtain "slices" of a particular area and study them separately to detect trauma, blood clots, or tumors (1, 9, 16).

Positron Emission Tomography

PET scans are used to detect metabolic activity (the amount of chemical activity) in organs. In this procedure, a radioactive isotope is added to a substance (such as glucose) and is injected into the bloodstream. The PET scan can detect the rate at which certain tissues absorb the tagged glucose. PET scans are particularly useful in studying brain activity. For example, monitoring glucose absorption in the brain shows areas damaged by stroke or Alzheimer's disease. PET scans can also be used to study healthy brains because they will identify areas of greatest brain activity when the person is doing a specific thing, such as talking or doing a math problem. This adds to our knowledge about what part of the brain controls various functions (1, 9, 16).

Magnetic Resonance Imaging

MRI uses a magnetic field 60,000 times stronger than Earth's magnetic fields to produce very clear anatomical pictures in different body planes and to detect areas of diseased tissue. MRI is particularly attractive because it does not use x-rays or radioactive tracer substances. The details are beyond the scope of this chapter, but the clarity of MRI sections has even discovered tumors not seen during exploratory surgery (1, 9, 16). MRI has been used extensively of late in research studies by exercise scientists. Figure 3.8 is a picture of an MRI machine, and Figure 3.9 presents a research abstract as an example of the use of MRI by exercise science researchers.

Dual Energy X-ray Absorptiometry

DXA uses an x-ray with more than one wavelength that passes through a special filter that varies the energy peaks, thus giving greater accuracy for estimating the amount of fat, muscle, and bone tissue. It is currently used in exercise science studies of body composition. Future studies will refine DXA's accuracy, and it may become a standard for the study of specific soft and hard tissues in the body, much as underwater weighing is considered the present standard (13) (Figure 3.10).

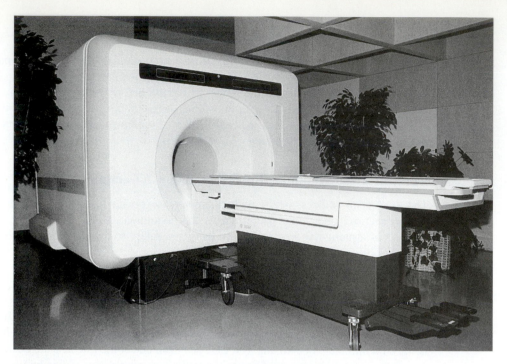

FIGURE 3.8   A magnetic resonance imaging (MRI) machine.

FIGURE 3.9   Abstract of an exercise science research study using magnetic resonance imaging (MRI).

Housh, D. J., T. J. Housh, J. P. Weir, L. L. Weir, G. O. Johnson, and J. R. Stout. Anthropometric estimation of thigh muscle cross-sectional area..
Med. Sci. Sports Exerc., Vol. 27, No. 5, pp. 784–791, 1995.

The purpose of this investigation was to derive and validate circumference and skinfold equations for estimating the anatomical cross-sectional area (CSA) of the quadriceps, hamstrings, and total thigh muscles. Forty-three adult male (X age $\pm$ SD = 25 $\pm$ 5 yr) volunteers underwent magnetic resonance imaging (MRI) to determine the CSA of the thigh muscles at the midfemur level as well as midthigh circumference and anterior thigh skinfold assessment. Multiple regression analyses were used to derive equations for predicting quadriceps, hamstrings, and total thigh muscle CSA of the dominant limb from the anthropometric dimensions on a random sample of 30 of the subjects. Cross-validation (CV) analyses were performed for each equation on: (a) the nondominant thigh of the derivation group (N = 30); (b) the dominant thigh of the CV group (N = 13); and (c) the nondominant thigh of the CV group (N = 13). The CV total error values for the quadriceps, hamstrings, and total thigh muscle CSA ranged from 5.4 to 14.4, 3.3 to 5.5, and 10.0 to 25.4 cm^2, respectively. The anthropometric equations are recommended for one-time estimates of muscle CSA values in healthy, well-nourished young adult males when more sophisticated procedures are not available.

Source: D. J. Housh et al., *Medicine and Science in Sports and Exercise* 27(5):784, 1995. Reprinted with permission.

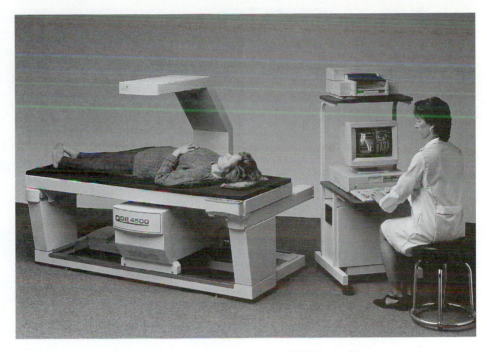

FIGURE 3.10   A dual energy x-ray absorptiometry (DXA) machine.
Photo courtesy of Hologic, Inc.

Ultrasound Imagery Sonography

Ultrasound sonography is a noninvasive technique. Sound waves sent into the body are reflected to different degrees by different types of body tissues. These waves cause echoes from which a computer constructs a picture of the tissue. Ultrasound is a very safe procedure and is often used to assess the age and/or health of a developing fetus. It has been used in exercise science research to estimate subcutaneous (under the skin) adipose (fatty) tissue (1, 9, 13, 15, 16) (Figure 3.11).

Employment Opportunities in Anatomy

It is always difficult to predict future employment opportunities in any field. There will likely always be a need for teachers of gross and microscopic anatomy at many different levels of sophistication, from medical, dental, and physical therapy schools to one-semester courses in universities, colleges, community colleges, and high schools. At major universities and medical schools, where both teaching and research are required for employment, a Ph.D. in anatomy will be necessary. In some cases, specializing in anatomical studies in exercise science doctoral programs will meet this requirement. A master's degree in anatomy or a degree in biology with some emphasis on anatomy is often sufficient to teach certain introductory courses. Requirements may vary, but the author believes that to successfully teach

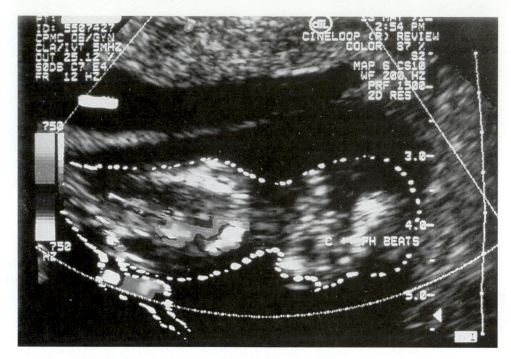

FIGURE 3.11 Ultrasound image of a fetus inside the uterus.
© Dr. Olan Timor/Peter Arnold Inc.

anatomy requires a minimum of at least premedical- or medical-level courses in gross anatomy, neuroanatomy, histology (including electron microscopy), embryology, human physiology, and chemistry through biochemistry. It is also essential, in the author's opinion, that an instructor of anatomy have considerable experience in dissection of human cadavers. Individuals interested in pursuing anatomical studies can obtain further information by writing or calling departments of anatomy at major universities or medical school facilities.

Professional Associations

The major professional association for exercise scientists is the American College of Sports Medicine (ACSM), described in other parts of this text. Considerable anatomically related research is presented at ACSM meetings. Examples of these would be the assessment of various types of exercise (or lack of exercise) on body tissues, such as muscle, bone, fat, tendons, and ligaments. Such studies may be done on either animals or humans using many of the aforementioned devices, such as MRI, DXA, ultrasound, or even anthropometry (measuring external boney structures and skin thickness). Exercise science anatomy specialists may also be members of and contribute research to the American Alliance for Health, Physical Education, Recreation, and Dance (AAHPERD) or specific medical specialties. Most anatomists in departments of anatomy belong to the American Association of Anatomists.

Prominent Journals

Considering the whole field of biology and its subspecialties along with the subspecialties in anatomy described at the beginning of this chapter, it would not be realistic to cite all the journals that publish anatomical research. Instead, a few major anatomical journals are presented along with some exercise science journals that publish anatomically related research.

Major Anatomical Journals

Acta Anatomica
Anatomical Record
Developmental Dynamics
Journal of Anatomy (published in Britain)
Journal of Clinical Anatomy
Journal of Histochemistry
Journal of Histochemistry and Cytochemistry

Exercise Science Journals that Publish Anatomically Related Studies

Journal of Sports Medicine and Physical Fitness
Journal of Strength and Conditioning Research
Isokinetics and Exercise Science
International Journal of Sport Biomechanics
Medicine and Science in Sports and Exercise
Pediatric Exercise Science
Research Quarterly for Exercise and Sport

Concluding Remarks and Future Trends

Without question, there will be future developments of new instruments and advances in current imagery techniques that will add to our knowledge about the human body. The beginning exercise scientist has an exciting future with respect to technological advances that will help us to better understand the human body and how it responds to various forms of exercise stress. What is "science fiction" today will be reality tomorrow.

The anatomy of the human body is an essential course of study for a variety of professional careers. Exercise science students, in particular, should have a solid preparation in human anatomy combined with other experiences that examine the effect of exercise on body tissues. Anatomy has a long, controversial history that parallels, to some degree, the history of medicine and, to a lesser degree, the history of exercise science.

Technological advances have increased our understanding of anatomy and how the body works. Future advances will certainly add to this understanding and provide us with better medical care and improved physical performance, along with improved exercise prescriptions. The future of anatomy and its contribution to exercise science is an exciting prospect.

Summary

A well-grounded knowledge of anatomy is crucial for exercise scientists. Without knowledge of the structure of the human body it is difficult to appreciate even the most basic concepts underlying physical activity.

Anatomy has a number of subspecialties including gross anatomy, histology, comparative anatomy, embryology, developmental anatomy, and pathological anatomy. Exercise science students should recognize the importance of these subspecialties to many professions including medicine, dentistry, physical and occupational therapy, and nursing.

Technological advances such as the electron microscope, X-rays, CT scan, PET scan, MRI imaging, DXA, and ultrasonography have greatly increased our knowledge of anatomy. These technologies are now frequently used in exercise science research and, in the future, will likely become even more common.

STUDY QUESTIONS

1. Define anatomy.

2. Name and describe the major subdivisions of anatomy.

3. Why is a knowledge of anatomy essential to the exercise scientist?

4. Present an example of a research study in exercise science that would involve anatomical knowledge.

5. Why is the study of the history of anatomy (or any subject) important?

6. What is the prescientific period?

7. What is meant by the scientific period?

8. Describe the major influence on the study of anatomy in ancient China.

9. What was a major philosophical difference between the Greek era and the era of the Roman Empire?

10. How did the Arabians contribute to the advance of anatomy?

11. Why was anatomy (and science) suppressed for nearly 1000 years after Claudius Galen?

12. What were the major contributions made to anatomy by Andreas Vesalius?

13. What was William Harvey's discovery and why is it considered one of the major anatomical–medical advancements?

14. What event in the 1450s was particularly influential to the advance of anatomy and science?

15. Who discovered the x-ray and why is it called an x-ray?

GLOSSARY

Anatomy   The study of the parts of an organism and their relationship to each other.

Alcmaeon (500 B.C.)   Greek scientist who wrote some of the earliest works on anatomy.

Aristotle (384–322 B.C.)   Greek scientist and philosopher considered the founder of comparative anatomy.

Arteriosclerosis   Hardening of the arteries; degenerative condition of the arteries resulting in a loss of their elasticity and the development of thicker walls.

CAT scan   Computerized-axial tomography, a body-imaging technique utilizing x-rays and computers to provide cross-sectional images of the body.

Comparative anatomy Type of anatomy that compares structural similarities and differences in animals, including humans.

Developmental anatomy Study of the anatomical changes that occur from birth to death.

DXA Dual energy x-ray absorptiometry; an x-ray using more than one wavelength and a special filter that varies the energy peaks. Useful for estimating amounts of fat, muscle, and bone.

Embryology The study of anatomical changes in tissues from conception to birth.

Erasistratus (310–250 B.C.) Greek physiologist and anatomist known as the Father of Physiology.

Galen, Claudius (129–199) The Prince of Physicians. His writings on anatomy and medicine dominated medical thought for over a thousand years.

Gross anatomy The study of body structures that can be seen without the aid of a microscope.

Hammurabi (1792–1750 B.C.) Babylonian king who published a set of laws for society known as the Code of Hammurabi.

Harvey, William (1578–1657) English anatomist who is credited with describing how the blood travels in a circle.

Herophilus (335–300 B.C.) Greek anatomist credited with being the Father of Anatomy.

Hippocrates (460–377 B.C.) Greek physician known as the Father of Western Medicine. Developed the Hippocratic Oath, still taken by some physicians, and known for the Hippocratic Collection, writings on medicine issued under his name.

Histology The microscopic study of cells and tissues.

MRI Magnetic resonance imaging, a medical diagnostic technique that uses a magnetic field to produce anatomical pictures of the living body.

Pathological anatomy The study of anatomical changes that occur in tissues as a result of disease.

PET scan Position emission tomography; a body-scanning procedure that used injected radioactive substances to help to measure the metabolic activity of a tissue or organ.

Roentgen, Wilhelm (1845–1923) Discovered the x-ray or Roentgen rays in 1895.

Ultrasound sonagraphy Use of sound waves to assess body tissues.

Vesalius, Andreas (1514–1564) Belgian physician known as the Reformer of Anatomy. Author of *De Humani Corporis Fabrica,* the first accurately illustrated anatomy text.

SUGGESTED READINGS

Chung, K. W. *Gross Anatomy* (3rd ed.). Philadelphia PA: Williams and Wilkins, 1995.

Hall-Craggs, E. C. D. *Anatomy as a Basis for Clinical Medicine* (2nd ed.). Baltimore MD: Urban and Schwarzeberg Inc., 1986.

Moore, K. L., and A. F. Dalley. *Clinically Oriented Anatomy* (4th ed.). Philadelphia PA: Lippincott, Williams and Wilkins, 1999.

REFERENCES

1. Carola, R., J. P. Harky, and C. R. Noback. *Human Anatomy.* New York: McGraw-Hill Book Company, 1992.

2. Chernow, B. A., and G. A. Vallasi (Eds.). *The Columbia Encyclopedia.* New York: Columbia University Press, 1993.

3. Chewning, E. B. *Anatomy Illustrated.* New York: Simon and Schuster, 1979.

4. Dorland's Illustrated Medical Dictionary (26th ed.). Philadelphia: W. B. Saunders Company, 1974.

5. Hixon, J. *The History of the Human Body.* New York: Cooper Square Publishers, 1966.

6. Karpovich, P. V., and W. C. Sinning. *Physiology of Muscular Activity.* Philadelphia: W. B. Saunders Company, 1971.

7. Knight, B. *Discovering the Human Body.* London: Imprint Books Limited, 1980.

8. Lyons, A., and R. J. Petrucelli. *Medicine, an Illustrated History.* New York: Harry N. Abrams, 1978.

9. Marieb, E. N., and J. Mallatt. *Human Anatomy.* Redwood City, CA: Benjamin/Cummings Publishing Company, 1992.

10. McMurrich, J. P. *Leonardo da Vinci, the Anatomist.* Baltimore: Williams and Wilkins, 1930.

11. Nuland, S. B. *Doctors.* New York: Random House, 1995.

12. Persaud, T. V. N. *Early History of Anatomy.* Springfield, IL: Charles C Thomas Publisher, 1984.

13. Roche, A. F., S. B. Heymsfield, and T. G. Lohman. *Human Body Composition.* Champaign, IL: Human Kinetics, 1996.

14. Saunders, J. B. de C. M., and C. D. O'Malley. *The Illustrations from the Works of Andreas Vesalius of Brussels.* New York: Dover Publications, 1973.

15. Singer, C. *A Short History of Anatomy and Physiology from the Greeks to Harvey.* New York: Dover Publications, 1957.

16. Van De Graaff, K. M. *Human Anatomy.* Dubuque, IA: William C. Brown Publishers, 1995.

CHAPTER

4 Athletic Training: The Profession

RONALD P. PFEIFFER

History of the National Athletic Trainers' Association
  Role Delineation Study of Athletic Training
  Description of the Profession
Definition of an Athletic Trainer
  NATA Membership Categories
NATA Board of Certification
  History of the BOC Examination
  NATABOC Examination Eligibility Today
  NATABOC Examination Format
  NATABOC Continuing Education
    Unit Requirements
  State Regulation of Athletic Trainers
Employment Settings
  Hospital-based Sports Medicine and
    Industrial Clinics
  High School Settings
  College and University Settings
  Professional Sports Settings
NATA Today
  NATA National Office, Administrative,
    and Leadership Structure

  Research and Education Foundation
  NATA District and National Meetings
  NATA on the World Wide Web
Professional Education of Athletic Trainers
**History of the NATA Professional
Education Committee**
**American Medical Association Recognition as
an Allied Health Profession**
From NATA Approved to CAAHEP Accredited
  Undergraduate Education: CAAHEP Accredited
  Graduate Education
  Synopsis of the Recommendations of the NATA
    Educational Task Force
The Future of Athletic Training
Professional Journals and Related Publications
Summary
Study Questions
Glossary
Suggested Readings
References

Historical records indicate that some of the earliest known athletic trainers were associated with the athletes of the ancient Greek civilization. In those days the athletic trainers were known as *paidotribi* (literal interpretation meaning "youth, or boy, rubbers") (1). Although it is doubtful that these early athletic trainers provided much more than simple massages and basic nutritional advice to their athletes, they were, no doubt, greatly appreciated. The modern version of the athletic trainer first evolved in association with the growth of inter-collegiate athletes in the late nineteenth and early twentieth centuries within the United States. As sports programs grew in size, it was inevitable that the numbers of injuries would increase as well. This is particularly true in the sport of tackle football for which safety equipment was extremely crude and offered little protection from the forces of the game. As intercollegiate athletic programs grew in popularity during the first half of the twentieth century, there was parallel growth in the numbers of athletic trainers associated with these programs. Because no formal professional education programs for athletic trainers existed, much of their knowledge was learned on the job and borrowed from the medical community. It was not until the 1950s that a professional association for athletic trainers emerged.

History of the National Athletic Trainers' Association

The need for a professional association for athletic trainers became apparent during the 1940s when a number of regional athletic training associates began to meet on a regular basis. Thus, the stage was set for the establishment of a professional association of athletic trainers at the national level. On June 24–25, 1950, the first national meeting of athletic trainers was held in Kansas City, Missouri, and the National Athletic Trainers' Association (*NATA*) was formed. This first meeting was attended by 101 athletic trainers from across the United States (11). The following year, the first organized meeting of the newly formed association was held on June 22–24, again in Kansas City, Missouri (11).

Five years later NATA approved the publication of its professional journal, entitled the *Journal of the National Athletic Trainers Association,* which was published quarterly. Many changes occurred within both the NATA and the profession of athletic training during the next several decades. A number of committees were formed to oversee such functions as professional education, certification, and membership. On June 21, 1967, the American Medical Association (*AMA*) first recognized the role of the athletic trainer as an important part of the health care team of the athlete. In essence, the AMA recognized that the athletic trainer formed an extremely valuable link between the athlete, coach, and physician.

Role Delineation Study of Athletic Training

In 1993 the National Athletic Trainer's Association Board of Certification (*NATABOC*), along with Columbia Assessment Service (CAS), conducted an extensive role delineation study to determine the work that an athletic trainer performs (4). Two thousand surveys were mailed to a randomly selected group of NATABOC-certified athletic trainers within the United States (certification indicates that the individual has passed the required examination; see the section on certification). Of those, 810 usable surveys were returned to CAS. The findings of this latest NATABOC role delineation study were subsequently published in a document entitled *The National Athletic Trainers' Association Board of Certification, Inc.—Role Delineation Study.* (4).

Description of the Profession

The results of the NATABOC role delineation study indicated that in the 1990s NATABOC certified the athletic trainer's scope of practice to include the following domains:

Prevention of athletic injuries
Recognition, evaluation, and immediate care of athletic injuries
Rehabilitation and reconditioning of athletic injuries
Health care administration
Professional development and responsibility

Obviously, not all certified athletic trainers spend the same amounts of time on each of these domains in their day-to-day practice. For example, an athletic trainer employed in a sports medicine clinic setting may spend most of his or her time in the third domain, rehabilitation and reconditioning. The modern sports medicine clinic is typically equipped with an array of exercise machines, both *isokinetic* and *isotonic* (see Figure 4.1). State-of-the-art isokinetic machines such as Cybex and Biodex are highly sophisticated rehabilitation devices that typically include computer hardware and software used to both assess and record patient progress. In addition, athletic trainers receive extensive training in the proper application of electrotherapeutic devices such as transcutaneous electrical nerve stimulation (TENS), ultrasound, galvanic stimulators, neuromuscular electrical stimulation (NMES), shortwave and microwave diathermy, and interferential electrical muscle stimulation. All these devices can be utilized during the injury recovery process. Athletic trainers receive formal education in the proper application and protocols used in exercise rehabilitation and reconditioning.

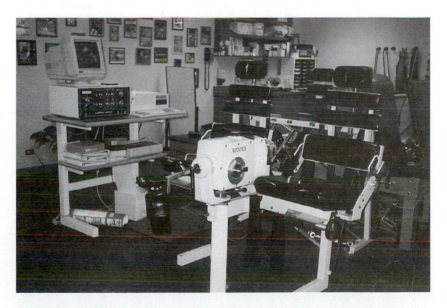

FIGURE 4.1   Biodex isokinetic dynamometer.

An athletic trainer employed in the more traditional setting (Figure 4.2) of a collegiate athletic program may find that his or her time is distributed completing tasks in all five of the domains listed above. It should be noted that, as a profession, athletic training has been and continues to be an evolving profession with respect to scope of practice, location of professional employment, and the population being served.

Definition of an Athletic Trainer

According to the National Athletic Trainers' Association, an *athletic trainer* is defined as "a highly educated and skilled professional specializing in athletic health care. In cooperation with physicians and other allied health personnel, the athletic trainer functions as an integral member of the athletic health care team in secondary schools, colleges and universities, sports medicine clinics, professional sports programs, and other athletic health care settings" (8).

As can be seen by this definition, the athletic trainer may practice within a wide array of professional settings. Although these settings are many, all athletic trainers are similar in both their professional education and certification process.

NATA Membership Categories

The NATA offers a variety of different membership categories: certified (open only to those individuals who possess current NATABOC certification), associate (other professionals without NATABOC certification), student (may be either non-NATABOC certified or may possess the credentials; typically graduate students), international (non-NATABOC

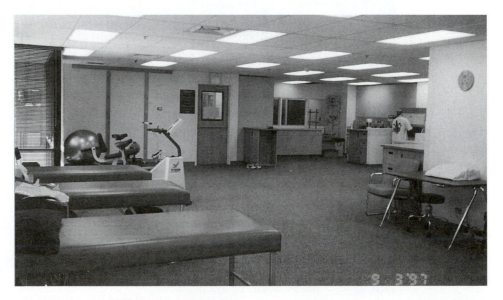

FIGURE 4.2   Typical athletic training room.

certified without an address in the United States), and supplier (open only to corporations that manufacture products that are used by athletic trainers). The bulk of the membership annually is made up primarily of the certified members, followed by the student membership category.

NATA Board of Certification

December 31, 1969, the date of the first NATA certification examination, was a historic date within the profession. Prior to this date, no form of standardized examination existed for the purposes of establishing a minimal competency level for the entry-level athletic trainer. In 1970 a formal NATA Board of Certification was established to oversee the examination process.

History of the BOC Examination

The first certification examination was given in 1969. Designed to verify what were at the time considered to be the essential cognitive and psychomotor skills for an athletic trainer, this test consisted of both a written and oral–practical component. With the inception of the certification exam, all previously practicing athletic trainers were allowed to be "grandfathered" (automatically certified). Thus, only those individuals wishing to enter the profession were required to sit for the examination.

The first NATA certification examination was developed with the help of the Professional Examination Service (PES) of the American Public Health Association. In 1973, the following general requirements were established by NATA in order to sit for the certification examination.

1. College graduate with a teaching license
2. Work under a NATA certified trainer
   Approved curricula (two years)
   Physical therapy degree (two years)
   Apprenticeship (two years)
3. One-year NATA membership prior to examination

NATABOC Examination Eligibility Today

Since the early days of the NATA certification examination, the profession of athletic training has changed significantly with respect to virtually all aspects of the field. Whereas the majority of the entry-level jobs in the 1970s were in the high school and collegiate settings, initial placement shifted to a new venue in the 1980s, the sports medicine clinic. In addition, educational requirements have evolved, with more emphasis on specialized course work, more structure of the practical hours, and the dropping of the teaching certificate requirement. Thus, the certification examination process has also been modified significantly to better reflect the changes within the profession.

Several major structural changes that took place during the 1980s also had a significant impact on the certification testing process. First, the Certification Committee formally separated from the NATA in 1989 to become an independent, incorporated certification body, the NATA Board of Certification (NATABOC). This change was seen as an important step in improving the professional status and recognition of the certification examination process. The headquarters for NATABOC are currently located in Raleigh, North Carolina, where a full-time staff provides a number of services to athletic trainers related to certification and continuing education. The NATABOC is a member of the National Organization of Competency Assurance (NOCA) in Washington, D.C.

Second, a new professional testing agency was brought into the process in an effort to make the examination more appropriate. Columbia Assessment Services, Inc., of Raleigh, North Carolina, presently is charged with the development and administration of the NATABOC certification examination.

Third, the test itself has been modified significantly and now consists of three major components, the written, the practical, and a new section, the written simulation. These three components are designed to test the candidate on his or her mastery of the essential cognitive, affective, and psychomotor skills that have been identified as necessary for the entry-level athletic trainer. The NATABOC presently requires completion of one of the following education options in order to sit for the certification examination.

1. *Internship route* (formerly known as the apprenticeship route), to be eliminated in 2004.   Graduate with a minimum of a bachelor's degree from an accredited institution of higher learning and completion of the seven required classes: health (nutrition, drugs and substance abuse, health education), human anatomy, kinesiology–biomechanics, human physiology, physiology of exercise, basic athletic training, advanced athletic training, and 1500 practical hours (1000 hours must be attained in the traditional setting).

2. Graduate of an accredited curriculum in athletic training, as accredited by the Commission on Accreditation of Allied Health Education Programs (*CAAHEP*). Accredited curriculum graduates are required to have earned a minimum of 800 practical hours under the direct supervision of a clinical instructor. Presently, there are approximately 100 colleges and universities within the United States that offer either NATA approved, or CAAHEP accredited curricula in athletic training. A list of these colleges and universities can be found at the website http://www.nata.org/approved/index.htm.

■ As of 1993, all existing NATA-approved curricula wishing to continue their programs, as well as any universities wishing to initiate a curriculum, were required to do so under the new guidelines as set forth by the Commission on Accreditation of Allied Health Education Programs (CAAHEP). For more details, refer to the section in this chapter on the professional education of athletic trainers.

■ The NATABOC provides a detailed description of the certification examination application process, including application criteria and specific requirements. This information can be obtained by contacting NATABOC, Inc., 3725 National Drive Suite 213, Raleigh, NC 27612, (919)787–2721.

NATABOC Examination Format

The first certification examination consisted of both a written and an oral–practical component. The written examination was 150 multiple-choice questions covering content from the required courses. The oral–practical portion consisted of a set of questions designed to assess the applicant's practical skills and knowledge.

At present, the NATABOC certification examination consists of three components: (1) the written (150 multiple-choice questions), (2) the practical (administered by two certified athletic trainers), and (3) the written simulation (designed to evaluate the candidate's real-life decision-making skills). The test is designed to test for competency in all the major domains identified as comprising the knowledge and skills required for the entry-level athletic trainer. The examination is offered four times per year at different sites throughout the United States. In the event that a candidate fails to pass one or more portions of the examination, he or she can reapply to take the portion(s) failed at a later date.

Upon successful completion of the NATABOC certification examination, the candidate can legally claim the title of Athletic Trainer Certified (ATC) or Certified Athletic Trainer (CAT).

NATABOC Continuing Education Unit (CEU) Requirements

Once the certification examination has been passed, the candidate carries the credential ATC. However, this credential represents entry-level competence only. To remain certified by the NATABOC, all certified athletic trainers must complete a minimum of eight continuing education units (CEUs) every three years. *CEU*s can only be earned if they have been preapproved by the NATABOC. They fall into one of four categories based on their format. Categories A and B are formal events, such as seminars, conferences, symposiums, and home study courses that have been approved by the NATABOC. Category C includes postgraduate education, specifically college courses that reflect one or more of the five domains identified in the most recent role delineation study. Category D includes formal training in CPR, EMT, or first aid. To receive credit for any CEU, the athletic trainer must document having completed the work in any of the four categories, and the official CEU reporting form must be sent to the NATABOC prior to the CEU deadline. Furthermore, all evidence of the specific CEUs earned for a given reporting period must be kept on file by the athletic trainer in the event of an audit by the NATABOC.

State Regulation of Athletic Trainers

Although having a well established process for professional certification assures the general public of some level of quality control (minimum level of competence) for anyone claiming to be an athletic trainer, it does little with respect to defining the specific procedures and/or services that can be performed and the population that can legally be treated. This is due to the fact that the real mechanisms for professional standards and scope of practice in the medical and allied health professions are virtually always regulated at the state level. Practice acts are the end result of legislative action resulting in the passage of a bill that defines a profession in terms of who may legally claim to be in the profession, what services may legally be provided, and to whom the services may be provided. The specific mechanism is most often a state license, or registration, that is typically monitored, either directly or indirectly, by the Board of Medicine in that particular state.

According to Rello,

> state licensure not only ensures that only those credentialed may refer to themselves as ATs (ATCs), it also provides guidance as to where and how the AT may practice, by placing limitations on approved settings, clarifying proper medical supervision, and restricting client population. For example, ATCs should not be caring for stroke patients in a hospital but should be allowed to care for athletes in a sports medicine clinic. (13)

Getting such legislation started, shepherded through the legislative process, voted on, passed, and finally enforced is a complex and often expensive process, both in monetary terms and time invested. However, practicing athletic trainers, regardless of professional setting, stand to benefit from having such state regulation in place. Virtually all other medical and allied health professions, including medical doctors, nurses, physical therapists, occupational therapists, dentists, and others, operate under such statutes.

Although it is debatable as to which type of statute is more beneficial (license or registration), either is generally considered as better than no regulation at all. To date, 33 states have enacted some type of regulatory mechanism governing the practice of athletic training within the confines of their borders. It is important for anyone planning to seek employment as an athletic trainer in a particular state to check with the Board of Medicine in that state to see if such a practice act is in place and if they are in compliance with the law. A complete listing of all states with athletic training regulations in place can be obtained by contacting NATA (see the subsection NATA on the World Wide Web for information on how to contact NATA).

Employment Settings

Before specific employment settings are described, the following short description of "a typical day" for the certified athletic trainer should help the reader gain insight into the professional duties of an athletic trainer.

> The typical athletic day for a certified athletic trainer varies with the level of competition and other institutional requirements. Some high school athletic trainers are hired by school systems and may also teach. These individuals must manage their time carefully to ensure that students receive professional academic instruction in the classroom and quality health care in athletic endeavors.
>
> Before practice, the athletic trainer tapes, bandages, wraps, braces, and completes similar preventive measures. During practice, the athletic trainer evaluates injuries and determines whether to refer athletes to a physician or follow standing orders and manage minor injuries. The athletic trainer must ensure continual communication between the injured athlete, physician, coach, and family on when and how the athlete can return to practice and competition.
>
> As specialists in the prevention, recognition, and rehabilitation of injuries incurred by athletes, athletic trainers administer immediate emergency care and, under the supervision of the family or team physician, use their knowledge of each athlete's injuries and the factors influencing them to develop a treatment program based on medical, exercise, and sports sciences. (*Source:* The Certified Athletic Trainer, brochure, 1996, NATA)

The history of the athletic trainer in the United States is directly related to the intercollegiate athletic setting. For the better part of this century the bulk of the certified athletic trainers in this country have found employment within the college or university setting or within secondary schools. However, as the field of sports medicine grew in the late 1970s and early 1980s, a major shift occurred in employment trends for the athletic trainer. It has been reported that since 1980 there has been a 300% increase in the number of sports medicine centers within the United States (14). This trend has played significantly into the employment market for the certified athletic trainer.

Hospital-based Sports Medicine and Industrial Clinics

The explosive growth in the field of sports medicine and in the number of sports medicine clinics throughout the country is nothing short of remarkable. This growth has been directly related to the fitness boom that swept through the United States beginning in the 1970s. A large number of the patients coming to a typical sports medicine clinic are adult aged, recreational athletes. In addition, many sports medicine clinics also establish contractual agreements with public schools to provide athletic training services (outreach services) for their student athletes. Hospitals have not ignored the tremendous growth in sports medicine, and many have established sports medicine centers that provide outpatient services to both the recreational and interscholastic athlete. Additionally, larger corporations that provide in-house exercise and recreation activities for their employees have become a potential market for certified athletic trainers.

As of July, 1995, 41.5% of all certified athletic trainers were working in a hospital, industrial clinic, or high school setting. (see Table 4.1). Moss reported that the 1996 projected annual salary for an entry-level athletic trainer in the clinic/hospital settings would be $25,698 (BS degree) and $30,300 (MS degree). See Table 4.2 (7).

The future of employment in the clinic/high school (outreach) and hospital-based settings is unclear because of recent changes in the health care industry. Clinics and hospitals rely greatly on third-party billing for reimbursement for their services. Reimbursement for the services of an athletic trainer is just beginning to be accepted on a limited basis and is directly related to state regulations and practice acts.

High School Settings

Of the approximately 22,000 high schools within the United States, fewer than 2200 employ an athletic trainer. That computes to 15% of all certified athletic trainers. Schools have several options available to them regarding the employment of an athletic trainer. These include the *teacher/athletic trainer* combination, whereby the athletic trainer provides classroom instruction as well as serving as the athletic trainer in the afternoons and evenings. This option is the most common due to the fact that the administration is in essence killing two birds with one stone; they are filling a need in the classroom as well as providing athletic training services to their student athletes. Available data suggest that the majority of athletic trainers who graduate with a teaching degree are credentialed in either physical education or health education (3). Another option is the hiring of a full-time athletic trainer with no teaching assignments. The advantage in this situation is that the athletic

TABLE 4.1   NATA Certified Members, July 1995

Setting	No. of ATCs	%
Clinical/industrial	2,814	20
Clinic/high school	2,382	17
Hospital	632	4.5
High school	2,157	15
College/university	2,446	17
Junior college	221	2
Professional sports	444	3
Other professional	927	7
Retired	1	0
Certified students	1,828	13
No data	162	1
Unemployed	66	0.5
Total	14,080	

Source: Curtis, N. (1996). Job Outlook for Athletic Trainers. *Athletic Therapy Today* 1(2), pp. 7.

TABLE 4.2   Entry-level Salary Projections (Based on % Increases from 1994 Salaries)

Position	X% Salary Increase per Year	1996 Projected Salaries	
		Bachelor's	Master's
Hospital/clinic			
Athletic trainer	+3.81	$25,698	$30,300
Athletic trainer/athletics	+4.72	26,282	28,273
Total	+4.62	26,213	28,493
College/university			
Head athletic trainer	+3.64	24,813	27,611
Athletic trainer/teacher	+3.96	23,924	27,907
Assistant athletic trainer	+3.06	23,331	25,147
Total	+3.55	23,871	26,844
High School			
Athletic trainer	+3.32	23,041	24,552
Athletic trainer/teacher	+3.39	27,753	29,949
Total	+3.38	26,603	29,331
Salary Summary			
Total	+4.01	25,128	27,437

Source: Moss, C. L. (1996). 1994. Entry-level Athletic Training Salaries. *Journal of Athletic Training* 31(1), pp. 27.

trainer has more time to concentrate on providing services to the student and athletes and is not forced to spend time preparing for classes. The down side of this option is that many administrators are not able to justify the expense of hiring a full-time athletic trainer. The entry-level salary for 1996 for the high school teacher/athletic trainer with a BS degree was $27,753 and with an MS degree, $29,949. The salary projections for the nonteaching athletic trainer are approximately $4,000 less at both degree levels (see Table 4.2) (7). The average annual salary for the high school athletic trainer has been reported to be $31,730 nationally (12).

Clearly, the potential employment market for the high schools is tremendous; however, the growth in this area has been slow in recent years due to budgetary constraints in many school districts around the country. The NATA continues to promote the need for certified athletic trainers within the schools through its various public relations campaigns and by funding sports injury research.

College and University Settings

For many aspiring athletic trainers, the dream job is working with a big-time intercollegiate athletic program. Available data suggest that this venue provides opportunities for a relatively small number of athletic trainers. As of July, 1995, 2667 athletic trainers were employed in this setting (2). The college and university positions take several forms, ranging from a full-time head or assistant athletic trainer to an athletic trainer with some teaching responsibilities. Data in Table 4.2 indicate that the highest salary is earned by the head athletic trainer, both at the B.S. and M.S. degree level. The future employment potential in this venue is not clear due to the fact that growth in the number of available positions appears to be stagnant. The data support this premise. Over the 3-year span from 1993 to 1995, there were approximately 2600 certified athletic trainers employed in these settings during each of those three years (2). Students interested in a career in athletic training at the college and university level should consider earning a graduate degree in athletic training or a related field and, if possible, should serve as a graduate assistant athletic trainer while completing their graduate studies. Graduate assistantships in athletic training provide an excellent opportunity to gain on-the-job experience at the college and university level. Many graduate assistantships in athletic training are available throughout the country each year at colleges and universities. To qualify, a student normally needs to be NATABOC certified or ready to sit for the examination and, in addition, may be required to complete the Graduate Record Examination (GRE). Graduate assistantships usually provide the student with a tuition waiver as well as a monthly stipend.

Professional Sports Settings

For many students in athletic training, the lure of professional sports is most compelling. The prospect of providing health care for multimillion dollar, high-profile athletes sounds almost too good to be true. The available data suggest that this dream remains just that for the majority of athletic trainers. As of 1995, 444 certified athletic trainers were employed in the professional sports setting, or 3% of the total certified membership. The number of jobs in the professional sports venue is not expected to change significantly in the near future. A typical National Football League team will employ as many as three athletic trainers, while profession baseball and basketball teams typically employ two or less. Some growth may occur with respect to the new professional soccer league that is developing within the United States and the new women's professional sports teams (basketball, softball, soccer, and others). For now, however, it appears that finding employment in professional sports will not be possible for the vast majority of new athletic trainers entering the job market.

NATA Today

The year 1950 was significant to the profession of athletic training, as it was then that the National Athletic Trainers' Association was organized. With fewer than 200 members in 1950, the NATA has since grown into a professional association with over 21,000 members today, approximately 50% of which are female. In 1990 the American Medical Association granted formal recognition as an allied health profession to athletic trainers. NATA membership is represented by 10 districts that include all 50 states and the District of Columbia, nine Canadian Provinces, Puerto Rico, and the Virgin Islands.

NATA Mission Statement.   "The mission of the National Athletic Trainers' Association is to enhance the quality of health care for the physically active through education and research in prevention, evaluation, management and rehabilitation of injuries" (NATA Membership Directory, 1996, NATA).

NATA National Office, Administrative, and Leadership Structure

The NATA national office is located in Dallas, Texas, where a variety of membership services is coordinated, including marketing, meetings coordination, publications, governmental relations, continuing education, management, research and education foundation, placement, conventions/meetings/exhibits, and accounting. The national office is staffed by a number of full-time personnel, including an executive director.

NATA operates under a constitution and an extensive set of bylaws with an administrative structure, consisting of an executive director and a board of directors; the board includes a president and the district directors from the 10 NATA districts. In turn, each of the 10 NATA districts maintains a similar administrative structure: district director (member of NATA board of directors), district president, vice-president, secretary, and treasurer. Depending on the size of the membership, individual districts may combine some of these offices.

NATA maintains a large number of standing committees that serve a variety of functions, such as advising the NATA board of directors and the membership on matters related to the profession. Examples of such committees include Audio-Visual Committee, Clinical/Industrial/Corporate Athletic Trainers' Committee, College/University Athletic Trainer's Committee, Convention Committee, History and Archives Committee, Honors and Awards Committee, and the Joint Review Committee on Athletic Training (**JRC-AT**) just to name a few.

NATA has also established professional liaisons with a large number of allied organizations, such as the American Academy of Family Physicians; American Academy of Pediatrics; American Alliance for Health, Physical Education, Recreation and Dance (AAHPERD); National Collegiate Athletic Association (NCAA); National Association of Intercollegiate Athletics (NAIA); and National Federation of State High School Associations.

NATA continues to receive major corporate sponsorship from companies such as Johnson & Johnson, Inc., Cramer Products, Inc., Gatorade, and others.

Research and Education Foundation

In keeping with its mission statement, NATA established the Research and Education Foundation (REF) in 1991 to "advance the knowledge base for injury awareness and prevention and the science of athletic training" (10). The mission of the NATA-REF "is to encourage and support research and educational programs that will advance the quality of athletic health care and promote athletic injury prevention" (10). A number of REF research grants are available to the membership on a competitive basis. The REF also serves to disseminate the results of scientific inquiry when a sufficient body of knowledge is accumulated. For example, the publication entitled "Proceedings: Mild Brain Injury in Sports Summit" was published by the NATA-REF after it sponsored a summit on this topic in Washington, D.C., on April 16–18, 1994. The NATA-REF also provides annual training grants, postgraduate fellowships, and undergraduate scholarships.

NATA District and National Meetings

Along with the NATA Annual Meeting, each of the 10 NATA Districts also holds district meetings for its members. The purpose of these meetings is to provide continuing education opportunities for certified members, to hold a general business meeting to keep the membership appraised of the financial status of both the national organization and individual districts, and to provide a forum for feedback directly to the members of the NATA board of directors regarding NATA policies and procedures and general business of the association.

In addition to the 10 NATA districts, athletic trainers in many states have established state athletic training associations. These state associations serve similar functions as the NATA districts; however, in addition, state associations are essential in the development and implementation of state regulation of athletic trainers in a particular state (licensing or registration). State associations also provide an avenue for effective public relations at the state and local levels through such activities as offering educational workshops, symposia, and in-service seminars for public school personnel, local emergency medical service personnel, and other members of the medical community.

NATA on the World Wide Web

In an effort to make services more available to the membership and to serve as a public relations tool, NATA recently established an extensive home page on the WWW at http://www.nata.org/. A great deal of information is available at this site, including descriptions of NATA, careers in athletic training, NATABOC certification, NATA leadership, and description of the profession, as well as links to other interesting sites.

NATA also offers another useful service called NATA Fax-on-Demand, which is essentially a 24 hour a day service whereby a caller with a fax machine can phone in to order a wide variety of informational documents, free of charge. For a complete listing of the documents available, phone 1-888-ASK-NATA from a Touch-Tone phone, follow the automated voice instructions, and then hang up and turn on your fax machine. You will receive the requested material within minutes of placing your order.

Professional Education of Athletic Trainers

During the same time period that the certification examination was first being developed, another NATA subcommittee, the professional advancement committee, was developing guidelines for the structure of future academic programs in the study of athletic training. It was determined that the NATA would grant approved curriculum status to programs meeting the minimum requirements (these are listed below). In 1969 only two schools had met the requirements for NATA approval of their curriculums in athletic training, the University of New Mexico and Mankato State College (11). Interest in such programs was quick to develop, however, and by 1979 there were 23 NATA-approved undergraduate curricula. Requirements for the NATA Approved Curriculum in Athletic Training at that time were the following:

> Teaching certificate in the area of choice
> Specific required courses:
>> Anatomy
>> Physiology
>> Physiology of Exercise
>> Applied Anatomy and Kinesiology
>> Psychology (two courses)
>> First Aid and Safety
>> Nutrition
>> Remedial Exercise
>> Personal, Community, and School Health
>> Techniques of Athletic Training
>> Advanced Techniques of Athletic Training
>> Laboratory Practice (six semester hours or 600 clock hours)

An alternative route to qualify for the NATA certification examination, dubbed the apprenticeship route, was also recognized during this time period. The apprenticeship route placed a heavy reliance on the educational benefits of practical experience gained under a NATA-certified athletic trainer. Initially, applicants for the NATA certification examination who completed the apprenticeship route were required to complete 1600 hours of practical work. Additionally, a college degree was required, typically in physical education or health.

History of the NATA Professional Education Committee

A number of significant changes have occurred with respect to the professional education of athletic trainers since the professional advancement committee developed curriculum guidelines in the late 1960s. In 1973, Sayers "Bud" Miller was appointed to a 2-year term as chairman of the newly created NATA Professional Education Committee (PEC). The major purpose of this important committee was to continue to evaluate the educational programs for athletic training and to make recommendations for their improvement to the NATA board of directors. The NATA-PEC developed guidelines for both undergraduate and graduate curricula in athletic training. PEC also developed an approval process for athletic training programs, including the development of procedures for the on-site evaluation of such programs. During this time period, three different educational options were available to students wishing to become certified athletic trainers: (1) graduate from an NATA-approved undergraduate curriculum, (2) graduate from an NATA-approved graduate curriculum, and (3) graduate and qualify for the NATA certification examination by the apprenticeship route.

In 1980 a resolution was passed by the NATA board of directors that required all existing NATA-approved programs to become academic majors or major equivalents by 1990 or sooner (3). The impact of this resolution was that many programs that were most often degrees in physical education with either a minor or emphasis in athletic training would need to change their curricula to become full-fledged majors, or their equivalent, in Athletic Training.

Once a program was granted NATA-PEC-approved status, it was valid for 5 years, at which time the program was required to apply for reapproval. All NATA-PEC-approved programs were required to have a designated program director (NATABOC-certified athletic trainer), NATABOC-certified clinical instructors, a designated team physician, and support faculty. The program director was in charge of the day-to-day operation of all aspects of the athletic training education program. In addition, the program director was required to complete an annual report verifying compliance with the guidelines to the NATA-PEC. Programs found not to be in compliance with the guidelines were placed on probation for 1 year in order to correct the problem(s).

American Medical Association Recognition as an Allied Health Profession

On June 22, 1990, a major milestone was achieved by the chairman of the NATA-PEC, Robert Behnke, and former chairman Gary Delforge, NATA vice-president, John Schrader, NATA executive director, Alan A. Smith, and a small group of other NATA members. It was on this date that the American Medical Association's Council on Medical Education (CME) formally recognized athletic training as an allied health profession (9). AMA recognition brought with it not only a significant amount of prestige for the athletic training profession, but also signaled a transition in the process of professional education for athletic trainers.

From NATA Approved to CAAHEP Accredited

Effective in 1993, all entry-level athletic training programs were no longer evaluated under the NATA-PEC guidelines, but rather by the AMA's Committee on Allied Health Education and Accreditation (CAHEA). Professional accreditation by an outside agency (that is, the AMA) was a major step in the professional advancement of athletic training. The CAHEA was replaced by the Committee on Accreditation of Allied Health Education Programs (CAAHEP), which accredits 28 allied health professions. The NATA-PEC no longer serves in the capacity of approving undergraduate athletic training education programs. They continue to grant approval status to graduate programs in athletic training designed to provide advanced instruction in the field of athletic training.

Undergraduate Education: CAAHEP Accredited

All NATA-approved curricula in athletic training that existed at the time that the CAAHEP was brought online were treated as "new" programs when their 5-year NATA approval period expired. At the time of the transition there were 73 existing undergraduate and 13 graduate programs in the United States. CAAHEP accreditation is the culmination of a lengthy application process, by some estimates a process that takes two or more years to complete. In the CAAHEP format, the NATA-PEC was essentially replaced by a new review committee, the Joint Review Committee-Athletic Training (JRC-AT). The JRC-AT is a standing committee that meets several times annually to review athletic training education programs that are in the final stage of the application process for CAAHEP accreditation. CAAHEP-accredited programs are required to have personnel similar to the NATA-PEC-approved programs, that is, designated program director, clinical instructors, medical advisor, and the like. It is important to note that CAAHEP accreditation applies to entry-level education programs, that is, professional programs that provide education and training that is sufficient to meet the requirements for entry into a given professional field such as athletic training. The following outline provides an overview of the application process.

1. *Request of all application materials from JRC-AT office.*   These materials consist of a copy of the Standards and Guidelines for an Accredited Educational Program for the Athletic Trainer, an application for accreditation, and a self-study report.

2. *Development of a self-study committee.*   This committee, normally spearheaded by the curriculum director, consists of a number of key personnel, including the medical advisor (team physician), athletic training clinical instructors, key faculty members, the department chairperson, and others. This committee meets on a regular basis to discuss and review all aspects of the athletic training education program. Normally, each team member is charged with collecting necessary information, such as the budget, equipment, facilities, required and elective classes required, course syllabi, admission, retention, graduation procedures, verification of teaching of all required competencies (191 cognitive, affective, and psychomotor skills), NATABOC examination passing rates, placement data, and a number of other pieces of information. In addition, program weaknesses are identified and a plan for their correction is developed and implemented. Once this material is collected, it is placed in the self-study document and forwarded to the JRC-AT office for initial review. It should be noted that the self-study document is typically a bound volume consisting of several hundred pages of materials.

3. *CAAHEP accreditation application and self-study document review.*   The JRC-AT reviews all documents provided by the institution to determine if they will be granted an on-site visitation by a review team from the JRC-AT. Once the site visit is granted, the next step is the on-site visit.

4. *JRC-AT on-site visitation.*   The purpose of the on-site visit is to verify what has been reported in the self-study document. The visiting team consists of two NATA-BOC-certified athletic trainers who have attended JRC-AT training sessions at the NATA annual meetings. There is a chief review officer and an assistant review officer on each visit. The visiting team interviews a large number of faculty, staff, administrators, medical personnel, and students during the visit, which normally lasts two to three days. At the conclusion of the visit the review team compiles a listing of program strengths and weaknesses, as well as any areas where there appears to be a noncompliance or partial compliance with the required program standards as set forth by CAAHEP. There is an exit meeting with the athletic training program director, department chair, and the review team at which all initial findings of the review team are discussed. At this point the site visit is concluded and the review team departs and later submits a written report of their findings to the program director. The program director is allowed to respond in writing to any aspect of the site visit report. At this time the review team's written report, along with the program director's written response, if any, is forwarded to the JRC-AT office for review.

5. *JRC-AT review of site visit report.*   The JRC-AT meets several times a year to review all programs that have undergone an on-site visit during the preceding period from the last JRC-AT meeting. The purpose of this meeting is to determine if a program has complied with all the CAAHEP essentials for an athletic training education program. The committee reviews the self-study documents and the site visitors' report. At this time a decision is made regarding the program, with three possible options: program is deemed (1) fully compliant, (2) partially compliant, or (3) noncompliant. These recommendations are then forwarded to CAAHEP for a final decision.

6. *CAAHEP review and recommendation.*   CAAHEP takes the recommendations forwarded by JRC-AT and makes the final decision on each program. If the program is found to be fully compliant with all the essentials, it may be granted accreditation for a duration of up to 7 years. If the program is found to be partially compliant, it may be granted a shorter period of accreditation with the stipulation that the program must undergo another on-site visit in order to verify that the deficiencies have been corrected. A program found to be noncompliant is denied accreditation and required to resubmit an application and self-study document and undergo another on-site visit before being considered again for accreditation.

The process of developing and maintaining a CAAHEP-accredited athletic training education program is a complex endeavor that requires a considerable amount of effort by a large number of personnel. In spite of this, however, institutions are eager to engage in the process, and having accreditation from an outside agency such as CAAHEP is seen as a prestigious accomplishment. Students also benefit by having the assurance that the program in which they are enrolled meets the rigid requirements for accreditation that ensures that they receive a quality educational experience.

A survey of athletic training program directors regarding their perceptions of the transition from the NATA-PEC approval process to the CAAHEP accreditation process concluded that overall the transition would not have a major impact on existing NATA-approved programs. The major changes were seen as positive, such as more involvement in the program by both faculty and administration, a greater emphasis on educational outcomes, and more time required for the self-study process (5).

Model Program Based on CAAHEP Standards and Guidelines. CAAHEP-accredited educational programs in athletic training are competency-based programs, rather than course based. The competencies represent specific cognitive (knowledge), affective (attitude), and psychomotor (skill) outcomes that the entry-level athletic trainer needs to master in order to be successful. The competencies are derived from the role delineation study mentioned earlier and must be accounted for either in the classroom instruction component or the clinical instruction component, or in both. CAAHEP does not require specific courses; rather, general subject matter areas are listed and required. However, individual programs can choose to devote either one or more full college courses to a subject matter area or, if possible, may devote a portion of one class to a given area. Programs are given a great degree of flexibility to tailor the construction of an athletic training curriculum based on the unique aspects of each institution. The following is a list of the required subject matter areas as stated in the CAAHEP document "Essentials and Guidelines for an Accredited Educational Program for the Athletic Trainer":

1. Prevention of athletic injuries/illnesses
2. Evaluation of athletic injuries/illnesses
3. First aid and emergency care
4. Therapeutic modalities
5. Therapeutic exercise
6. Administration of athletic training programs
7. Human anatomy
8. Human physiology
9. Exercise physiology
10. Kinesiology/biomechanics
11. Nutrition
12. Psychology
13. Personal/community health

Again, it should be noted that CAAHEP does not require a course in each of these areas; rather, each area must be accounted for either by way of classroom instruction or in the clinical education component of the athletic training education program. The typical program, however, will offer one or more courses for each of the above subject matter areas.

Clinical Instruction Component. Since athletic training is an allied health profession that deals with people in a medical setting, any educational program must also include a clinical instruction component. As was described earlier in this chapter, even in its infancy, athletic training education programs required a specific number of clinical hours for graduation.

CAAHEP does not specify a specific minimum number of clinical hours; however, NATABOC requires a minimum of 800 hours for a CAAHEP-accredited program graduate in order to sit for the certification examination. In reality, most existing programs require more than 800 hours. The clinical instruction components consist of hands-on instruction within the athletic training room settings on campus or, in some cases, in the high school setting. A clinical instructor (NATABOC-certified athletic trainer) provides direct supervision to the student on a daily basis. Specific skills are taught and mastered prior to graduation. Students generally are given specific assignments to a team or teams and may eventually travel with the team for off-site events. In addition, students typically view surgeries, complete injury evaluations with the team physician(s), and perform many administrative tasks, such as updating medical files, completing insurance forms, and working on inventory. For most students, the clinical component of the program is the most rewarding and interesting. Although no specific criteria for the number of years required for the clinical component are specified by CAAHEP, the typical program spreads the clinical experience out over a 2- to 3-year period.

In conclusion, a CAAHEP-accredited athletic training education program will offer a major, or major equivalent, in athletic training and, in addition, will require that the student complete at least 800 clinical hours in the training room setting. Individual programs may vary greatly in the specific classes required to meet the subject matter and competencies as stipulated by CAAHEP. As of June 1998 there were 82 CAAHEP-accredited undergraduate, entry-level programs in the United States. A sample curriculum from Boise State University, a CAAHEP-accredited program, is shown in Table 4.3.

Graduate Education

With the transition to CAAHEP accreditation of all entry-level athletic training education programs, the existing graduate programs in athletic training were forced to consider if they wanted to pursue accreditation through CAAHEP. This would require that they meet the same requirements as an undergraduate athletic training education program in the required subject matter areas and clinical instruction. The other option would be to offer a graduate degree, masters or doctorate, in athletic training with the intent to offer advanced instruction in the field of athletic training. As of the 1996–97 academic year, there were no CAAHEP-accredited graduate programs in athletic training. There are, however, a number of excellent graduate programs in athletic training, the majority of which are at the master's degree level. Sample graduate programs at the master's (University of Oregon) and doctoral (University of Virginia) levels are shown in Figures 4.3 and 4.4, respectively.

Synopsis of the Recommendations of the NATA Educational Task Force

As a result of growing pressure from within the membership of NATA, a 15-member panel, called the Educational Task Force (ETF), was appointed by the board of directors in December 1994 (6). The membership of the ETF was comprised of athletic training educators,

TABLE 4.3 Undergraduate Curriculum at Boise State University for the Bachelor of Science Degree in Athletic Training

Course Number and Title	Credits	Course Number and Title	Credits
E101, 102 English Composition	6	PE 142 Taping and Wrapping Techniques in Athletic Training	1
Area I		PE 230, 231 Applied Anatomy and Lab	3
Area I core course in one field	3	PE 236 Introduction to Athletic Injuries	3
Area I core course in a second field	3	PE 284 Microcomputers in PE	3
Area I core in a third field	3	PE 306, 308 Human Growth and Motor Learning and Lab	3
Area I core course in any field	3	PE 309 Evaluation in Physical Education	3
Area II		PE 310, 312 Exercise Physiology and Lab	3
CM III Fundamentals of Speech Communication	3	PE 313 Conditioning Procedures	2
P 101 General Psychology	3	PE 351, 352 Kinesiology and Lab	3
Area II core course in a third field	3	PE 401 Psycho/Social Aspects of Activity	3
Area II core course in any field	3	PE 402 Advanced Athletic Training	3
Area III		PE 403 Training Room Modalities	2
Z 111, 112 Human Anatomy and Physiology	8	PE 406 Theory and Application of Therapeutic Exercise	3
PH 101 General Physics	4	PE 411 Athletic Training Clinical Instruction I	2
C 107, 108, 109, 110 Essentials of Chemistry and Labs	9	PE 412 Athletic Training Clinical Instruction II	1
H 101 Medical Terminology	3	PE 413 Athletic Training Clinical Instruction III 2	2
H 207 Nutrition	3	PE 414 Athletic Training Clinical Instruction IV	1
PE 100 Health Education	3	PE 417 Health Promotion	3
PE 101 Foundations of Physical Education	3	PE 422 Injury Evaluation	2
PE 114 Fitness Foundations	1	PE 451 Adapted Physical Education	3
PE 120 Training Room Procedures	1	Upper-division electives to total 40 credits	3
PE 121 Standard First Aid and CPR	1	Electives to total 128 credits	10
		Total	128

Note: Prephysical therapy students should take C 131, 132, 133, 134 instead of C 107, 108, 109, 110 and should also take M 111 and PH 102. Students planning to apply to physical therapy schools should check those schools' prerequisite course requirements and select their BSU courses accordingly.

FIGURE 4.3   Sports Medicine Studies (Master's Degree Program) at the University of Oregon

---

CURRICULUM

MASTER'S DEGREE PROGRAM* (with thesis or research publication)

AREA OF CONCENTRATION (18–24 credits)

EMS	610	Clinical Anatomy
EMS	663	Sports Medicine I: Exercise and Development
EMS	664	Sports Medicine II: Exercise, Adaptation, and Pathology
EMS	665	Sports Medicine III: Exercise as Medicine
EMS	507	Special Topic in Sports Medicine
EMS	607	Seminar
EMS	601	Research***
EMS	609	Practicum***

SUPPORT AREA (18 credits)

Support Area Options

- Exercise Physiology
- Biomechanics
- Social Psychology of Sport
- Motor Learning/Motor Control

Option 1: Three graduate courses in each of two EMS areas of concentration other than sports medicine.

Option 2: Two graduate courses in each of three EMS areas of concentration other than sports medicine.

Option 3: Two graduate courses in each of two EMS areas of concentration other than sports medicine, and two graduate courses in the College of Arts and Sciences outside of exercise and movement science.

RESEARCH

EMS	691	Statistical Methods I
EMS	610	Statistics Laboratory
EMS	693	Critique and Interpretation of Research
PSY	611	Data Analysis I**
EMS	503	Thesis***
EMS	601	Research***

*Accredited by the National Athletic Trainers Association.
**Required for thesis and research publication options.
***Requires instructor's consent.

FIGURE 4.4   Physical Education Program with Emphasis in Sports Medicine (Doctoral Degree Program) at the University of Virginia

PROGRAM DESCRIPTION

The program is offered through the Department of Human Services, Health and Physical Education Program Area and is subject to the requirements of the Graduate School of Arts and Sciences (Ph.D.) and Curry School of Education (Ph.D. & Ed.D) of the University, in addition to any specific requirements of the Program Area of Health and Physical Education. The Ph.D. is designed for the individual primarily interested in teaching and research, and the Ed.D for the person most interested in clinical practice with an ancillary interest in teaching and research.

Admission to the program is competitive and is subject to satisfactory review of all requirements. Candidates with an accredited undergraduate degree (and in most case a master's degree) are nominally eligible. Successful applicants will generally have previous outstanding academic preparation in Athletic Training, Biomechanics, Exercise Physiology, Physical Therapy, or Sports Medicine. Prior experience in clinical practice and teaching is highly desirable. Appropriate score of above 1500 on the combined verbal, quantitative and analytical sections of the Graduate Record Exam and a minimum GPA of 3.0 on the undergraduate and master's degree levels are necessary for admission.

PROGRAM OF STUDY

Selection of courses from among those listed in the various areas will be made in consultation with the student's advisor and subject to committee approval. The emphasis will be on competencies rather than quantity of coursework.

Sample Coursework (54 hours)

Sports Medicine

Coursework	Credit Hours	Coursework	Credit Hours
EDHS 758 Anatomical Basis of	3	EDHS 542 Motor Learning	3
Sports Medicine	3	EDHS 749 Sports Psychology	3
EDHS 743 Adv. Exercise Physiology	3	EDHS 558 Sports Psychology Conf.	3
EDHS 850 Sem. in Sports Medicine	3	EDHS 554 Therapeutic Modalities	3
EDHS 741 Adv. Athletic Training	3	EDHS 841 Orthopaedic Basis of	
EDHS 850 Sem. in Athletic Training	3	Athletic Training	3
EDHS 750 Pract. in Athletic Training	3+	EDHS 853 Supervised Research	3
EDHS 557 Sports Medicine Conf.	3	EDHS 552 Emergency Medical Care	4
EDHS 751 Nutrition for Athletes			
Biomedical Science			
BIOM 603 Mammalian Physiological		BIOM 728 Skeletal Biomechanics	3
Systems I	3		
BIOM 604 Mammalian Physiological			
Systems II	3		

Research and Statistics

EDHS 561 Computer Applic. in PE	3	EDHS 835 Multivariate Statistics	3
EDHS 589 Sem. Research & Writing	3	EDHS 733 Single-Subject Design	3
EDHS 730 Intro. to Ed. Research	3	EDHS 836 Sem. in Adv. Statistics	3
EDHS 731 Education Design	3	GSAS 803 Biostatistics	3
EDHS 830 Experimental Design	3	EDLP 849 American Proffessoriate	1–3
EDHS 831 Correlation & Regression	3		

Dissertation (minimum of 12 semester hours)

EDHS 999 Dissertation	12

RESEARCH OPPORTUNITIES

Doctoral students in sports medicine are expected to become involved in research by assisting faculty with ongoing projects, pursuing their own interests, and assisting with M.Ed. athletic training student theses. The Athletic Training/Sports Medicine Research Laboratory is equipped with contemporary instrumentation for assessment of human performance, joint laxity, and postural sway (balance). Collaborative research is also available with Medical Center faculty in orthopaedics, radiology, rehabilitation engineering and other areas.

FINANCIAL ASSISTANCE

Graduate assistant stipends are available through athletic training assignments to local private schools, athletic training/physical therapy assignments to the UVA athletic training room, and through teaching assignments in Health and Physical Education. A limited number of out-of-state tuition waivers are available for doctoral students in sports medicine.

members of the NATA board, and athletic trainers from internship route schools. The purposes of the ETF were (1) to examine all aspects of professional education in athletic training, including undergraduate entry-level programs and graduate programs, (2) to query the NATA membership with respect to their concerns and recommendations for change, and (3) to develop a list of recommended changes to be submitted to the NATA board of directors for final approval or rejection.

Richard Ray, Ed.D., ATC, Hope College, Michigan, and John Schrader, H.S.D., ATC, Indiana University co-chaired the ETF. Perhaps the strongest incentive to evaluate the entire educational process was the fact that many NATA members expressed confusion and concern about the fact that NATA continues to offer two very different routes leading to NATABOC certification. The most recent track is the NATA-PEC-approved/CAAHEP-accredited undergraduate program, and the older is the less structured internship route, which involves significantly less specialized course work but more practical experience in clinical hours. For many, this system of having two different tracks leading to the same credential was confusing to potential employers and to state regulatory agencies such as boards of medicine.

The ETF initially developed a list of 120 ideas for changes in the educational process, eventually reducing this list to 18 potential recommendations. The ETF then sent a representative to each of the 10 NATA district meetings during 1996 in order to share these recommendations with the membership and to solicit feedback. After this process the final revised recommendations were presented to the NATA board of directors. Although a complete discussion of all the recommendations is beyond the scope of this chapter, arguably the most significant of the 18 recommendations does warrant a brief description here. Recommendation 1 reads as follows: "The NATA should work with the NATABOC to institute a requirement, to take effect in 2004, that in order to be eligible for NATABOC certification, all candidates must possess a baccalaureate degree and have successfully completed a CAAHEP accredited entry-level athletic training education program" (6). The rationale for this recommendation is relatively simple: there is a growing opinion within the athletic training community that the internship route to NATABOC certification is no longer adequate in preparing students for careers in athletic training. This premise is supported by the fact that the NATABOC examination results, when compared between curriculum students and internship route graduates, indicate clearly that the internship route graduates pass significantly less often. This is not to say, however, that no effective internship route programs exist. To the contrary, many of the successful athletic trainers in practice today graduated from an internship route program. The reality is, however, that the body of knowledge in the field of athletic training continues to grow at a phenomenal rate. It seems obvious that a program that requires only seven specific college courses, 1500 hours of practical experience, and a baccalaureate degree in virtually any field, cannot adequately prepare a student in all the necessary areas.

In December 1996 the NATA board of directors met and approved the 18 recommendations put forth by the ETF. To facilitate their implementation, the next step in the process involved a major restructuring of professional education within NATA. A new standing committee known as the education council was formed with 45 members and a chair. This committee is charged with supervising graduate education, entry-level education, and continuing education for NATA. In addition, the education council serves as a clearinghouse for information on all aspects of professional education and continuing education for athletic training.

The Future of Athletic Training

Predicting the future of any professional group, especially in the health care arena, is at best a nebulous endeavor. However, recent trends in health care reform may be useful in speculating about the immediate future for those entering the field of athletic training. The primary employment settings for entry-level athletic trainers have historically been sports medicine and hospital-based sports medicine clinics, high schools, colleges and universities, and professional sports. The latter two categories have seen little growth over the past 5 years.

It has been predicted that a slow but steady increase in employment of athletic trainers will be seen in the high school venue (2). There are approximately 23,000 high schools in the United States, with fewer than 3000 employing full-time athletic trainers or teacher/ athletic trainers. Obviously, there is tremendous potential for future employment in this setting. Athletic training students should recognize that many high schools will demand that the athletic trainer be able to teach at least a partial load and serve as the athletic trainer. Thus, athletic training students should earn teaching credentials in teaching fields that are in high demand, such as math, science, or English, while also completing their athletic training studies.

Recent changes in the health care system within this country have resulted in major changes in how health care services are delivered. For example, health insurance companies that pay for medical services are demanding that costs be reduced. Although many new models of health care delivery are being developed to address this situation, one model that seems to favor the athletic trainer is the physician extender paradigm. A *physician extender* is an allied health care professional who is trained to perform many of the duties previously provided by a physician, such as the following:*

> Take initial patient histories and documenting them for physicians
> Apply casts
> Order and apply custom or ready-made braces
> Determine body composition
> Provide nutritional counseling
> Give exercise instruction for home programs
> Conduct injury rehabilitation
> Do gait analysis
> Foot orthosis fabrication
> Assist with in-office minor surgery

A major factor that will contribute to more athletic trainers becoming physician extenders will be an increased willingness on the part of health insurance companies to reimburse for the services of athletic trainers. This is already beginning to occur in isolated regions across the country, and it is anticipated that this trend will increase as the value of athletic trainers in the health care setting becomes more well recognized. It is anticipated that more athletic trainers will find employment in private practice medical settings as physician extenders.

Two areas that will likely see little or no employment growth for athletic trainers in the immediate future will be the college–university and professional sports settings. Given the financial constraints presently being experienced by many states, funding for higher education is predicted to continue to decline. Thus, available dollars for adding additional staff in the athletic training area are not expected. Future positions will become available primarily through retirements as career athletic trainers conclude their tenure at given institutions.

The professional sports venue has never represented a large market for athletic trainers because there are relatively small numbers of professional sports and teams available in relation to the number of entry-level athletic trainers seeking employment. The only exception to

Source: T. E. Koto, Athletic therapists as physician extenders, *Athletic Therapy Today* 1:21, 1996.

this may be professional soccer if it continues to grow in popularity within the United States. Even so, it is not likely that this new market would significantly increase the number of available jobs at the professional level.

Professional Journals and Related Publications

NATA publishes a quarterly professional journal, *Journal of Athletic Training* (JAT) and a monthly newsletter, *NATA News.* Both of these publications are provided to NATA members as a member benefit.

JAT serves as the research journal for the profession of athletic training and regularly features a variety of scientific, clinical, and pedagogically based research manuscripts. A sample abstract from a recent issue is given next.

Journal Abstract

Temperature Changes during Therapeutic Ultrasound in the Precooled Human Gastrocnemius Muscle

Stephanie J. Rimington, MS, ATC David O. Draper, EdD, ATC Earlene Durrant, EdD, ATC Gilbert Fellingham, PhD. *Journal of Athletic Training,* 29:325–327, 1994.

Abstract: Therapeutic ultrasound is frequently employed as a deep heating rehabilitation modality. It is administered in one of three ways: (a) ultrasound with no preceding treatment, (b) ultrasound on preheated tissues, or (c) ultrasound on precooled tissues. The purpose of this study was to investigate the effect of ultrasound treatments on the tissue temperature rise of precooled human gastrocnemius muscle. Sixteen male subjects had a 23-gauge hypodermic needle microprobe inserted 3 cm deep into the medial aspect of their anesthetized gastrocnemius muscles. Data were gathered on each subject for one of two randomly assigned treatments: (a) ultrasound treatment on precooled tissue, or (b) ultrasound with no preceding treatment. Each treatment consisted of ultrasound delivered topically at 1.5 watt/cm^2 in a continuous mode for 10 minutes. Ultrasound was applied in an overlapping longitudinal motion at 4 cm/s, with temperature readings recorded at 30-second intervals. We discovered a deference between the two treatment methods [$t(14) = 16.16$, $p < .0001$]. Ultrasound alone increased tissue temperature an overage of 2°C, whereas ultrasound preceded by 15 minutes of ice did not increase tissue temperature even to the original baseline level. We concluded that, at a depth of 3 cm, ultrasound alone provided a greater heating effect than ultrasound preceded by an ice treatment.

Professional journals related to athletic training include the following:

American Journal of Sports Medicine
Athletic Therapy Today
Journal of Orthopedic and Sports Physical Therapy
Journal of Sports Medicine and Physical Fitness
Medicine and Science in Sports and Exercise
Sports Medicine
The Physician and Sportsmedicine

Summary

Athletic training is an area of exercise science which specializes in the health care of athletes, and includes the following domains: prevention of athletic injuries; recognition, evaluation, and immediate care of athletic injuries; rehabilitation and reconditioning of athletic injuries; health care administration; and professional development and responsibility. Athletic trainers are highly educated and skilled professionals who are employed in a number of settings, including hospitals, clinics, schools, colleges and universities, and professional sports. The particular setting in which an athletic trainer is employed determines, to a large degree, the amount of time spent in each of the above domains. For example, an athletic trainer employed in a sports medicine clinic may spend a majority of his/her time in the rehabilitation and reconditioning domain. Athletic training is an evolving profession with a wide scope of practice, employment opportunities, and populations being served.

STUDY QUESTIONS

1. The first national meeting of the National Athletic Trainers' Association was in the year:

   a. 1950
   b. 1969
   c. 1927
   d. 1972
   e. 1894

2. According to the most recent NATABOC role delineation study, the athletic trainers' scope of practice includes all but which one of the following?

   a. Prevention of athletic injuries
   b. Professional development and responsibility
   c. Health care administration
   d. Rehabilitation and reconditioning of athletic injuries
   e. Diagnosis of athletic injuries

3. The first certification examination in athletic training was given in the year:

   a. 1950
   b. 1959
   c. 1972
   d. 1969
   e. 1927

4. The majority of new entry-level jobs for athletic trainers shifted from high schools in the 1970s to ____ in the 1980s.

   a. hospitals
   b. junior high schools
   c. professional sports teams
   d. college and university programs
   e. sports medicine clinics

5. The NATA board of certification formally separated from the NATA in the year:

   a. 1969
   b. 1950
   c. 1989
   d. 1972
   e. 1927

6. Athletic training students completing the internship route are required to complete ____ practical (clinical) hours by the NATABOC in order to sit for the NATABOC certification examination.

   a. 800
   b. 1200
   c. 5000
   d. 1500
   e. 600

7. As of 1993, all existing NATA-approved curricula in athletic training wishing to continue their programs were required to do so under new standards as set forth by the:

   a. AMA
   b. NATABOC

c. CAHEA
d. CAAHEP
e. PES

8. The NATABOC certification examination is a three-part test that includes an oral–practical component, a written simulation, and a written exam that consists of ___ questions.

a. 500
b. 150
c. 75
d. 200
e. 300

9. Once certified, athletic trainers must continue their education by earning a minimum of ___ continuing education units (CEUs) every ___ years.

a. 8, 3
b. 3, 8
c. 5, 5
d. 3, 3
e. 8, 8

10. Of the major employment settings for athletic trainers, the ___ continues to be the largest single employment setting.

a. high school
b. professional sports
c. college or university
d. corporate or industrial
e. sports medicine clinic

11. The AMA Council on Medical Education formally recognized athletic training as an allied health profession in the year:

a. 1969
b. 1950
c. 1989
d. 1990
e. 1972

12. The NATA board of directors, in December 1996, accepted 18 recommendations made by the Education Task Force regarding professional education in the future. One of the more significant recommendations requires that the internship route to NATABOC certification be discontinued after the year___.

a. 2001
b. 2004
c. 1999
d. 2010
e. 2020

13. List five electrotherapeutic devices that athletic trainers are trained to use in the treatment of injuries.

14. Describe the four continuing education categories as set forth by the NATABOC and list a specific activity from each category.

15. Briefly describe the different types of athletic training positions that can be created within the public school setting.

GLOSSARY

AMA   American Medical Association.

Athletic trainer   A highly educated and skilled professional specializing in athletic health care. In cooperation with physicians and other allied health personnel, the athletic trainer functions as an integral member of the athletic health care team in secondary schools, colleges and universities, sports medicine clinics, professional sports programs, and other athletic health care settings.

CAAHEP   Committee on Accreditation of Allied Health Education Programs.

CEU   Continuing education unit.

Clinical instruction   Hands-on education in the traditional athletic training room setting (college and university, high school) that focuses on psychomotor skills such as taping and bracing, application of therapeutic modalities, injury recognition and evaluation, exercise, rehabilitation, and record keeping. Clinical education must be supervised by an NATABOC-certified athletic trainer.

Electrotherapeutic Devices   Machines that use electrical energy in the treatment of disease or injury. Those commonly used by the athletic trainer include transcutaneous electrical nerve stimulation (TENS), ultrasound, galvanic stimulators, neuromuscular electrical stimulation (NMES), shortwave and microwave diathermy, and interferential electrical muscle stimulation.

Isokinetic machine   A resistive device that allows for controlling the velocity of movement of the extremity while simultaneously providing accommodating resistance.

Isotonic machine   A resistive device that allows for an extremity to move through a complete range of motion while the muscles actively contract against a constant resistance.

JRC-AT   Joint Review Committee-Athletic Training

NATA   National Athletic Trainers' Association

NATABOC   National Athletic Trainers' Association Board of Certification

Teacher/Athletic Trainer   An individual who has completed the requirements for both a teaching credential and on entry-level athletic training.

SUGGESTED READINGS

Arnheim, D. D., and W. E. Prentice. *Principles of Athletic Training,* 9th ed. St. Louis, MO: Mosby Year Book, 1997.

Pfeiffer, R. P., and B. C. Mangus. *Concepts of Athletic Training.* Boston: Jones & Bartlett, 1995.

REFERENCES

1. Arnheim, D. D., and W. E. Prentice. *Principles of Athletic Training,* 8th ed. St. Louis, MO: Mosby Year Book, 1993.

2. Curtis, N. C. Job outlook for athletic trainers. *Ath. Therp. Today* 1:7–11, 1996.

3. Curtis, N. C. Teacher certification among athletic training students. *J. Ath. Training* 30:349–351, 1995.

4. Heavner, S. (Ed.). *The National Athletic Trainers Association Board of Certification, Inc.—Role Delineation Study* (3rd ed.). Philadelphia: FA Davis, 1995.

5. Mathies, A. L., C. R. Denegar, and R. W. Arnhold. Changes in athletic training education as a result of changing from NATA-PEC to CAAHEP. *J. Ath. Training* 30:129–132, 1995.

6. McMullan, D. Renewing athletic training education—A step into the future. *NATA News,* February:17–27, 1996.

7. Moss, C. L. 1994 entry-level athletic training salaries. *J. Ath. Training* 31:25–28, 1996.

8. NATA. The Certified Athletic Trainer [World Wide Web]. Available at http://nata.org/trainer/index.html, 1996.

9. NATA. AMA endorses athletic training as allied health profession. *NATA News* 2:1, 1990.

10. NATA-REF. *Proceedings—Mild Brain Injury In Sports Summit,* Washington, DC, April 16–18, 1994. National Athletic Trainers Association–Research and Education Foundation, 1994.

11. O'Shea, M. E. *A History of the National Athletic Trainers Association,* 2nd ed. Greenville, NC: NATA, 1980.

12. Rankin, J. M. Financial resources for conducting athletic training programs in the collegiate and high-school settings. *J. Ath. Training* 27:344–349, 1992.

13. Rello, M. N. The importance of state regulation to the promulgation of the athletic training profession. *J. Ath. Training* 31:160–164, 1996.

14. Weidner, T. G. Sports-medicine centers: Aspects of their operation and approaches to sports-medicine care. *Ath. Training* 23:22–26, 1988.

CHAPTER

5

Biomechanics

DANIEL J. BLANKE

NICK STERGIOU

What Is Biomechanics?

History of Biomechanics

**Techniques and Technologies Used
in Biomechanics**

   Areas of Biomechanical Inquiry
      Developmental Biomechanics
      Biomechanics of Exercise and Sport
      Rehabilitative Biomechanics
      Occupational Biomoechanics
   Simple and Complex Biomechanical Instruments

Advanced Expertise in Biomechanics
   Education in Biomechanics

Employment Opportunities in Biomechanics

Professional Associations in Biomechanics

**Professional Journals and Related Sources
in Biomechanics**

Summary

Study Questions

Glossary

Suggested Readings

References

What Is Biomechanics?

Biomechanics is the study of the human body in motion. By applying principles from mechanics and engineering, biomechanists are able to study the forces that act on the body and the effects that they produce (4). Hay (12) describes biomechanics as the science that examines forces acting on and within a biological structure and the effects produced by such forces, whereas Alt (1) describes biomechanics as the science that investigates the effects of internal and external forces on human and animal bodies in movement and at rest. Each of these definitions describes the essential relationship between humans and mechanics found in biomechanics.

   Kinesiology, the parent discipline of biomechanics, is a science that investigates movement. It can be divided into the mechanical and anatomical aspects of human movement. The mechanical aspects can be further subdivided into statics and dynamics. *Statics* is a branch of mechanics that investigates bodies, masses, and forces at rest or in equilibrium. *Dynamics* investigates bodies, masses, and forces in motion. Dynamics consists of temporal analysis, kinematics, and kinetics. *Temporal analysis* uses time as the sole basis for analysis. *Kinematics* investigates motion without reference to masses or forces. *Kinetics* investigates the actions of forces in producing or changing the motion of masses.

In the United States, the use of mathematical and mechanical principles to study human movement was initially called kinesiology; in Europe, it was called biomechanics (15). There has been considerable controversy over the years as to the correct name for this area of study. This controversy seems to have been settled with biomechanics as the most accepted term worldwide.

Biomechanics is a discipline. A discipline deals with understanding, predicting, and explaining phenomena within a content domain. In biomechanics, movement is studied in order to understand the underlying mechanisms involved in the movement or in the acquisition and regulation of skill. The uniqueness of biomechanics as an area of study evolves not from the unique body of knowledge, but from the questions that are asked relative to understanding human movement (4). Techniques and methods from other scientific disciplines, such as physics and engineering, are used to examine human movement. In this way, biomechanics involves mechanical measurements used in conjunction with biological interpretations (14).

The study of movement involves the explanation and understanding of the structural and functional mechanisms underlying human performance, in all its presentations, from fundamental motor skills to demanding exercise. Higgins (13) proposed that skill is a movement that allows the organism to respond or act effectively within the environment and to integrate past and present. To become skillful requires mastery of the redundant degrees of freedom (5). These degrees of freedom or constraints are morphological, biomechanical, environmental, and task specific (13). The study of these constraints is required in order to explain and understand the underlying mechanisms of movement. Thus, movement must be approached from an interdisciplinary perspective. Movement, as a very broad phenomenon, appears in many different forms: play, dance, sport, work, and daily living activities. This is why a biomechanist can not study meaningful questions without adequate preparation in areas such as motor control, physics, exercise physiology, and engineering.

History of Biomechanics

The history of biomechanics can be traced back to the ancient Greeks. According to Nigg and Herzog (16), the contribution to biomechanics during the period from 700 B.C. to A.D. 200 included separation between facts and fiction, development of mechanical and mathematical models, development of anatomical models, and the first attempt to examine the human body biomechanically.

Aristotle (384–322 B.C.) was the first to examine and write about complex movements such as running and walking. He said, "The animal that moves makes its change of position by pressing against that which is beneath it. Hence, athletes jump farther if they have the weights in their hands than if they have not, and runners run faster if they swing their arms, for in extension of the arms there is a kind of leaning upon the hands and wrists." Archimedes (287–212 B.C.) was the first to examine floating bodies and their movements in the water. Hippocrates (460–370 B.C.) advocated that humans should base observations on and draw conclusions from only what was perceived through the senses. Galen (131–201) was the physician of the gladiators. He developed anatomical descriptions and the present-day terminology in use in certain biological science fields.

During the Renaissance, Leonardo da Vinci (1452–1519) examined the structure and function of the human body in a variety of movements. Vesalius (1514–1564) laid the foundation of modern anatomy. The contribution of the Renaissance period from 1450 to 1527 to biomechanics included the awakening of science, the foundation of modern anatomy and physiology, and an early examination of movement and muscle action (16).

During the modern era, another group of scientists contributed to the growth of biomechanics. Galileo Galilei (1564–1642) studied the action of falling bodies and laid the basis for the mechanical analysis of movement. Alphonso Borelli (1608–1679), a student of Galileo, examined muscular movement and mechanical principles. His work *De Motu Animalium* is the first biomechanical "textbook," in which he combined the sciences of mathematics, physics, and anatomy. Isaac Newton (1642–1727) developed his famous mechanical laws and was the founder of calculus, statics, and dynamics. The contribution of this time period to biomechanics included Newtonian mechanics, which provided us with a theory for mechanical analysis, and an improvement in science through the development of the process of theory and experimentation (16).

During the nineteenth century the contribution to biomechanics included the foundation of electromyography, the development of measuring techniques to examine the kinematics and kinetics of movement, and the beginning of the use of engineering principles in biomechanical analysis (16). The Weber brothers (around 1836) investigated the influence of gravity on limb movements in walking and running and were the first to study the path of the center of gravity during movement. Eadweard Muybridge (1830–1894) was the first to develop cinematographical serial pictures to study animals (horses) and humans. Étienne Jules Marey (1830–1904) used various photographical methods to examine movement. Christian Wilhelm Braune (1831–1892) and Otto Fischer were the founders of the scientific method to study human movement, which resulted in the development of the prosthesis.

During the twentieth century, biomechanics became a discipline with graduate programs and faculty positions; biomechanical research influenced applications in industrial, medical, and other practical areas; and biomechanics evolved as a necessary discipline-based method in the study of human and animal movement (16). During this time period, Jules Amar summarized the physical and physiological aspects related to industrial work. His book *The Human Motor* was translated into English in 1920 and set the standards for human engineering in the United States and Europe. Nicholas Bernstein (1896–1966) examined walking, running, and jumping. He laid the foundation of motor control and coordination. A. V. Hill (1886–1977) investigated efficiency and energy cost in human movement, and in 1931 W. O. Fenn published the first biomechanical works in the exercise and sport science literature, a cinematographical analysis of sprint running (10, 11).

In the 1960s the term *biomechanics* began appearing with more frequency in the literature, and biomechanics finally became a graduate specialization, first at Pennsylvania State University and second at the University of Indiana. Richard Nelson developed a laboratory for biomechanical research at Penn State in 1966, and it was the first that was identified with the term *biomechanics* (2). His first graduates were Doris Miller and Charles

Dillman. Following his graduation, Charles Dillman went to the University of Illinois to establish a biomechanics program. John Cooper developed a similar laboratory at the University of Indiana in 1967. The first graduate of this program was Barry Bates, who later developed the biomechanics program at the University of Oregon. From these pioneer programs and their graduates, many programs around the country were developed. Others who made tremendous contributions to the development of biomechanics programs around the nation were James Hay (University of Iowa), Stanley Plagenhoef (University of Massachusetts), and Carol Widule (Purdue University).

The period from 1966 to the present is an era of great growth in biomechanics. It includes the development of a number of new societies, journals, and professional meetings, such as the First International Seminar on Biomechanics, which was held in Zurich, Switzerland, in 1967 (19) and the origination of the *Journal of Biomechanics* in 1968. In the United States, the first North American meeting in biomechanics was organized by John Cooper at Indiana University in 1970 (8). Furthermore, the fourth international seminar on biomechanics was held at Penn State University in 1973 (3). This marked the foundation of the International Society of Biomechanics (ISB). In 1975, the fifth international seminar on biomechanics in Jyvaskyla, Finland, marked the conceptualization of the American Society of Biomechanics (ASB), which was founded the following year in Chicago, Illinois. This society included members from physical education, medicine, ergonomics, biology, and engineering (19).

Another important meeting was held in 1977 at the University of Illinois: the first national conference on teaching kinesiology. At this conference the differences between the terms *biomechanics* and *kinesiology* were discussed at length. Kinesiology was found to vary from a name of a course to a title of a college department (9). It was also found that in the United States the use of mathematical and mechanical principles to study human movement was initially called kinesiology, whereas in Europe it was called biomechanics (15). *Kinesiology* was defined as the parent discipline of biomechanics and generally of the science that investigates movement. *Biomechanics* was defined as a discipline to study the forces that act on the body and the effects that they produce.

In 1982, the International Society for Biomechanics in Sport (ISBS) was founded in San Diego, California (18). More recently, an international electronic mail communication list with the name BIOMCH-L (Biomechanics-List) was established at the University of Calgary, Canada, to help biomechanists from all over the world exchange ideas, problems, information, and the like (6). Finally, in 1989 the Academy of Physical Education was renamed the Academy of Kinesiology and Physical Education, because kinesiology was defined as the overall science of human movement (7). As a result, in 1993 the Kinesiology Academy of the American Alliance for Health, Physical Education, Recreation, and Dance (AAHPERD), which was representing the biomechanics section, was renamed the Biomechanics Academy to more clearly identify its role (19).

Table 5.1 provides a summary of important events in the history of biomechanics.

Techniques and Technologies Used in Biomechanics

Areas of Biomechanical Inquiry.   Using similar techniques and instruments, biomechanists work in a variety of areas. Each of these areas can be identified and the type of research

TABLE 5.1   **Important Dates in Biomechanics**

Date	Event
384–322 B.C.	Aristotle examined and wrote about complex movements such as running and walking.
1452–1519	Leonardo da Vinci examined the function of the human body.
1608–1679	Alphonso Borelli wrote the first biomechanical text, *De Motu Animalium.*
1642–1727	Sir Isaac Newton developed calculus and his mechanical laws.
1830–1894	Eadweard Muybridge developed cinematographical serial pictures to study animals and humans.
1920	Jules Amar's book *The Human Motor* was translated into English.
1931	W. O. Fenn published a cinematographical analysis of sprint running.
1966	Richard Nelson developed the first laboratory for biomechanical research at Penn State.
1967	First International Seminar on Biomechanics, Zurich, Switzerland
1968	Origination of the *Journal of Biomechanics*
1973	Foundation of the International Society of Biomechanics
1976	Foundation of the American Society of Biomechanics
1982	Foundation of the International Society of Biomechanics in Sports
1993	The Kinesiology Academy of AAPHERD was renamed the Biomechanics Academy of AAPHERD.

described. The four areas described here include developmental biomechanics, biomechanics of exercise and sport, rehabilitative biomechanics, and occupational biomechanics.

Developmental Biomechanics.   Biomechanical research in this area focuses on evaluating essential movement patterns across the life-span. Individuals of many ages have been examined while performing a variety of daily-living motor skills. The activities can then be quantified, described, and analyzed. Biomechanical analysis has been specifically important in quantifying the developmental motor skills and movement patterns in walking, kicking, jumping, throwing, and catching. This research has resulted in the description of a typical pattern for the activity for each age group. This pattern can then be compared to an individual's performance to determine his or her level of ability at any age. This type of analysis has also been done for a variety of other activities of daily living across the life-span, including ascending and descending stairs, raising from and lowering to a different level such as a chair or bed, lifting and carrying objects, pushing and pulling objects, and working with short- and long-handled implements. Again, evaluation and quantification of each type of activity at a variety of age levels have allowed comparisons to be made between age levels and have made it possible to evaluate an individual's skill or ability in a specific activity at a particular age.

The cause of slips, trips, and falls are often evaluated by the biomechanist. In one case a biomechanist was asked by a law firm to determine the possible causes of a fall while descending a stairway. The primary reason was to determine whether small deviations in riser heights and tread slopes could alter performance sufficiently to result in a claimed fall. Biomechanical evaluation suggested that the fall resulted from other factors. Evaluations have also been done to determine if a slip and fall accident can result from poorly designed and constructed shoes. Site and product examination verified that the shoe construction was such that over time a deterioration took place, resulting in a hazardous product when worn on selected surfaces. Investigation of a fall from a kitchen stool being used on a linoleum surface was also done. Biomechanical evaluation of the stool–surface system showed that a "typical" movement by the user was sufficient to cause the stool to slide, resulting in the fall.

Biomechanics of Exercise and Sport.   Biomechanical research in the area of exercise and sport has focused on exercise postures and movement patterns that minimize the risk of injury during exercise and improve performance. Among the contributions of biomechanics are the development of exercise machines for improving strength, endurance, flexibility, and speed; the development of new exercise modes such as plyometrics and isokinetics to improve performance; the design of exercise and sports equipment to minimize injuries; and the development of exercise and sport techniques to optimize performance.

The design of sports footwear is an example of the use of biomechanics to improve performance and reduce injury. Until the beginning of the 1970s, changes in the design of sport shoes were based on the subjective observations of athletes and coaches. Because the movements of the lower extremities were too fast to be evaluated with the naked eye or even standard film cameras, a new technology needed to be developed. A welcome invention was high–speed cinematography (100 to 300 pictures per second). Sixteen-millimeter film taken at high speed could be displayed at normal speed or evaluated frame by frame for detailed examination of the movement of the foot and leg during contact with the ground while walking or running.

The amount of force that is applied to a surface or an individual during a sport activity is also important to the biomechanist. To determine this force, biomechanists have developed special scales, known as *force platforms* (Figure 5.1), that can measure the impact forces between the shoe and the ground. By measuring these forces, we know today that the foot and the shoe must absorb two to three times the body's weight with each running step.

Another recently developed device is an insole that can be worn in a shoe under the foot, where it measures the pressure between the shoe and the foot. With this device, biomechanists can determine the extent that each part of the sole plays in a specific activity. This information can then be used to determine which bones will sustain most of the load while the foot is in contact with the ground. By knowing the amount of force that each bone receives, the sport shoe manufacturer can adjust the amount of support and cushion in the shoe to best support the foot and reduce the chance of injury.

Currently, the majority of biomechanical shoe research is directed toward the cushioning and stability of the sport shoe. Some other important considerations in shoe design are the flexibility and density of the sole, as well as the weight, durability, and "breatheability" of the

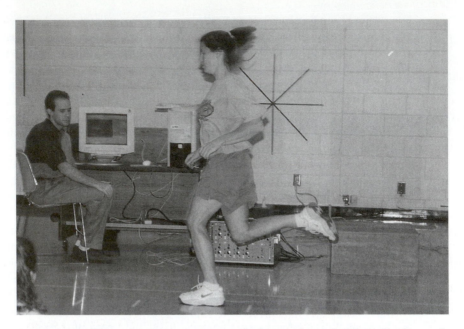

FIGURE 5.1   **Biomechanists can measure the impact forces between the shoe and the ground using a force platform.**

upper. Furthermore, using the techniques previously described, biomechanists analyze the demands of a specific sport (for instance, basketball or volleyball) in relation to the shoes that are designed for that sport. This research has dramatically improved the design of all sport shoes.

An example of biomechanists' involvement with the development of exercise equipment to improve strength and endurance can be found in stair-stepping machines and exercise bicycles. Biomechanists have evaluated posture and the ability to produce force while reducing the potential for injury on each of these devices. The result has been the evolution of both the stair-stepping machine and the exercise bicycle. These devices have become more comfortable and easier to use, while providing safe and effective resistance for improving strength and endurance.

Biomechanists have also been involved in the development of sport equipment to improve the safety of participation and the ability to be competitive. Biomechanists have been involved in the development and testing of protective devices, such as eye guards and football helmets and pads, and in the development and testing of sport equipment that helps the player improve performance. Recent innovations include large-head golf clubs and tennis racquets.

An example of the use of biomechanics to improve sport performance can be found in the golf-swing analysis now available from many golf teaching professionals. With a high-speed video camera and speed-measuring device, the golf teacher can determine a player's position and movement throughout the golf swing. The speed and path of the golf club head, as well as the speed and path of the ball after contact, can also be determined.

These data provide the teacher with the information needed to describe the player's actions that result in the path of the golf ball. By adjusting the player's actions, the teacher can alter the path of the ball and perhaps improve performance. This type of analysis can be helpful to the beginner as well as the highly skilled player.

Rehabilitative Biomechanics. Biomechanical research has focused on studying the movement patterns of injured and disabled people. Included among the enormous developments in this area are the development of sound exercises and exercise machines to train injured individuals back to normal functioning; the development of supplement devices such as canes, crutches, walkers, and orthotics; and the development of substitution devices such as prostheses and wheelchairs.

Some of the most common services that biomechanists provide are scientific investigations, technical reports, and expert testimony for a broad range of human-performance-related-incidents involving personal injury. The expert-witness work always involves a human element or component interacting with various aspects of the environment. Most accidents typically involve an initial perceptual component, some form of expectation, and an action, which typically results in a biomechanical consequence. Also, there is often a need to match the resulting injuries with the actions.

In one incident a biomechanist was asked to determine which of two occupants involved in a fatal auto accident was driving. Vehicle and site inspection data, in addition to the evaluation of injuries, were incorporated in the analysis to show that the driver was likely to be thrown from the auto during the progress of the accident. In another incident an analysis and evaluation was done to determine the potential effects of lap belt and shoulder harness restraint systems on the injuries suffered by a passenger in an auto accident. Various forces on the spine were calculated using a computer simulation program to demonstrate the differential effects of the restraint systems and body positions. A number of cases involving low-speed, rear-end impacts were also evaluated. Cases are typically evaluated using a computer simulation program that estimates movement and forces of the head and neck. Investigations of possible causes for auto accidents involving unexpected accelerations, which involved the human elements of perception and expectation regarding the function of the gas and brake pedals, have also been done. In addition, biomechanical analyses were conducted on the system designs to determine their adequacy.

Occupational Biomechanics. Biomechanical research often focuses on providing a safer and more efficient environment for the worker. The development of better safety equipment (helmets, shin guards, footwear, and the like) to protect the body from the effects of falling or colliding with other objects is an important area of biomechanical research. In addition, the development of safer or more mechanically efficient tools and improvement in the design of transportation modules (airplanes, spacecrafts, trains, boats, and automobiles) are major contributions by biomechanists to various work environments.

As with other areas of biomechanical inquiry, biomechanists are often involved with legal cases of industrial design and safety. In one case a biomechanist was asked to determine factors contributing to two nail-gun accidents. Issues assessed included the adequacy of the design relative to human performance capabilities, expected use patterns, and use and effect of warnings. The adequacy of machine design relative to safety of cleaning and operating was also a concern. Site and product examination coupled with an analysis of human perceptions and expectations suggested that the design was unsafe and a contributing cause of the accidents.

Product liability is another area in which biomechanists are ask to testify. Product evaluation and design effects on a performance injury are common in this area. In one case a woman playing softball severely injured her ankle as a result of sliding while wearing an improperly designed shoe. The analysis demonstrated the high probability that the specific injuries were caused by the improper shoe design even though the slide was properly executed. In another case, an evaluation of the possible causes of a knee injury while playing golf was done to determine the likelihood that poorly designed shoes were the cause.

Simple and Complex Biomechanical Instruments

Biomechanists use a large number of pieces of equipment to measure and record time, motion, and force. These devices are essential to the ability of the biomechanist to collect and analyze a large amount of information (17).

Timing devices, including watches and digital clocks, are used in biomechanics to provide temporal data. Temporal data can be combined with movement data to provide kinematic data. Temporal data can be used to determine such things as the performance of a sprinter.

Optical recording devices used in biomechanics include photography, cinematography, videography, and magnetic resonance imaging. These devices provide kinematic data from which kinetic data can be calculated. They provide permanent recorded images of movement that can be evaluated with more precision than can be done with the naked eye (see Figure 5.2). The human eye operates at a speed of only 30 frames per second. Therefore, many activities, such as the contact of the foot with the ground while running, happen

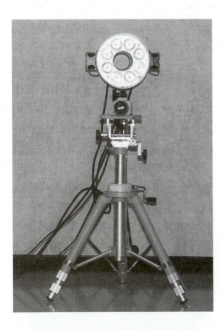

FIGURE 5.2 Optical recording devices, such as this high-speed camera, provide permanent recorded images for evaluation.

so quickly that they need to be analyzed by specialized equipment that can capture the activities in many more frames per second. In this way, a biomechanist can more precisely analyze such things as foot injuries that may occur while running.

Photographs provide permanent still images of one instant during a performance that can then be analyzed and described. A photograph can also be used to record the location of equipment used to collect research data. A 35mm camera with a variable focal length lens and adjustable shutter speed and aperture provides the most flexibility in photographing a performance or the data collection environment.

Cinematography provides a sequence of images that can be displayed as a motion picture or viewed one by one. Filming can be done at nearly any speed, from less than one frame per second to more than five million frames per second. By filming at high frame rates, motion that is too fast to see with the naked eye can be captured and viewed in slow motion or as individual images, which can then be analyzed with a digitizer. Sixteen-millimeter film cameras with variable focal length lenses and adjustable shutter speeds and apertures, capable of adjustable frame rates of up to 500 frames per second, provide the most flexibility in data collection.

Videography also provides a sequence of images that can be displayed as a motion picture or viewed individually. The images are recorded on videotape and are most commonly taken at a rate of 30 frames per second. High-speed video can be taken at 60 or more frames per second. Videography provides most of the features of cinematography with the convenience of instant viewing and the ability to reuse the videotape. The most common videotape cameras and recorders capture images at 30 frames per second using variable focal length lenses and adjustable shutters and apertures.

A *digitizer* is a device that is capable of acquiring planar coordinates in numerical form from a projected image. In biomechanics, the most frequent use of a digitizer is to convert the location of body markers on a projected image into coordinates that can be processed by a computer. From the coordinates, displacements, velocities, and accelerations can be calculated. See Figures 5.3 and 5.4.

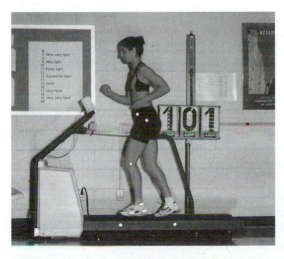 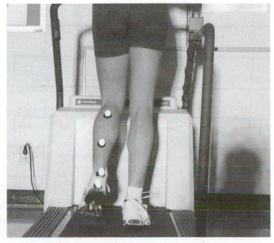

FIGURE 5.3   Body markers are placed in various positions for later analysis using a digitizer.

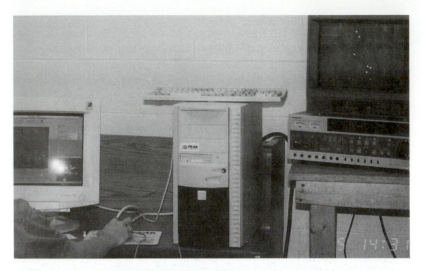

FIGURE 5.4   A digitizer is used to convert the location of body markers on a projected image into planar coordinates.

Magnetic resonance imaging (MRI) provides a computer-generated image of any body part. After an image is acquired, it can be manipulated to be viewed on a video monitor. MRI provides a noninvasive means of viewing the structures under the skin. Thus, a better evaluation of an injury or a muscle adaptation to training can be acquired.

Goniometers provide kinematic data on joint positioning. They are used to measure static positions of limb segments with respect to a joint axis. An electrogoniometer (elgon) is a goniometer with a potentiometer (variable resistor) at its axis of rotation. The electrogoniometer provides an indication of joint position during movement and can be calibrated to determine the speed of movement. The device is most often attached to the body with the axis of the potentiometer aligned with the joint axis. The elgon provides an output voltage, proportional to joint angle, that can be measured, scaled, and recorded. The information can be used to assess flexibility for diagnosis, rehabilitation, and exercise prescription.

Electromyography (EMG) provides data on muscle activity. An electromyograph records electrical changes that occur in a muscle during or immediately before contraction. This electrical activity can be captured, amplified, filtered, and recorded as an indication of muscle activity during a performance.

Dynamography provides kinetic data. A dynamograph is a device used for measuring forces produced during an activity. An example of one type of dynamograph is a force platform, an electromechanical device that provides electrical signals proportional to the components of force acting on it. The most common use of a force platform is to measure the reaction forces and center of pressure between the foot and the floor during locomotor activities. The resultant force is usually resolved into three orthogonal components. Force transducers used in a force platform are usually either strain gauges, which change their electrical resistance with strain, or piezoelectric elements, which generate charge when stressed. A transducer is a measuring device that converts one form of energy into another.

An electrical displacement transducer, for example, converts kinetic energy from movement into electrical energy. The electrical energy can then be measured and recorded as an indication of the amount of movement demonstrated. Force platforms can be used to assess the forces generated during contact with the ground in a variety of activities, such as running, walking, jumping, landing, and hopping.

A *pressure platform–pressure insole* is a device that consists of a matrix of elements that are small force transducers of known area. If this area is sufficiently small, the force on each element can be considered uniformly distributed and thus an estimate of pressure is available. This device gives more information concerning load distribution than a force platform because the pressure acting on individual anatomical regions can be measured, rather than just the resultant force acting on an entire region, for example, the whole foot. This information is especially important in shoe design, diabetic foot evaluation, and pathological gait.

An *accelerometer* is a transducer that measures acceleration. It usually consists of an inertial mass that exerts a force against an element, such as a beam, whose resulting strain is then measured. Since we know from Newton that force is the product of mass and acceleration and that mass is a constant, by knowing accelerations we can estimate forces. Therefore, accelerometers have been used where other force measurement devices could not be. For example, it is very difficult to use a force platform on a treadmill. However, an accelerometer can provide information about the forces generated during treadmill running.

Modeling and *simulations* provide a prediction of kinematic and kinetic data. These techniques are used to provide insight into specific activities or events. For example, muscles can be modeled as springs and bones as rigid bodies and then internal forces can be measured. Such information can be valuable for estimating forces, such as those acting at the lower back during lifting.

Advanced Expertise in Biomechanics

Education in Biomechanics

Because of the diversity of the areas related to the field of biomechanics, a broad range of knowledge is required to be a successful biomechanist. In 1997 the entrance requirements for the doctoral program in Biomechanics at the University of Calgary, under the direction of Benno Nigg, included coursework in mechanics (statics and dynamics), mathematics (calculus, linear algebra, and differential equations), computers (competent in one language), measuring techniques (force measuring systems, accelerometers, electromyography, cinematography–videography, goniometers), and gross anatomy and mechanical properties of human tissues (bone, cartilage, joints, tendons, muscles). In 1997, course requirements for entry into the doctoral program, under the direction of Barry Bates, at the University of Oregon included study in the areas of mathematics, computer science, physics, and motor control and learning.

Although the general course requirements for entry into a doctoral program in biomechanics and those required to complete a doctoral program in biomechanics are similar from one university to another, there are specific courses and activities that each university provides that sets that program apart from all others. These courses are often tied to the focus of the research coming out of the biomechanics lab at the university. Since biomechanics is a broad and diverse field, there should be variety in the training of the individuals working in the field. The training for someone working in rehabilitative biomechanics will be distinctly different from that of someone working in sport biomechanics or industrial biomechanics. Therefore, if there is a question about who is the best trained person in the field, the answer depends on the job requirements.

Sample Biomechanics Curricula (University of Oregon, June 1997).   The Department of Exercise and Movement Science at the University of Oregon offers a master of science (M.S.) degree and/or a doctor of philosophy (Ph.D.) degree with specialization in a variety of areas of concentration, including biomechanics, motor control, physiology of exercise, social psychology of sport and exercise, and sports medicine. An integral part of the graduate program is the exchange of information and inquiry with other disciplines throughout the university, such as the biological, physical, and social sciences.

I. Master's Program

   Requirements. Applicants to the master's program must have:

   1. A minimum cumulative undergraduate GPA of 2.75 for the last 90 quarter credits or 60 semester credits
   2. Minimum qualifying Graduate Record Examinations (GRE) scores of 470 verbal, 500 quantitative, or a combined score of 1000 with neither portion below 450
   3. A minimum score of 550 on the Test of English as a Foreign Language (TOEFL) if the applicant's native language is not English

   Prerequisites. Master's degree candidates must complete all undergraduate major requirements or their equivalents. These courses may be taken concurrently with master's degree requirements.

   Program of Study. Each student must complete a minimum of 12 credits in one area of concentration and a minimum of 18 credits in the support area of integrated exercise science. At least two graduate-level courses must be taken in each area of concentration. Candidates may choose one of the following options:

   a. Three graduate courses in each of two additional areas of concentration
   b. Two graduate courses in each of three additional areas of concentration
   c. Two graduate courses in each of two additional areas of concentration and two courses in a related department

   All students must satisfactorily complete Statistical Methods I and Critique and Interpretation of Research. Thesis students must also complete Data Analysis I.

   The master's degree requires a thesis, a published research paper, a research project, or a comprehensive examination. The department decides whether a master's degree student will write a thesis, publish a research paper, complete a research project, or take a comprehensive examination.

II. Doctoral Program

Requirements. Admission to the doctoral program is based on the applicant's academic record and the following:

1. Favorable recommendation from the area coordinator in the desired area of concentration and by the department's graduate admissions committee.
2. Minimum qualifying Graduate Record Examinations (GRE) scores of 520 verbal, 560 quantitative, or a combined score of 1100 with neither portion below 500
3. A minimum score of 550 on the Test of English as a Foreign Language (TOEFL) if the applicant's native language is not English
4. Candidate's statement of up to 500 words that indicates goals and objectives for pursuing the doctoral degree and the reason for selecting the prospective area of concentration
5. At least two letters of recommendation from individuals who can attest to the applicant's potential for doctoral study

Prerequisites. Doctoral candidates must complete the equivalent of the support area of integrated exercise science that is required for the master's degree program. These courses may be taken concurrently with doctoral courses and integrated into program requirements.

Program of Study. Doctoral degrees are granted primarily for the achievement and proven ability. The Graduate School requires at least three years of full-time study beyond the bachelor's degree, of which at least one academic year (three consecutive terms) must be spent in continuous residence on the UO campus. It should be noted, however, that most students take three to four years of full-time study beyond the master's degree to complete their doctoral degree. Graduate courses completed with grades of A, B, or P (pass) from other approved institutions may be accepted if they are relevant to the program of study.

Completion of Master's Thesis. Before taking doctoral comprehensive examinations, candidates who have not written a master's thesis must complete one or be first author on a research paper accepted for publication in a peer-edited journal. Every candidate must complete a dissertation.

Tools of Research. Prior to taking the doctoral comprehensive examination, the Tools of Research requirement must be met by completing one of four options. Credits earned for these courses do not count as part of the 135-credit minimum degree requirement.

Option 1: Foreign Language. Pass two languages on the Graduate School Foreign Language Test (GSFLT) with a scaled score equivalent to the 33rd percentile or one language with a scaled score equivalent to the 50th percentile or above, as reported in the current *GSFLT Program Score Interpretation Leaflet for Examiners.*

Option 2: Computer Science (minimum of three courses). Complete courses in computer science with programming emphasis, as determined by the candidate and approved by his or her adviser or advisory committee.

Option 3: Advanced Statistical and/or Research Design (minimum of three courses). Complete specific advanced statistics or research design courses in addition to the Research Area requirements. Sequences or courses are determined by the candidate and approved by his or her adviser or advisory committee.

Option 4: Combination. Complete a minimum of two courses in computer science (programming emphasis) and two courses in Advanced Statistical and/or Research Design as determined by the candidate and approved by his or her advisory committee.

Areas of Concentration. Each doctoral candidate must have a minimum of 30 credits in one area of concentration and 21 credits in a support area.

1. Biomechanics
2. Motor Control
3. Physiology of Exercise
4. Social Psychology of Sport and Exercise
5. Sports Medicine

Support Areas. Any of the areas of concentration and approved topics in other departments may be selected for the support area.

Other Areas of Study. A minimum of 20 credits must be earned in graduate courses outside the department. These credits may be applied to the area of concentration or the support area.

Final Examinations. Written and oral doctoral comprehensive examinations in the area of concentration and the support area are taken after completing substantial course work, a master's thesis or equivalent, and the research tools requirement. Upon passing these examinations the student is advanced to candidacy and may enroll in Dissertation. A final oral defense is held after completion of the dissertation and after all other degree requirements have been met.

Employment Opportunities in Biomechanics

Employment opportunities in the field of biomechanics are extremely varied as a result of the great variety of applications related to biomechanics. The opportunities can be arbitrarily classified into academic, postdoctoral, research and graduate assistant, and industry and government positions. An indication of the type and quantity of the positions available was determined by searching the advertisements on the BIOMCH-L over a 6-month period.

Between November 1996 and April 1997 there were 43 academic positions (faculty) posted on the BIOMCH-L. For more information on faculty positions contact http://www. kin.ucalgary.ca/isb/jobs/faculty.html. There were 28 postdoctoral position and 25 research and graduate assistantship position postings. There were also 32 industry and government postings. These jobs were for research assistants or technicians in various laboratories located in hospitals or companies that develop biomechanical-related products. Also included were positions for product specialists, sales representatives, and product designers for companies that design and produce equipment and apparel. The most notable include sport shoe companies and companies that specialize in exercise equipment.

Figures 5.5 and 5.6 provide examples of the workdays for two biomechanists.

Professional Associations in Biomechanics

There are a number of professional associations in the field of biomechanics. These associations have been in existence for a relatively short period of time, but have finally allowed biomechanists to come together to meet and discuss specific topical areas in biomechanics.

The American Society of Biomechanics (ASB) was founded in October 1977. The purpose of the ASB is to provide a forum for the exchange of information and ideas among

FIGURE 5.5 A day in the life of biomechanist Howard Davis

Howard Davis, Ph.D., teaches part-time at Washington State University (WSU) in Pullman, Washington and has his own business developing exercise testing equipment. He received his doctorate from the University of Oregon, where his advisor was Dr. Barry T. Bates. What follows is a typical workday for Dr. Davis.

April 28, 1997

7:15–8:45 A.M.	Lectured on kinematics in an undergraduate biomechanics course at WSU; specifically, the relationships among position, velocity, and acceleration.
8:45–10:30 A.M.	Office hours: worked with students who had questions about assignments.
10:30–10:45 A.M.	Traveled to business office.
10:45–1:00 P.M.	Business office: worked on sales-related projects, including calls to customers interested in his company's equipment, explanations to customers who had questions about the equipment, technical support for customers installing and testing the equipment.
1:00–1:15 P.M.	Traveled to a local clinic.
1:15–2:00 P.M.	Tested subjects at a local clinic that had purchased several pieces of equipment from his company. Davis assisted with the testing and examination of subjects at the clinic, whose typical subject population includes athletes and injured patients.
2:00–2:15 P.M.	Traveled back to WSU.
2:15–4:00 P.M.	Performed data analyses on data collected on patients at the local clinic. These analyses included statistical analyses and the generation of reports for the patients.
4:00–5:00 P.M.	Transferred e-mail messages and managed the web page of his business. Most of this was related to his preparation for travel to the American College of Sports Medicine Convention and to NASA headquarters to discuss ongoing research projects.

FIGURE 5.6   A day in the life of biomechanist Martyn Shorten

Martyn R. Shorten, Ph.D., received his doctorate in biomechanics from the Pennsylvania State University and works as a consultant in the field of sport biomechanics. Most of his clients are manufacturers of sport shoes and protective equipment, although he also undertakes projects involving biomechanical computer systems and software development. The projects on which he works vary greatly: some are basic research, some involve the development and testing of new products, and others are more esoteric, involving research management and strategy development. He lives in Portland, Oregon, but has clients scattered around the Untied States. What follows is a diary of a fairly typical day in the summer of 1997.

6:15 A.M.   Alarm. I am not an early morning person on the best of days, but today is even worse because I arrived home very late last night, returning from a business trip to San Antonio, Texas.

7:00 A.M.   Over breakfast, I work through the accumulated mail. One package contains background material for some software that I am developing with a colleague, Jim, from the University of North Dakota. The software does health and fitness assessments and will be distributed with undergraduate textbooks. This latest set of notes from Jim should help me to finish up the programming. Another letter, from Japan, invites me to chair a session on "Posture Control" at the forthcoming Congress of the International Society of Biomechanics (ISB) in Tokyo. "Posture Control" is something I know very little about. I accept the invitation anyway, because I know how hard it is to find session chairs. I will do my best to study the abstracts and find some intelligent questions to ask.

8:00 A.M.   The Office. In the office, there is more mail, e-mail and some faxes waiting. I am organizing a Symposium on Footwear Biomechanics at the ISB Congress and there are several related messages. One speaker, from Germany, wants to confirm that computer projection will be available. Another speaker asks for help preparing his extended abstract. I have already ordered a computer projector, but I send a quick e-mail reminder to Tokyo, just in case.

8:40 A.M.   Call Joe. Joe and I both work as consultants for a small start-up company in Texas. The company is developing new products based on a shock-attenuating material that Joe and I have patented. We dream of replacing all the foam that is commonly used in sports shoes and protective equipment. In reality, we have one licensing agreement and a long way to go. We are currently working on some new sports surface designs. I have been doing some testing and finite element modeling of prototypes and have some suggestions for Joe, who will organize the next round of prototype samples. We also reviewed yesterday's board meeting.

10:00 A.M.   Arrive at Nike. Nike is the world's largest sports and fitness company and one of my most important clients. Nike world headquarters campus is about 25 miles form my home and I am typically here twice a week, working on projects in the Nike Sport Research Laboratory (NSRL). The NSRL is a very well equipped biomechanics laboratory. A large central space is equipped with force plates and a pressure-distribution measuring system mounted in the floor. The five electronic cameras of a 3D motion analysis system stare unblinkingly at a large treadmill. Corners of the lab are filled with equipment for measuring impact shock, traction, and the morphology of the foot and lower leg. In my view, the most valuable assets in the building are the researchers and research assistants who work here. Nike employs a dozen sport biomechanists, more than any other private sector organization that I am aware of. Nike has retained me to develop and implement a program of research on sport shoe cushioning systems and has assigned three research assistants to work on my projects. Today we are planning to try our new protocol for measuring the pressure distribution inside basketball shoes. The equipment for measuring in-shoe pressures is commercially available. Our challenge is to collect data under conditions that are as close to actual playing conditions as possible. The four of us hold an impromptu meeting to review the situation. Bin and Dan have arranged a subject for another trial later this afternoon. I soon realize that they have everything under control and don't really need my help. I tell them that I will be there to observe the data collection, trying to make it sound more like a promise than a threat. I have a meeting in the early afternoon. Before then I have some Nike internal reports to review, and one to write. The report is a brief one, two and a half pages discussing the implications of a recent series of experiments.

12:00 noon   Lunch. Over lunch I make a few phone calls while munching on a sandwich. I call Jim to thank him for the package and to talk briefly about the software project. We agree that the user interface is very functional but a little dull. Where can we get some good graphics? I call my personal research assistant, Jennifer, and leave a message. She has been testing the stress–strain properties of some playground surfaces and I am eager to start working on the results.

3:00 P.M.   Meeting. Part of my role at Nike is to work with a cross-disciplinary team that focuses on the development of next-generation products. This afternoon, in our weekly meeting, we discuss the progress of a number of projects, one of which is the testing and development of a cushioning system that I have been working on. Most of the meeting is taken up with a discussion of field-testing protocols. After all the biomechanical research and testing are done, people have to actually like the products that we develop. Objectively measuring just how much they like them is a perennial problem. We have been trying a new perception measuring technique. It looks promising, but we still have to determine just how reliable it is.

3:30 P.M.   Back to the Lab. Bin and Dan have the Pedar in-shoe pressure measuring system calibrated and ready to go. They even have some prototype basketball shoes for the subject to wear. They have some time reserved on the basketball court at Nike's on-campus fitness center. They pack the equipment and head out. I promise to join them once I have caught up on some paperwork and finished off the report that I was working on.

4:30 P.M.   Bo Jackson Fitness Center. By the time I arrive they have been working with the subject for half an hour. Bin is working the computer and Dan is doing his best to challenge our volunteer basketball player in various one-on-one situations. They have already worked out some ways of collecting data while the two players are competing. I had hoped to be redundant, but Bin asks politely if I would mind holding a cable so that the players do not get tangled in it. I pick up the cable and try to look as though I am in charge, wondering when the wireless system we have on order will be delivered. I have a list of basketball drills that I want to work through. At a sample rate of 100 pictures per second, with each sample containing data from 99 pressure sensors inside the shoe, we can collect data for about 10 seconds. We work with our basketball player to package the skills into meaningful 8-second segments and to develop simple cues so that everyone knows when the action and the data collection will start.

6:00 P.M.   Things have gone better than expected and we seem to have a workable measurement protocol. Bin will process the data that he has collected and have it ready for my review in a few days. A quick look suggests data of appropriate quality. Most importantly, our subject said he felt like he was really playing basketball. We agree to start scheduling subjects for a pilot study.

7:00 P.M.   Home. Back at home, I have a few more messages. Jennifer has finished the surface testing and will bring the data files over tomorrow afternoon. Joe called to confirm that he has ordered molds for a new set of knee-pad samples, and Tokyo assures me that computer projection really will be available for the Symposium. Oh, and there is an e-mail from a professor at the University of Nebraska at Omaha. I will read it in the morning.

researchers in biomechanics. The society is affiliated with the *Journal of Biomechanics.* Meetings are held on an annual basis throughout the United States. For current information, contact http://www.usc.edu/dept/biom/main.html.

The Canadian Society of Biomechanics (CSB) was founded in 1973 by Canadian biomechanists. The purpose of the CSB is similar to the ASB. However, the CSB has successfully expanded internationally, as evidenced by the large participation of international scientists in the ninth biennial conference in Vancouver. In addition, at the same conference there were five symposia that featured 26 international speakers. The meetings are held biannually. For more information, contact http://www.biomech.uottawa.ca/index.html.

The International Society of Biomechanics (ISB) was founded in 1973 and today has about 1000 members. The purpose of the ISB is to promote the study of all areas of biomechanics at the international level, although special emphasis is given to the biomechanics of human movement. The ISB meetings are held on an biannual basis. For more information, contact, http://www.kin.ucalgary.ca/isb/aboutisb.html.

The International Society of Biomechanics in Sports (ISBS) was set up to provide a forum for the exchange of ideas for sport biomechanics researchers, coaches, and teachers; to bridge the gap between researchers and practitioners; and to gather and disseminate information and materials on biomechanics in sports. The first meeting took place in 1982, and a constitution was developed by 1983. Meetings are held on an annual basis. For current information, contact their web site at http://www.uni-stuttgart.de/isbs

Professional Journals and Related Sources in Biomechanics

Because of the breadth of scientific inquiry in the field of biomechanics, a large number of journals publish articles related to biomechanics. A list of those in which scientific articles are most common follows:

American Journal of Sports Medicine
British Journal of Sports Medicine
Clinical Biomechanics
Ergonomics
Foot and Ankle International
Gait & Posture
Human Factors
Human Movement Science
International Journal of Sports Medicine
Journal of Applied Biomechanics
Journal of Biomechanics
Journal of Biomedical Engineering
Journal of Bone and Joint Surgery
Journal of Electromyography and Kinesiology
Journal of Human Movement Studies

Journal of Orthopaedic and Sports Physical Therapy
Journal of Orthopaedic Research
Journal of Sports Medicine and Physical Fitness
Journal of Strength and Conditioning Research
Journal of the American Podiatric Medical Association
Medicine and Science in Sport and Exercise
Medicine, Exercise, Nutrition and Health
Physical Therapy
Research Quarterly for Exercise and Sport
Strength and Conditioning Research

The BIOMCH-L Newsgroup is an E-mail discussion group for biomechanics and human and animal movement science. To subscribe, send an e-mail message to SUBSCRIBE

FIGURE 5.7   Abstract of a biomechanical research study that examined the effect of the material composition of shoe inserts on foot and leg movements during running.

Benno M. Nigg, B. M., A Khan, V. Fisher, and D. Stefanyshyn.
Effect of shoe insert construction on foot and leg movement.
Med. Sci. Sports Exerc., Vol. 30, No. 4, pp. 550–555, 1998.

Purpose: The purpose of this study was to quantify changes in foot eversion and tibial rotation during running, resulting from systematic changes of material composition of five shoe inserts of the same shape. **Methods:** Tests were performed with 12 subjects. The inserts had a bilayer design using two different materials at the top and bottom of the insert. The functional kinematic variables examined in this study were the foot–leg in–eversion angle, β, and the leg–foot tibial rotation, p. Additionally, the subject characteristics of arch height, relative arch deformation, and active range of motion were quantified. The statistical analysis used was a two-way repeated measures MANOVA (within trials and inserts). **Results:** The average group changes resulting from the studied inserts in total shoe eversion, total foot eversion, and total internal tibial rotation were typically smaller than 1° when compared with the no-insert condition and were statistically not significant. The measured ranges of total foot eversion for all subjects were smallest for the softest and about twice as large for the hardest insert construction. Thus, the soft insert construction was more restrictive, forcing all feet into a similar movement pattern, whereas the harder combinations allowed for more individual variation of foot and leg movement and did not force the foot into a preset movement pattern. The individual results showed substantial differences between subjects and a trend: Subjects who generally showed a reduction of tibial rotation with all tested inserts typically had a flexible foot. However, subjects who generally showed an increase of tibial rotation typically had a stiff foot. **Conclusions:** The results of this study suggest that subject-specific factors such as static, dynamic, and neurophysiological characteristics of foot and leg are important to match specific feet and shoe inserts optimally.

FIGURE 5.8   **Abstract of a biomechanical research study that examined the effect of stride length on foot–ground impact.**

Derrick, T. R., J. Hamill, and G. E. Caldwell.
Energy absorption of impacts during running at various stride lengths.
Med. Sci. Sports Exerc., Vol. 30, No. 1. pp. 128–135, 1998.

Purpose: The foot–ground impact experienced during running produces a shock wave that is transmitted through the human skeletal system. This shock wave is attenuated by deformation of the ground/shoe as well as deformation of biological tissues in the body. The goal of this study was to investigate the locus of energy absorption during the impact phase of the running cycle. **Methods:** Running speed (3.83 m·s^{-1}) was kept constant across five stride length conditions: preferred stride length (PSL), +10% of PSL, −10% of PSL, +20% of PSL, and −20% of PSL. Transfer functions were generated from accelerometers attached to the leg and head of ten male runners. A rigid body model was used to estimate the net energy absorbed at the hip, knee, and ankle joints. **Results:** There was an increasing degree of shock attenuation as stride length increased. The energy absorbed during the impact portion of the running cycle also increased with stride length. Muscles that cross the knee joint showed the greatest adjustment in response to increased shock. **Conclusion:** It was postulated that the increased perpendicular distance from the line of action of the resultant ground reaction force to the knee joint center played a role in this increased energy absorption.

BIOMCH-L firstname lastname (affiliation) to LISTSERV@nic.surfnet.nl. For more information, contact http://www.kin.ucalgary.ca/isb/biomch-l.html.

The Biomedical Engineering Network is an Internet service that is maintained at Purdue University under a grant from the Whitaker Foundation. For more information, contact http://bme.www.ecn.purdue.edu/bme/.

Figures 5.7 and 5.8 are typical abstracts of articles published in professional journals.

Summary

Biomechanics is a discipline that uses a wide variety of instruments, techniques, and technologies to study movement. Biomechanists work in a number of areas, including developmental biomechanics, biomechanics of exercise and sport, rehabilitative biomechanics, and occupational biomechanics. Because of the diversity of the areas in biomechanics, a broad range of knowledge is required. Therefore, many students of biomechanics pursue advanced expertise in masters and doctoral programs. As a result of the variety of applications related to biomechanics, employment opportunities are extremely varied. These opportunities include positions in academia as well as industry and government positions.

STUDY QUESTIONS

1. Isaac Newton is best known for his study of the:

   a. Structure and function of the human body.
   b. Action of falling bodies.
   c. Efficiency and energy cost of human movement.
   d. Mechanical laws of motion.

2. Developmental biomechanics focuses on

   a. Exercise patterns and postures that minimize the risk of injury.
   b. Movement patterns of injured and disabled people.
   c. Evaluating movement patterns across the life-span.
   d. Movement patterns of skilled athletes.

3. The safety and mechanical efficiency of tools would most likely be evaluated by a(n) ___ biomechanist.

   a. Developmental
   b. Exercise and sport
   c. Rehabilitative
   d. Occupational

4. All the following are optical recording devices *EXCEPT:*

   a. Cinematography.
   b. Electromyography.
   c. Magnetic resonance imaging.
   d. Videography.

5. A digitizer is a device used for

   a. Counting the number of fingers or toes in the field of view.
   b. Acquiring planar coordinates from an image.
   c. Reducing the size of an acquired image.
   d. None of the above.

6. Define biomechanics.

7. Is biomechanics a discipline? Explain.

8. Why do we need to study movement from an interdisciplinary approach?

9. Identify the most important periods in the history of biomechanics along with one person who significantly contributed to the field of biomechanics during each of those periods.

10. What is the difference between biomechanics and kinesiology?

11. Define kinetics, kinematics, dynamics, and statics.

12. Identify the major areas of research in biomechanics.

13. Give five examples of biomechanical applications.

14. What is a force platform?

15. Name five journals in which biomechanists publish their research.

GLOSSARY

Accelerometer   A transducer that measures acceleration. It usually consists of an inertia mass that exerts a force against an element, whose resulting strain is then measured.

Biomechanics   The study of the human body in motion.

Cinematography   A technique that provides a sequence of images that can be displayed as a motion picture or viewed one by one.

Digitizer   A device that is capable of acquiring planar coordinates in numerical form from a projected image.

Dynamics   A branch of mechanics that investigates bodies, masses and forces in motion.

Dynamography   A technique that provides kinetic data. A dynamograph is a device used for measuring forces produced during an activity.

Electromyography   A technique that provides data on muscle activity. An electromyograph records electrical changes that occur in a muscle during or immediately before contraction.

Force platform   An electromechanical device that provides electrical signals proportional to the components of force acting on it.

Goniometer   A device that provides kinetic data on joint positioning. A goniometer is used to measure static positions of limb segments with respect to a joint axis.

Kinematics   A branch of mechanics that investigates motion without reference to masses or forces.

Kinesiology   The parent discipline of biomechanics, a science that investigates movement.

Kinetics   A branch of mechanics that investigates the actions of forces in producing or changing the motion of masses.

Magnetic resonance imaging   A technique that provides a computer generated image of any body part. MRI is a noninvasive means of viewing the structure under the skin.

Pressure platform/pressure insole   A device that consists of a matric of small force transducers. It provides detailed information concerning load distribution.

Statics   A branch of mechanics that investigates bodies, masses, and forces at rest or in equilibrium.

Temporal analysis   A technique that uses time as the basis for examining motion.

Videography   A technique that provides a sequence of images that can be displayed as a motion picture or viewed individually. The images are recorded on videotape and are most commonly taken at a rate of 30 frames per second. High-speed video can be taken at 60 or more frames per second.

SUGGESTED READINGS

Adrian, M. J., and J. M. Cooper. *Biomechanics of Human Movement,* 2nd ed. Dubuque, IA: William C. Brown & Benchmark, 1995.

Alexander, R. M. *The Human Machine.* New York: Columbia University Press, 1992.

Cavanagh, P. R. *Biomechanics of Distance Running.* Champaign, IL: Human Kinetics, 1990.

Chaffin, D. B., and G. B. J. Andersson. *Occupational Biomechanics,* 2nd ed. New York: John Wiley & Sons, 1991.

Hall, S. J. *Basic Biomechanics,* 2nd ed. St. Louis, MO: Mosby Year Book, 1995.

Hamill, J., and K. M. Knutzen. *Biomechanical Basis of Human Movement.* Media, PA: Williams & Wilkins, 1995.

Nordin, M, and V. H. Frankel. *Basic Biomechanics of the Musculoskeletal System,* 2nd ed. Philadelphia, PA: Lea and Febiger, 1989.

REFERENCES

1. Alt, F. *Advances in Bioengineering and Instrumentation.* New York: Plenum Press, 1967.

2. Atwater, A. E. Kinesiology/biomechanics: Perspectives and trends. *Res. Q. Exerc. Sport* 51:193–218, 1980.

3. Bates, B. T. The fourth international seminar on biomechanics. *J. Health Phys. Ed.Rec.* 45:69–70, 1974.

4. Bates, B. T. The need for an interdisciplinary curriculum. In: *Third National Symposium on Teaching Kinesiology and Biomechanics in Sports Proceedings.* Ames, IA, July 1991, pp. 163–166.

5. Bernstein, N. *The Coordination and Regulation of Movement.* New York: Pergamon Press, 1967.

6. Bogert, T. V., and K. Gielo-Perczak. Letter to the Editor: BIOMCH-L: An electronic mail discussion forum for biomechanics and movement science. *J. Biomech.* 25:1367, 1992.

7. Charles, J. M. *Contemporary Kinesiology: An Introduction to the Study of Human Movement in Higher Education.* Englewood, CO: Morton, 1994.

8. Cooper, J. M. Selected topics on biomechanics. Chicago: Athletic Institute, 1971.

9. Dillman, C. J., and R. G. Sears. *Proceedings of the National Conference on Teaching Kinesiology.* Urbana–Champaign, IL: University of Illinois, 1978.

10. Fenn, W. O. Mechanical energy expenditure in sprint running as measured in moving pictures. *Am. J. Physiol.* 90:343–344, 1929.

11. Fenn, W. O. A cinematographical study of sprinters. *Sci. Monthly,* 32:346–354, 1931.

12. Hay, J. G. *Biomechanics of Sports Techniques.* Englewood Cliffs, NJ: Prentice Hall, 1973.

13. Higgins, J. R. Human movement: An integrated approach. St. Louis, MO: C. V. Mosby, 1977.

14. Higgins, S. Movement as an emergent form: Its structural limits. *Hum. Mov. Sci.* 4:119–148, 1985.

15. Nelson, R. C. Biomechanics: Past and present. In: *Proceedings of the Biomechanical Symposium.* J. M. Cooper and B. Haven (Eds.) Bloomington, IN: The Indiana State Board of Health, 1980, pp. 4–13.

16. Nigg, B. M., and W. Herzog. *Biomechanics of the musculoskeletal system.* New York: John Wiley & Sons, 1994.

17. Rodgers, M. M., and P. R. Cavanagh. Glossary of biomechanical terms, concepts, and units. *Phys. Ther.* 64:1886–1902, 1984.

18. Terauds, J. *Biomechanics in Sports: Proceedings of the International Symposium of Biomechanics in Sports.* Del Mar, CA: Academic Press, 1982.

19. Wilkerson, J. D. Biomechanics. In: *The History of Exercise and Sport Science.* J. D. Massengale and R. A. Swanson (Eds.). Champaign, IL: Human Kinetics, 1997, pp. 321–365.

CHAPTER

6

Exercise Physiology

JOSEPH P. WEIR

What Is Exercise Physiology?

Parent Disciplines of Exercise Physiology

What Is an Exercise Physiologist?

History of Exercise Physiology
Establishment of the American College
of Sports Medicine
Scientific Journals

Areas of Study in Exercise Physiology
Areas of Basic Study
Areas of Applied Study

Research Tools Used in Exercise Physiology
Treadmills and Ergometers
Metabolic Measurements
Body Composition Assessment
Muscle Biopsy
Electromyography
Magnetic Resonance Imaging and Nuclear
Magnetic Resonance Spectroscopy

Academic Training in Exercise Physiology
Undergraduate
Graduate
Exercise Physiology as Part of a Preprofessional
School Degree

Professional Organizations
American College of Sports Medicine

American Society of Exercise Physiologists
American Physiological Society
American Alliance for Health, Physical
Education, Recreation, and Dance
National Strength and Conditioning Association
American Association of Cardiovascular and
Pulmonary Rehabilitation

Certifications
American College of Sports Medicine
National Strength and Conditioning Association

Employment Opportunities
Clinical Exercise Physiology
Health and Fitness
Sports Conditioning

List of Prominent Journals
Primary Journals
Associated Journals

Summary

Study Questions

Glossary

Suggested Readings

References

What Is Exercise Physiology?

Exercise physiology has been defined as "the study of how the body, from a functional standpoint, responds, adjusts, and adapts to exercise" (42). Two aspects of exercise physiology that form the core of the discipline are the responses to exercise and the adaptations to exercise. A response is distinguished from an adaptation in that a response is an acute or short-term change (adjustment) in the body that is associated with exercise. For example, as one jogs, the heart rate increases from the resting value. In contrast, an adaptation to exercise involves a long-term change in the body due to exercise training. For example, highly conditioned runners typically have lower resting heart rates than less fit individuals. This decrease in resting heart rate (bradycardia) occurs over time as a result of regular exercise training. It is the study of these types of responses and adaptations that provides the scientific basis for the field of exercise physiology.

In addition, exercise physiology has applied aspects, with many people trained to work in a hands-on environment with both healthy and patient populations. The application of the knowledge base of exercise physiology to clinics, health clubs, and athletic conditioning has the potential to significantly improve human performance and quality of life.

Parent Disciplines of Exercise Physiology

Exercise physiology has two primary parent disciplines: physiology and physical education. Academic training in exercise physiology typically crosses the boundaries of both disciplines. Physiology involves the study of the function of the body. That is, physiology is concerned with how the body works. Physiology itself is based on other disciplines such as anatomy, biochemistry, and cellular biology. Most academic training in exercise physiology focuses on the function of the body from a systems approach, that is, how the organ systems respond and adapt to exercise. Increasing emphasis, however, is being placed on the study of the cellular and molecular aspects of exercise (26, 90). To physiologists, exercise can serve as a stressor, thereby serving as a useful tool to challenge an organism and study its responses and adaptations to the stressor (26, 28). Indeed, since exercise can provide a potent stimulus to a variety of physiological systems simultaneously (the muscular, cardiovascular, thermoregulatory, and endocrine systems, for example) it can be a powerful tool to help further understand the function of the body (27).

The second parent discipline is physical education (26). To physical educators, the knowledge from the study of exercise physiology can be used to improve health and enhance human performance during physical activity and athletic events. Indeed, as early as the 1890s, exercise physiology was a part of the curricula in some university physical education programs (29), and a biological aspect has been a component of physical education since the inception of the field (55). Currently, most academic programs in exercise physiology are part of departments that are or were affiliated with the applied, professional field of physical education, which now usually involves the preparation of teachers for public and private schools. However, the scope of exercise physiology now extends beyond both physiology and physical education, because exercise physiology influences researchers and clinicians in other professions such as medicine, physical therapy, and gerontology. Further discussion of these topics will be included later in this chapter.

What Is an Exercise Physiologist?

The American College of Sports Medicine (ACSM) has defined an exercise physiologist as one who "studies the muscular activity and functional responses and adaptations during exercise" (2). Although this helps to define the parameters of what it is that people who are considered exercise physiologists actually do, there are no standards set down by a governing body regarding who is and who is not an exercise physiologist. Unlike physical therapists, nurses, physicians, and the like, there is, as of now, no license to practice exercise physiology. Academic programs vary to some degree in their requirements and course content (see Chapter 1). For example, some academic programs heavily stress clinical aspects of exercise physiology, in which students are trained to work in clinical environments such as cardiac rehabilitation and pulmonary rehabilitation. Other academic programs prepare students for research careers. Another complication is that there is no set standard for the amount of education required to become an exercise physiologist, that is, no bachelor's, master's, or doctoral degree. Similarly, there is no consensus as to what it is that every exercise physiologist should know.

Despite the lack of strict formulation regarding what it takes to be an exercise physiologist, exercise physiologists in the broadest sense are working in a variety of settings. Clinical exercise physiologists design, implement, and monitor exercise programs for individuals with cardiac, pulmonary, and metabolic disorders (for example, diabetes). Practitioners in the health and fitness industry perform exercise tests and design exercise programs for the general population in order to improve health, decrease clients' risk for disease, and improve well-being and self-esteem. Researchers study the mechanisms of response and adaptation that occur with exercise, as well as the practical aspects of exercise physiology, such as how to maximize the benefits of an exercise intervention.

Although most exercise physiologists work in an applied setting, that is, they work with real people in a clinical, athletic, or fitness setting, new information is continually being reported by researchers. Because of this continual information turnover, applied exercise physiologists have the responsibility of staying current with research. Similarly, researchers in exercise physiology have the responsibility of effectively disseminating new information to practitioners.

History of Exercise Physiology

Although the formal study of exercise physiology as a discipline is new to this century, interest in the physiology of physical activity dates back to the ancient Greeks (11, 21, 29–31, 33, 38, 39, 55, 62, 74, 90). DeVries has provided an account of the historical development of exercise science (including the major aspects of exercise physiology) in Chapter 2. Therefore, students are strongly encouraged to consult Chapter 2 to develop an appreciation for the rich history that has led to modern-day exercise physiology.

Establishment of the American College of Sports Medicine

Clearly, a significant event in the development of exercise physiology was the establishment of the American College of Sports Medicine (ACSM) in 1954. Indeed, Brooks (27) suggests that the closure of the Harvard Fatigue Laboratory corresponded with a loss of activity in exercise physiology in the United States and that formation of the ACSM was associated with a subsequent rebirth of study in exercise physiology. The founders of ACSM were physicians (notably cardiologists), physical educators, and physiologists. A common thread among these individuals was an interest in exercise and fitness (21). Although the scope of the ACSM goes beyond exercise physiology, this organization has become a preeminent exercise science organization, and many people who consider themselves exercise physiologists are members.

Recently, however, the lack of an organization that is specifically dedicated to the development and promotion of exercise physiology has led to the formation of the American Society of Exercise Physiologists (ASEP). The general goal of ASEP is to facilitate professionalization of the field of exercise physiology. Examples of specific goals of the organization are to develop standards for the training of exercise physiologists, promote increased research in exercise physiology, and enhance career opportunities for exercise physiologists. To date, the organization is in its infancy, but it has the potential to significantly improve the field of exercise physiology.

Scientific Journals

Because progress in any academic discipline depends on publication of research, the evolution of scientific journals associated with exercise physiology is an important part of its history. The *American Journal of Physiology* was an important venue for exercise physiology research in the first half of the 1900s. Although this is still an important source of exercise-physiology-related research, the publication of the *Journal of Applied Physiology* in 1948 was a significant event in that it became and remains a primary outlet for research in exercise physiology. European researchers also made use of *Internationale Zeitschrift fur angewandte Physiologie einschlieslich Arbeitsphysiologie* (currently *European Journal of Applied Physiology*) and *Acta Physiologica Scandinavia.* In 1969, the ACSM began publishing *Medicine and Science in Sports* (currently *Medicine and Science in Sports and Exercise*), which has grown into another primary journal for research in exercise physiology. As an indication of the growth of the field of exercise physiology, Costill (33) estimates that currently at least 25 scientific journals frequently publish research in exercise physiology.

Areas of Study in Exercise Physiology

In this section, a brief overview of the different areas of study that are a part of exercise physiology is presented. This section will be divided into basic and applied areas of study. For simplicity, the different areas are covered separately. It should be noted, however, that there is a great deal of overlap in the different areas of study. For example, it is difficult to adequately study the control of respiration without consideration of the nervous system (which controls the respiratory muscles) and the processes of bioenergetics and metabolism (which provide metabolites that influence respiratory control). Similarly, applied areas of study such as gerontology and diabetes involve all the areas of basic study.

Areas of Basic Study

Cardiovascular System.   The cardiovascular system is responsible for the transport of blood, and therefore oxygen and nutrients, to the tissues of the body. Similarly, the cardiovascular system facilitates removal of waste products such as carbon dioxide from the body. In addition, the cardiovascular system is centrally involved in the dissipation of heat, which is critical during prolonged exercise. The primary components of the cardiovascular system are the heart, which pumps the blood, and the arteries and veins, which carry the blood to and from the tissues. Clearly, the functions of the cardiovascular system are critical during exercise, and therefore a large proportion of study and research in exercise physiology focuses on the responses and adaptations of the cardiovascular system to exercise. Examples of areas of research regarding the cardiovascular system and exercise include the effect of exercise on coronary circulation (the blood supply to the heart itself), the effect of exercise on the size of the heart and the implications of changes in heart size, and the relationship between exercise and the neurological control of the heart.

From a health perspective, the study of the relationships between exercise and the cardiovascular system is critically important because cardiovascular disease is the leading cause of death in the United States (95). The primary cardiovascular disease is coronary artery disease, in which *cholesterol* and other blood lipids (fats) build up in the walls of arteries that supply blood to the heart itself. This process of *atherosclerosis* can lead to blockage of a coronary artery and ultimately to a heart attack. Physical activity and habitual exercise are associated with decreased risk of morbidity and mortality from cardiovascular disease (68). Important beneficial effects of exercise on the cardiovascular system include a decrease in resting blood pressure (an important risk factor in cardiovascular disease) and a decrease in blood cholesterol levels (reducing the risk for developing atherosclerosis). Furthermore, exercise is an important component of the cardiac rehabilitation process following a cardiac event such as a heart attack (95). Individuals with training in exercise physiology are playing important roles in the research and implementation of exercise programs for the prevention of cardiovascular disease and the rehabilitation of individuals with cardiovascular disease.

Pulmonary System.   The pulmonary system is important for the exchange of oxygen and carbon dioxide between the air and the blood. Exercise places a great deal of stress on the pulmonary system as oxygen consumption and carbon dioxide production are increased during exercise, thus increasing the pulmonary ventilation rate. The control and regulation of the pulmonary system during exercise are areas of much research. As with the cardiovascular system, the interplay of exercise and the neurological control of breathing is not completely understood. In addition, there is controversy as to whether the pulmonary system limits exercise performance in high-level athletes (36,79). Surprisingly, most evidence indicates that there are few, if any, adaptations to exercise in the pulmonary system itself by healthy individuals (62). However, adaptations in the musculature that controls breathing are apparent (37).

From a clinical perspective, exercise is an important component of pulmonary rehabilitation for individuals with diseases such as chronic obstructive pulmonary disease (COPD; includes diseases such as emphysema and asthma), and exercise physiologists may work with physical therapists, respiratory therapists, and pulmonologists as part of the pulmonary rehabilitation team. On the other hand, exercise can induce asthmatic events in some individuals (exercise-induced asthma), and the exact mechanisms of this phenomenon are under study. These events, in which exercise can precipitate airway constriction, shortness of breath, and wheezing, can occur in both asthmatic and nonasthmatic people; however, the incidence is much higher in asthmatics. Obviously, these events can lead to submaximal performance in athletes and likely reduce exercise compliance in nonathletes (49).

Nervous System.   *Voluntary.*   Among the many functions of the nervous system is the control of movement by way of the skeletal muscles, which are under voluntary (and reflex) control. Most of the study of the neural control of movement is considered the domain of motor control and motor learning (see Chapter 10). However, certain areas of inquiry are also of interest to exercise physiologists. Two notable areas are neuromuscular fatigue and neurological adaptations to strength training. With respect to neuromuscular fatigue, research suggests that under certain conditions the central nervous system may play an important role in the development of fatigue (22). For example, changes in brain levels of serotonin and dopamine may influence fatigue (35). In addition, the firing rate of motor units can change during fatigue (86), which may be due to an elegant interplay between peripheral receptors and the central nervous system (CNS; includes the brain and spinal cord). Similarly, strength training may influence the CNS control of muscle activation by increasing the number of motor units that the CNS will turn on during a contraction and the firing rate of the active muscle (63). Much of the data regarding neurological adaptations to strength training is contradictory, but this remains an important area of study. These areas of study are important not only to basic researchers in exercise physiology, but also new information in these areas may have implications in the rehabilitation of individuals with neuromuscular disorders.

Autonomic.   The *autonomic nervous system* is involved in the involuntary control of bodily functions. The autonomic nervous system has two divisions. The *sympathetic nervous system* becomes active during situations of increased stress, such as during exercise. The *parasympathetic nervous system* is more active during resting conditions. Most notable in exercise physiology is the autonomic control of the cardiovascular system. For example, during exercise an increase in sympathetic activity and a decrease in parasympathetic activity result in an increase in activity of the heart and an increase in blood pressure. In addition, the autonomic nervous system is involved in the redistribution of blood flow away from inactive tissues, such as the gastrointestinal tract, and toward the active tissues during exercise.

Adaptations also occur in the autonomic nervous system following exercise training. For example, the decrease in resting heart rate and heart rate at a submaximal exercise load in trained individuals is believed to be a result, at least in part, of altered autonomic function, that is, elevated parasympathetic activity (81, 83, 100). These adaptations have important clinical implications as a shift in the balance toward sympathetic and away from parasympathetic tone is associated with increased risk of heart attack and sudden death (23, 92). Therefore, the adaptations in autonomic balance following aerobic exercise training, especially after a first heart attack, may decrease risk. Recent technological advances allow for the noninvasive assessment of autonomic nervous system function and should further our understanding of the effects of exercise on the autonomic nervous system.

Muscular System.   Exercise is about movement, and the muscular system is primarily responsible for creating movement. Therefore, the responses and adaptations of the muscular system to exercise are important parts of exercise physiology. During exercise, a variety of changes takes place in skeletal muscle, such as changes in temperature, acidity, and ion concentrations. These changes affect muscle performance and may lead to fatigue. Indeed, the mechanism(s) of muscle fatigue is an important area of inquiry in exercise physiology (60). In addition, the adaptations of the muscular system to exercise lead to long-term changes in exercise capability. Depending on the type of exercise, changes in enzyme concentrations, contractile protein content, and vascularization affect the ability of the muscle to perform work. For example, endurance exercise increases concentrations of enzymes in skeletal muscle that are involved in the aerobic production of energy (43, 48).

In contrast, strength training is associated with increases in the size of the muscle due to increased synthesis of contractile proteins, with little change in anaerobic enzyme content (88). These types of adaptations are appropriate for a certain type of activity in that these adaptations will improve muscle performance in the type of activities that stimulated these adaptations. The muscle biopsy procedure has been and continues to be an important tool to study these adaptations. In addition, technology such as electromyography (EMG), nuclear magnetic resonance spectroscopy (NMR), and magnetic resonance imaging (MRI) are helping to further our understanding of muscle function with exercise.

A variety of neuromuscular conditions, such as multiple sclerosis, postpolio syndrome, and Guillain–Barré syndrome, affect skeletal muscle. The effect of exercise on individuals with these conditions may be important for improving quality of life. Unfortunately, relatively little is currently known about the beneficial and harmful effects of exercise in many of these diseases (34). Future research may create new roles for exercise physiologists in the rehabilitation of neuromuscular disease.

Bioenergetics and Metabolism.   With respect to exercise, the area of bioenergetics and metabolism involves the study of how the body generates energy for muscular work. The energy for exercise, in the form of *adenosine triphosphate* (ATP), is derived from the breakdown of food from the diet. Originally in the form of protein, fat, and carbohydrate, the energy is made available by different enzymatic pathways that break down food and ultimately lead to ATP formation. The specific metabolic pathway used and the associated food broken down for energy are affected by the type of exercise that a person is performing and have implications for the ability of the person to perform that exercise. These are important issues in exercise physiology because they affect decisions that exercise professionals make regarding the type, intensity, and duration of exercise to be prescribed to a client.

Tools that are described later in the chapter, such as indirect calorimetry, muscle biopsy, and magnetic resonance spectroscopy, are used in research to study these processes.

Exercise biochemists use muscle biopsy and magnetic resonance spectroscopy to study the biochemical changes that occur in skeletal muscle during exercise. Figure 6.1 presents an abstract of a research study that utilized muscle biopsies to examine the effect of sprint cycle training on muscle enzyme activity. The whole body metabolic response to exercise is studied with *indirect calorimetry,* which involves the collection and analysis of oxygen and carbon dioxide levels in expired air. The study of whole body metabolic responses and adaptations to exercise has application to topics such as exercise and obesity, because this type of metabolic information can be used to maximize the fat-burning effects of exercise.

Endocrine System.   The endocrine system is the system of *hormones,* which are chemicals released into the blood by certain types of glands called *endocrine glands.* Many hormones are important during exercise and may affect performance. For example, during exercise the hormone called growth hormone increases in concentration in the blood. This hormone is important in regulating blood glucose concentrations. Similarly, other hormones, such as cortisol, epinephrine, and testosterone, increase during exercise. Their effects may be short term in that they affect the body during the exercise bout. Other effects are prolonged and may be important in the long-term adaptation to regular exercise. The effects of exercise on the hormonal responses to exercise and the effects of these hormones on the responses and adaptations to exercise are areas of intense study.

FIGURE 6.1   Abstract of a research study that utilized muscle biopsies to examine the effect of sprint cycle training on muscle enzyme activity.

Hellsten, Y., F. S. Apple, and B. Sjodin.
Effect of sprint cycle training on activities of antioxidant enzymes in human skeletal muscle.
J. Appl. Physiol., Vol. 81, No. 4, pp. 1484–1487, 1996.

The effect of intermittent sprint cycle training on the level of muscle antioxidant enzyme protection was investigated. Resting muscle biopsies, obtained before and after 6 wk of training and 3,24, and 72 h after the final session of an additional 1 wk of more frequent training, were analyzed for activities of the antioxidant enzymes glutathione peroxidase (GPX), glutathione reductase (GR), and superoxide dismutase (SOD). Activities of several muscle metabolic enzymes were determined to assess the effectiveness of the training. After the first 6-wk training period, no change in GPX, GR, or SOD was observed, but after the 7th week of training there was an increase in GPX from 120 ± 12 (SE) to 164 ± 24 µmmol·min^{-1} ($P < 0.05$) and in GR from 10.8 ± 0.8 to 16.8 ± 2.4 µmol·min^{-1}.g dry wt^{-1} ($P < 0.05$). There was no significant change in SOD. Sprint cycle training induced a significant ($P < 0.05$) elevation in the activity of phosphofructokinase and creatine kinase, implying an enhanced anaerobic capacity in the trained muscle. The present study demonstrates that intermittent sprint cycle training that induces an enhanced capacity for anaerobic energy generation also improves the level of antioxidant protection in the muscle.

Source: Hellstern, Y., Apple, F. S., and Sjodin, B., Effect of sprint cycle training on activities of antioxidant enzymes in human skeletal muscle. *J. Appl. Physiol.,* 81(4)·1484–1487, 1996.

Another aspect of exercise endocrinology is the study of exogenous (produced outside the body) hormone supplementation on both short- and long-term exercise. For example, supplemental testosterone (the primary male sex hormone) and associated anabolic steroids have been used by athletes for many years to enhance performance in athletic events that require strength and power. This is a type of ergogenic aid (discussed later). Although the use of anabolic steroids is against the rules of most athletic governing bodies and may have detrimental health consequences, the use of such substances may have significant therapeutic effects for those with limited exercise capacity, such as the frail elderly (20, 93).

Immune System.   The immune system fights off pathogens and infections. The study of the effect of exercise on the immune system is a relatively new phenomenon. Indeed, the first exercise physiology textbook to include a specific chapter on exercise and the immune system was published in 1994 (37). Currently, the relationship between exercise and the immune system is under intense study; however, much more research is needed to fully understand the implications of exercise on the ability of the body to fight disease. Some evidence indicates that exercise may have a deleterious effect on the immune response under certain conditions, whereas it may enhance the immune response under other conditions (37), which depends on the immune parameter being measured (67). Specifically, very intense or exhaustive exercise may result in short-term immunosuppression (37, 67). For example, marathon running has been associated with increased incidence of upper respiratory tract infection (66). In contrast, submaximal exercise may result in increases in immune system parameters (37). Clearly, more detailed information must be obtained in order for applied exercise physiologists to be able to optimally design exercise programs that enhance rather than suppress immune function.

Skeletal System.   The skeletal system serves as a structural framework and provides the lever system by which muscle contraction can lead to movement. In addition, the skeletal system acts as a depot of important minerals such as calcium. Interest in the skeletal system with respect to exercise has largely focused on the effects of exercise, or lack thereof, on bone mass. The importance of this area is reflected in the fact that there is a relationship between bone density and risk of fracture, as well as the fact that bone mass decreases with time in the elderly (14). In postmenopausal women, the decrease in estrogen production that occurs following menopause is implicated in the development of *osteoporosis.* Exercise may help slow the process of osteoporosis, especially if applied in conjunction with estrogen-replacement therapy, and weight-bearing exercise prior to the onset of menopause may enhance the development of bone mass so that the effects of menopause on the skeletal system are diminished (4). In younger women, exercise training may lead to menstrual dysfunction, hormonal disturbances, and possible deleterious effects on bone mineral density (10). In the future, individuals with training in exercise physiology may help to design exercise programs that maximize the beneficial effects of exercise on the skeletal system and minimize the deleterious effects.

Areas of Applied Study

Microgravity and Space Flight.   Space flight and the associated microgravity cause a variety of changes in humans, including decreases in muscle and bone mass (86) and orthostatic hypotension (low blood pressure upon standing). In addition, decrements in motor function also occur that compromise the ability of astronauts to function effectively, especially upon initial return to Earth. With the potential for more long-term exposure to microgravity (for example, in a space station), some of the deleterious effects of microgravity may have significant health and performance implications. In the case of loss of bone mass, some long-term effects may be irreversible.

Exercise during space flight is one form of countermeasure used to combat these effects. However, under conditions of microgravity, it is difficult to design effective exercise programs because weight-bearing exercise is not possible. Exercise devices designed specifically for space flight have been developed (32), and future research will need to be performed to take best advantage of these devices. In addition, most early attempts at exercise in microgravity have focused on endurance exercise. Future research and implementation of exercise countermeasures will also involve other types of exercise, most notably resistance exercise (15).

Gerontology.   Exercise has great potential to enhance the quality of life of elderly individuals and possibly to extend life. Much research is currently being performed to more clearly understand the unique responses and adaptations to exercise in the elderly. Some of these areas of exercise physiology and gerontology will be discussed now.

Some of the consequences of the aging process are a decrease in resting metabolic rate, loss of muscle mass, and an increase in body fat percentage (41, 71). These effects are associated with increased incidence of conditions such as cardiovascular disease. Exercise may be a powerful tool to retard and perhaps stop these processes. For example, endurance or *aerobic exercise* can directly improve body composition by the increased use of energy during the exercise sessions. In addition, aerobic exercise may also help increase resting metabolic rate (71).

An exciting area of study is strength training for the elderly. While the strength levels of the sedentary elderly have been reported to be quite low, recent research has shown that the elderly are capable of significantly increasing both muscle size and strength with strength training (77). Increased muscle strength makes the performance of the activities of daily living easier, and increased muscle mass may increase metabolism and help in maintaining appropriate body composition (99). Although more research needs to be performed, it seems likely that both aerobic and strength training will be increasingly utilized by exercise physiologists to improve the quality of life of the elderly.

Spinal Cord Injury.   Approximately 11,000 individuals experience a spinal cord (SCI) injury every year in the United States (80). Depending on the severity and site of the lesion, paralysis can result. Paralysis of both the upper and lower body results in quadriplegia; paralysis of the lower body is referred to as paraplegia. Among the many effects of paralysis, the decrease in physical activity can lead to increases in risk factors for cardiovascular disease (75,85). Although strength training and range of motion exercises are common in the rehabilitation of individuals with SCI, there is great potential for the inclusion of aerobic exercise in the rehabilitation following SCI. Figure 6.2 presents an abstract from a research study which examined the effect of exercise in subjects with quadriplegia. Individuals with paraplegia can exercise their upper bodies with the use of arm crank ergometers and wheelchair exercise. In addition, recent research has examined the use of artificial electrical

FIGURE 6.2   **Abstract of a research study that examined the effect of exercise in subjects with quadriplegia.**

McLean, K. P., P. P. Jones, and J. S. Skinner.
Exercise prescription for sitting and supine exercise in subjects with quadriplegia.
Med. Sci. Sports Exerc., Vol. 27, No. 1, pp. 15–21, 1995.

Although in able-bodied individuals heart rate (HR) indicates exercise intensity, the linearity of the HR/oxygen uptake (VO_2) relationship has not been established in persons with quadriplegia with impaired sympathetic function. The HR/VO_2 relationship and four ACSM recommended methods of exercise prescription were evaluated in 11 individuals with quadriplegia during intermittent progressive peak exercise tests. Tests were conducted in either a supine or sitting position using an arm ergometer. The HR response was highly variable, with HR/VO_2 correlation coefficients ranging from 0.22 to 0.99. A 2 × 2 ANOVA revealed an interaction between injury level, high-level (above C7) vs. low-level (C7 and below) and exercise position, with the high-level group exhibiting the lower coefficient (0.68) between the HR/VO_2 relationship in the sitting position. For all subjects, the target of 55–90% peak HR (mean = 72.5%) corresponded to 34% peak power output (PO) in sitting and 44% peak PO in supine. Similarly, 70% peak VO_2 corresponded to 46% and 50% of peak PO (sitting and supine, respectively). A rating of perceived exertion (RPE) of 10–12 corresponded to 50–60% peak PO and was associated with a higher PO than that predicted by the HR or VO_2 methods. The results of this study indicate that exercise intensity for quadriplegics be based on 50–60% peak PO and/or an RPE of 10–12.

Source: McLean, K. P., P. P. Jones, and J. S. Skinner. Exercise prescription for sitting and supine exercise in subjects with quadriplegia. *Med. Sci. Sports Exerc.,* 27(1):15–21, 1995.

stimulation to allow for lower-body aerobic exercise in both paraplegics and quadriplegics (85). Although the research is at an early stage, this type of intervention has the potential to allow individuals with SCI to experience the beneficial effects of aerobic exercise.

Stroke.   An estimated 500,000 individuals experience a stroke in the United States every year (72). A stroke, or cerebrovascular accident (CVA), occurs as a result of a disruption of blood flow to an area of the brain, resulting in death of the tissue supplied by the now disrupted blood flow. There are a variety of effects of a CVA, and the effects depend on the severity and location of the lesion. Common motor consequences of CVA include hemiparesis and spasticity. *Hemiparesis* is a loss of motor control (including strength) and sensation on one side of the body, whereas *spasticity* is a condition of excessive muscle tone and resistance to stretch. Recently, the effects of strength training and aerobic exercise by stroke patients with hemiparesis and spasticity have begun to be studied (40,73). Indeed, in the past, strength training was avoided in many patients with stroke because of fear of making certain stroke complications such as spasticity even worse. Although much more research needs to be performed, the rehabilitation of patients with stroke may require increased participation by professionals with training in exercise physiology.

Cardiac Rehabilitation.   The primary tasks of exercise physiologists in cardiac rehabilitation are to design, implement, and monitor exercise programs. Functions related to these activities include exercise testing and client education. Exercise testing is useful in diagnosing disease and measuring exercise capacity (44). The diagnosis of cardiac disease is performed under physician supervision and focuses on electrocardiogram (ECG) monitoring, which provides information about blockage in the arteries that supply blood to the heart. Determination of exercise capacity is useful in designing exercise programs and monitoring progress. Client education focuses on topics such as self-monitoring of exercise, proper nutrition, stress management, and weight management.

Traditional cardiac rehabilitation programs are separated into three to four phases. Phase I is in-patient (hospital-based) rehabilitation and is usually conducted for patients who have recently experienced a heart attack (called a myocardial infarction), had cardiac surgery, or have been hospitalized for another cardiac condition, such as heart failure or peripheral vascular disease. Although exercise physiologists may perform phase I cardiac rehabilitation, it is more typically performed by the nursing staff or physical therapists. Phases II through IV are outpatient services and are more likely to be performed by clinical exercise physiologists than phase I. Phase II occurs from just after discharge from the hospital for up to 12 weeks and involves close supervision, with electrocardiogram monitoring of the patients' exercise sessions. The transition from phase II to III involves less supervision and limited ECG monitoring during exercise. Similarly, phase IV differs from phase III in that supervision is minimal and ECG monitoring is discontinued.

Although many students think of cardiac rehabilitation as focusing on patients who have had a myocardial infarction or bypass surgery, other cardiovascular conditions are also treated with cardiac rehabilitation. In heart failure, the heart is unable to adequately pump blood through the circulatory system. This may be secondary to a heart attack, but it may also occur from conditions such as damage to the heart valves. Exercise is limited in its effects on the damaged hearts per se, but can significantly increase exercise tolerance in these patients, presumably because of adaptations in the skeletal muscle. Peripheral artery disease (PAD) is analogous to atherosclerosis of the arteries supplying blood to the locomotor muscles, such as the calves. A common symptom of PAD is pain and cramping in muscles during tasks such as walking or climbing stairs (76). Exercise training improves exercise tolerance in these patients largely by increasing local muscular endurance in the locomotor muscles.

Pulmonary Rehabilitation.   The primary purposes of pulmonary rehabilitation are to minimize the complications of pulmonary disease and to educate patients regarding maximizing their ability to perform activities of daily living (9). Exercise is an important component in the process of pulmonary rehabilitation because one of the primary consequences of pulmonary disease is a decrease in functional abilities. Indeed, most pulmonary patients initially seek medical attention because of breathlessness during physical exertion (1). Exercise physiologists perform clinical exercise tests and design and implement exercise programs for these patients.

Exercise testing provides information that is more correlated with functional abilities than even lung function testing (12). The information from clinical exercise testing in the suspected pulmonary patient can be used for diagnostic purposes, to provide information for decision making regarding therapeutic intervention, and to monitor the progress of the rehabilitation.

The primary purpose of exercise training in pulmonary rehabilitation is to increase functional capacity, resulting in an increase in the ability to perform activities of daily living. Of these, increased endurance for walking is essential. Endurance, strength, and flexibility exercises are all components of the rehabilitation process. Endurance exercise training should increase the amount of work that a person can perform without shortness of breath. Because lung disease often leads to weight loss and weakness, strength training exercises increase the ability of patients to do work with less fatigue. Similarly, alterations in posture and mobility that occur as a consequence of pulmonary disease can be corrected or minimized with flexibility training (18). An added benefit of exercise is the component of emotional support (provided by additional human contact), which may also contribute to improvement in patient function (82). It should be noted that, although exercise, and pulmonary rehabilitation in general, can significantly improve quality of life and enhance performance in activities of daily living, it has not been established that these factors can slow down the pulmonary deterioration associated with disease or extend life-span in pulmonary patients (9).

Body Composition and Weight Control.   Obesity is defined as an excess amount of body fat. The current estimate is that approximately one-third of Americans are overweight, and the trend is increasing (56). Because obesity has important implications for health, reducing the incidence of obesity is considered an important national health goal. Diseases that are associated with obesity include development of heart disease, Type II diabetes, and cancer (69). In addition, obesity and lack of physical activity are both independent risk factors for coronary artery disease (45, 69).

Exercise can facilitate fat loss in a comprehensive weight-management program (100); however, there is still controversy regarding the importance of physical activity in the treatment of obesity, and researchers in exercise physiology are studying different aspects of exercise and fat loss. Important questions remain to be answered regarding the most beneficial approach to using exercise in treating obesity. One important consideration is the type of exercise to be used. Aerobic exercise has traditionally been used to burn fat, but the role and effectiveness of resistance exercise needs further study. However, it has been shown that resistance training helps to maintain lean body weight during weight-loss diets (16) and can increase resting metabolic rate (78). Questions remain regarding the optimal mix of exercise intensity versus exercise duration for facilitating fat loss. Clearly, long-term exercise adherence needs to be a consideration. Gender differences may play an important role in the interaction between exercise and fat loss and need further study.

The importance of physical activity in the prevention of obesity is a new area of inquiry. Fat cells accumulate in childhood and adolescence (62), and exercise may be important in preventing obesity during these years, especially since obesity at these ages is a significant predictor of obesity in later life. Similarly, as people get older their resting metabolic rate tends to decrease and percent body fat tends to increase. Increasing physical activity may help prevent or slow this process. As can be seen, researchers in exercise physiology have many questions to answer regarding exercise and obesity. Because new information is being reported, applied exercise physiologists in both clinical and health and fitness areas need to stay current in order to adequately serve their clients.

Exercise and Diabetes.   *Diabetes* is a disease that involves the disruption of blood glucose regulation due to dysfunction of the body's insulin system. *Insulin* is a hormone secreted from the pancreas and serves to facilitate glucose transport from the blood to the cells. There are over 13 million diabetics in the United States (84), and complications from diabetes (for example, heart disease or stroke) are among the major causes of death. Diabetes is classified as Type I or Type II. Individuals with Type I diabetes usually develop the disease in childhood, and almost all require exogenous insulin to supplement pancreatic production. Those with Type II diabetes usually develop insulin resistance in later life and most do not require exogenous insulin (102).

High fitness levels have been shown to decrease the risk for developing diabetes (59); thus exercise training may help individuals avoid developing Type II diabetes. For those with diabetes, exercise has been shown to have a beneficial effect on glucose regulation. This effect is in part due to the fact that exercise promotes glucose transport from the blood to muscle cells (94). Although this effect is largely beneficial, exercise physiologists who work with those with insulin-dependent diabetes must be aware of the potential for the combined effects of exercise and exogenous insulin manipulation to result in hypoglycemia (low blood sugar) or hyperglycemia (high blood sugar) (94). Beyond the effects of exercise on blood glucose regulation per se, exercise can have a beneficial effect on risk factors associated with diabetes, such as obesity, elevated blood cholesterol, and high blood pressure. Because of the high incidence of diabetes, applied exercise physiologists should be aware of all current information regarding exercise and diabetes.

Exercise and Pregnancy.   There is as yet no conclusive evidence indicating that exercise during pregnancy facilitates the process of labor and delivery; however, a clear benefit of maternal exercise is maternal health and a more rapid return to prepregnancy levels of fitness. Applied exercise physiologists may work with pregnant clients and need to be aware of the exercise modifications necessary for safe and effective exercise during pregnancy.

The effect of exercise on both the mother and the infant has received increased research attention since 1984, when the first guidelines regarding exercise and pregnancy were published by the American College of Obstetrics and Gynecology (ACOG). Two of the primary considerations were the effect of elevation in maternal core temperature on the unborn child and the effects of maternal exercise on fetal blood flow. Because there was relatively little published research at that time, the initial guidelines were conservative in that it was recommended that exercise heart rate not exceed 140 beats per minute and core temperature not exceed 38°C.

The second set of guidelines was published in 1994 and were based on more research conducted over that 10-year period. The newer guidelines provide more flexibility in that higher exercise intensities may be reached, but still caution against exercising to exhaustion and inducing large increases in core temperature (70). These latest ACOG guidelines have been incorporated into the *ACSM's Guidelines for Exercise Testing and Prescription* (1).

Muscle Soreness and Damage.   The soreness that occurs 24 to 48 hours following strenuous exercise (especially if it is a new type of exercise) is familiar to all who exercise. The specific cause(s) of this soreness is (are) still being investigated, but much evidence suggests that it is associated with muscle damage and is more severe with *eccentric contractions* (contractions in which the muscle actively lengthens, such as when lowering a weight or walking down a hill). Although muscle soreness may be only a nuisance for healthy individuals, it may have important health implications for individuals with neuromuscular disease who wish to exercise, because some evidence suggests that muscle damage from overwork may exacerbate some diseases.

Environmental Exercise Physiology.   There are many aspects of environmental exercise physiology. These include issues such as exercise in cold environments and exercise and pollution. In this section, a brief overview of two frequently studied areas, altitude and heat–humidity, will be presented.

Altitude.   As one moves from sea level to high altitudes, barometric pressure decreases, which decreases the amount of oxygen that is driven into the blood to bind to *hemoglobin* (hemoglobin is the protein in red blood cells that carries oxygen and carbon dioxide). The decreased oxygen content leads to decreased performance in endurance exercise at the elevated altitude. Prolonged exposure to high altitude, however, results in increased synthesis of hemoglobin and red blood cells. These adaptations increase the oxygen-carrying capacity of the blood and theoretically may improve exercise performance at sea level. To date, however, there is little research support to suggest that exercise training at altitude results in improved performance at sea level, but topics such as these remain important areas of research.

Altitude exposure also poses health risks and unique problems for those who exercise. For example, mountain climbers must perform work at altitudes that may lead to mountain sickness and even death. Therefore, the study of the physiological adaptations to altitude and the associated exercise consequences is an important area of research. Projects such as Operation Everest II (87), in which a hypobaric chamber allowed for the simulation of high altitude, have made important contributions to our understanding of these issues.

Heat and Humidity.   Thermal adjustments are a very important aspect of exercise in a hot and/or humid environment, where exercise without adequate thermal adjustments can lead to serious health consequences, including death. In general, the most important heat-dissipating mechanism during exercise is sweating. The evaporation of sweat from the skin results in a transfer of heat from the skin to the environment, resulting in cooling. This process, however, can lead to a loss of body water and electrolytes (for example, sodium). Therefore, both the increase in body temperature and the effect of the water and electrolyte loss can affect performance and lead to short-term medical problems such as heat stroke. Humidity is an especially important problem because high humidity minimizes the amount of sweat that can evaporate; thus sweat is wasted.

Research by exercise physiologists has led to important recommendations regarding exercise in the heat. Many of these are presented in reference 5. Current areas of research focus on issues such as the proper method of fluid replacement during exercise in the heat.

Many sports drinks are commercially available and many have been developed in part from research conducted by exercise physiologists.

Ergogenic Aids. In athletic competition, the difference between winning and losing can be vanishingly small. For example, at the 1992 Olympics the average margin of performance difference between first and second place in the track and field sprint events was 0.86% (53). Because of this, athletes and coaches will try many things in order to gain a competitive advantage. The term *ergogenic aid* refers to any substance, device, or treatment that can or is believed to improve athletic performance. In contrast, *ergolytic* refers to practices that can impair performance. Many nutritional products and practices (for example, carbohydrate loading) are used to gain a competitive advantage. Some techniques can be beneficial, but most don't work. Drugs such as amphetamines and anabolic steroids are used illegally and may have dangerous side effects. Other aids can be mechanical, such as knee wraps in power lifting.

A large amount of research in exercise physiology has been conducted to evaluate the efficacy of different ergogenic aids. The research into ergogenic aids is important not only for the immediate effect of the data on athletic practices, but also because examination of these issues can provide insight into the limiting processes and mechanisms involved in human performance. In addition, because ergogenic aids are an important issue in athletic competition, applied exercise physiologists need to be up to date regarding efficacy, safety, and ethical issues regarding ergogenic aids that may be used by clients. Of special concern is the potential health consequences of some ergogenic aids. A few of these aids are discussed next.

Anabolic steroids are artificial derivatives of the male sex hormone testosterone. Because testosterone is involved, among other functions, in skeletal muscle development, anabolic steroids are primarily used by athletes to facilitate strength and power development. Therefore, they have been most frequently used in sports such as weight lifting, throwing events in track and field, and football (47, 101). Although the research data are not unequivocal, the general consensus is that anabolic steroids do seem to be effective in this regard. However, because of relatively recent changes in drug laws, illegal use of anabolic steroids can have significant legal implications. In addition, their use is against the rules of almost all athletic governing bodies. Moreover, a variety of health consequences is associated with the use of these drugs.

Caffeine is a drug commonly found in coffee, tea, chocolate, and many carbonated soft drinks. It also appears to be effective as an ergogenic aid. Caffeine can affect arousal levels and alter metabolism. It may have a beneficial effect in endurance activities due to its role in increasing fat utilization, with subsequent sparing of carbohydrate (98). The influence of caffeine on strength and power events seem to be minimal (97). Whereas low levels of caffeine are not grounds for disqualification, high levels can lead to disqualification and sanctions from athletic governing bodies.

An ergogenic aid that is receiving much attention recently in both the research and lay literature is *creatine supplementation.* Creatine phosphate is involved in ATP restoration in skeletal muscle, and some studies show that creatine supplementation can increase intramuscular concentrations of both free creatine and creatine phosphate (17). Creatine supplementation has also been shown to enhance performance and recovery from high-intensity exercise, but not endurance events, where it may in fact decrease performance. Future research will further delineate the role of creatine loading in improving performance.

Sodium bicarbonate, an alkalizing substance (neutralizes acids), has been studied for use as an ergogenic aid because increased acidity is one possible mechanism of muscle fatigue. Sodium bicarbonate ingestion is theorized to buffer acids during exercise and delay fatigue. Although the results of many studies are conflicting, a recent review suggests that this procedure may be beneficial for high-intensity exercise of 1 to 7 minutes duration (58). However, side effects include gastrointestinal distress.

Blood doping refers to two techniques used to increase red blood cell content for enhancement of endurance performance. One technique involves the infusion of red blood cells, either from a sample taken at an earlier time from the same subject or from another donor. The second technique involves exogenous administration of a drug called erythopoietin, which stimulates red blood cell production by the bone marrow. Research generally shows that blood doping may enhance endurance performance, but both techniques violate current International Olympic Committee rules and can have negative health consequences (6).

Pediatric Exercise Physiology. Pediatric exercise physiology is concerned with children and adolescents. Clearly, this area of exercise physiology has a direct bearing on the field of physical education. This is especially true considering the relatively poor state of physical fitness in American youth. In addition, the topic of pediatric exercise physiology has important clinical and health implications. As with adults, clinical exercise testing in children is used in the diagnosis of cardiovascular and pulmonary disease (91). The growth of the area of pediatric exercise physiology is evidenced by the publication of a new journal entitled *Pediatric Exercise Science,* which was first published in 1989. Because most of the subdisciplines addressed previously have application to pediatric exercise physiology, in this section we will address only a few select areas.

The relationship between bone mineral density and physical activity in children has important implications for the prevention of the loss of bone mass in later years. Most bone mass is laid down during childhood and adolescence, with peak bone mass occurring at about 30 years of age (14). Vigorous weight-bearing exercise appears to increase bone growth during these years, which may be protective during adulthood. In contrast, poor diet, menstrual irregularities, and lack of physical activity may minimize the development of bone tissue and result in increased risk for fracture in later life.

Strength training for children and adolescents may pose unique risks. In addition, the question of whether children can increase their strength with resistance training has received considerable examination. With respect to risks, because the growth plates at the ends of long bones are fragile and damage to these growth plates can affect growth, safety is of paramount concern. Although reports of growth plate injuries with strength training are rare, conservative guidelines have been developed and can be found in the position paper by the National Strength and Conditioning Association (65). In general, children are to avoid "weight lifting"; that is, children should not attempt to lift as much as they can. Rather, strength training can be used to help to improve strength levels. Research evaluating the use of strength training in children has generally shown that children can increase strength levels with resistance training, but the amount of change in muscle mass is limited until after puberty, at which time the endocrine system develops to the point that adequate hormone concentrations exist to support muscle mass development (24).

The effect of exercise on the rate and amount of growth in children and adolescents has important implications for the prescription of exercise in children. Exercise provides conflicting signals for growth in children. On the one hand, the increased metabolic demands of physical activity can potentially divert nutrients away from growth processes. On the other hand, exercise stimulates endocrine responses that facilitate growth (25). Comparing growth in active versus sedentary subjects is problematic due to selection bias; that is, any differences in growth and development in active versus less active subjects may be due to a tendency for individuals with a specific body type to gravitate toward certain activities and athletic pursuits. Malina (61), in a review of growth and maturation data in young athletes, concluded that most athletic training did not affect these processes in the long term. However, inadequate nutritional support, as may be associated with sports like wrestling and gymnastics, may have effects. Clearly, female gymnastics is associated with short stature and delayed menarche (time of first menstruation), but the factors driving these observations (for example, selection bias, stress, nutrition, and training) are difficult to untangle. In wrestling, where "making weight" is common in young athletes, recent data indicate that growth patterns are similar between high school competitors and a national sample of nonathletes (51).

Exercise and Human Immunodeficiency Virus.   Human immunodeficiency virus (HIV) is the virus that causes AIDS (acquired immune deficiency syndrome). It is believed that HIV attacks specific types of immune cells, which ultimately leads to decreases in the ability of the body to fight infection. As of now there is no cure, but important strides are being made with respect to increasing both the life-span and quality of life for individuals who are HIV positive.

Of interest here is the relationship between exercise and HIV. Exercise may have beneficial effects for individuals with HIV. For example, strength training may help maintain muscle mass, which may help to slow down the loss in lean body mass associated with AIDS wasting (57). Aerobic exercise will similarly improve cardiorespiratory endurance and quality of life. As noted previously regarding exercise and immunology, however, exercise also has the potential to be immunosupressive, and current guidelines suggest that exercise be submaximal in order to avoid immunosupression (57). Indeed, effective exercise along with stress management may enhance immune function in those who are HIV positive. Because the study of exercise and HIV is still in its infancy, more specific guidelines for applied exercise physiologists are likely to be forthcoming.

Research Tools Used in Exercise Physiology

The tools used by exercise physiologists for conducting research are numerous, and a comprehensive review is beyond the scope of chapter. However, in this section a brief outline of some common tools is presented. Emphasis has been given to noninvasive techniques.

Treadmills and Ergometers

The treadmill and cycle ergometer are the basic tools used by exercise physiologists to induce exercise in research subjects. The treadmill is very common in the United States, where walking and jogging are familiar forms of exercise. In Europe, where bicycling is more common, the use of cycle ergometers is more prevalent. However, both devices are in frequent use.

With treadmills, the intensity of exercise is controlled by manipulating the speed of the treadmill belt and the grade of the treadmill (for example, the steepness of the slope). The disadvantage of the treadmill is that it is difficult to precisely measure the exact work output by a subject because of differences in mechanical efficiency between people. In contrast, because cycle ergometers support the subject's body weight, the work by the subject is just a function of the resistance of the machine. Most cycle ergometers have resistance applied by a friction belt. When the exercise intensity is to be increased, the resistance by the belt is increased. However, the pedal rate affects the intensity of the exercise; therefore, subjects must maintain a constant pedal rate. More expensive electronically braked cycle ergometers use an electromagnet to provide resistance. These devices have the advantage of allowing the power output of the subject to be manipulated independently of pedal rate, so subjects can choose the pedal rate that is most comfortable for them.

Although less common than either the treadmill or the cycle ergometer, other types of ergometers, such as those for arm cranking, allow for exercise testing with modes of exercise other than running or cycling. The arm-crank ergometer is a modified cycle ergometer for which the arms are used to "pedal" the device. These devices are important for exercise testing and training of individuals such as those with paraplegia who are unable to use the lower body. Sports physiology laboratories may have access to sport-specific ergometers, such as rowing ergometers, cross-country skiing ergometers, and swim flumes. In the training and testing of high-level athletes, these devices provide information that is more specific to the types of events in which the athletes will be competing (89).

Metabolic Measurements

Probably the most common physiologic measurement in exercise physiology is the determination of oxygen consumption and carbon dioxide production for the purpose of measuring metabolic activity using indirect calorimetry. This is most often performed during exercise on a treadmill or cycle ergometer. These measurements, obtained by collecting and analyzing expired gases from the lungs, allow for the determination of a variety of factors, including the amount of energy (calories) used during an activity, the relative amount of fat versus carbohydrate burned, and the fitness status of a given individual. The maximal rate of oxygen consumption, or VO_2 *max,* is the primary standard for determining aerobic fitness. Prior to the development of fast and inexpensive computers, performance of these metabolic measurements was labor intensive and time consuming. Currently, however, computerized and automated metabolic carts allow the metabolic exercise tests to be performed quickly and with fewer technicians.

Body Composition Assessment

Measurement of body composition is an important tool for studying the effects of various exercise and/or dietary interventions. The most common model of body composition is the two-component model, which divides the body into fat weight and fat-free weight components. The fat-free weight component includes tissues such as muscle, bone, and various organs. The fat weight component is primarily adipose tissue (fat tissue), but also includes some neurological tissue. Newer multicomponent models further delineate body composition components into smaller subcomponents. These approaches are likely to improve measurement of body composition, especially for different racial groups (46).

Hydrostatic weighing, or underwater weighing, is the primary gold standard for assessing body composition. New technology such as dual-energy x-ray absorptiometry (DEXA; also used to study bone mineral content) is expanding the assessment of body composition and may displace underwater weighing as the gold standard. Currently, however, the widespread use of these new technologies is limited. Other techniques, such as the use of skinfold calipers, bioelectrical impedance analysis (BIA), and near infrared reactance (NIR) provide predictions of what a person's body composition would be if assessed with underwater weighing. These latter techniques, while less accurate than underwater weighing, do allow for more convenient and therefore widespread use of body composition assessment (46).

The practical utility of body composition assessment is that it facilitates the design of exercise and dietary programs for fat loss. Body composition data are used to set fat-loss goals for clients. In addition, continued measurement of body composition allows for the monitoring of progress over time.

Muscle Biopsy

The muscle biopsy procedure has been in use since the 1960s and can be traced to Bergstrom (19). In this procedure, a needle is inserted into the belly of a muscle and a small piece of tissue is removed. From this procedure, an exercise physiologist can make a variety of observations. For example, comparison of pre- versus postexercise biopsy samples has been used to study substrate utilization and metabolite accumulation during exercise. In addition, the muscle biopsy procedure is a technique by which muscle fiber type (fast-twitch versus slow-twitch percentages) can be determined in humans. Research employing muscle biopsies has led to many advances in our understanding of the physiology of exercise. Because of its invasive nature, however, use of the procedure requires extensive training, which limits its use to a relatively small number of research laboratories.

Electromyography

Electromyography (EMG) involves the measurement of muscle electrical activity. Because the stimulus for a muscle to contract is electrical, the measurement of this electrical activity provides information regarding the activation of the skeletal muscles involved during exercise. In general, there are two types of EMG measurement procedures. Intramuscular EMG involves placing recording electrodes into the belly of the muscle itself, most typically in the form of a needle electrode. This is a common clinical tool for the diagnosis of neuromuscular diseases, but also has some utility in studying exercise. More common, however, is the use of surface electrodes to record the EMG signal. Surface EMG provides information about the relative strength of a muscle contraction because, in general, the larger the amount of muscle activated, the larger the amount of electrical activity produced. Changes in the amount of electrical activity recorded have been used to study the neurological effects of strength training (64). In addition, as a muscle fatigues, there occur changes in the EMG signal that provide insight into the rate of fatigue of the muscle, as well as the mechanisms of fatigue.

Magnetic Resonance Imaging and Nuclear Magnetic Resonance Spectroscopy

Magnetic resonance technology has been a tool used for studying muscle and exercise since the early 1980s and is therefore a fairly recent addition to the tools of exercise physiology. Both magnetic resonance imaging (MRI) and nuclear magnetic resonance spectroscopy (MRS) are based on the application of strong magnetic fields to the tissue of interest. MRI has been used to examine changes in muscle size following strength training, because the MRI images offer advantages over ultrasound and computerized tomography (CT) scans in visualizing muscle tissue and other soft tissues (50). Two newer applications involve the use of MRI to study body composition and activation patterns of skeletal muscle during different tasks. For body composition, a series of cross-sectional scans can be made from head to toe. This allows for the assessment of not only the amount of fat versus lean tissue, but also the distribution of fat in different areas of the body, most notably in the abdominal cavity versus under the skin (subcutaneous). This is important because intraabdominal fat appears to be more related to disease risk than does subcutaneous fat. Although the use of MRI for this purpose is likely to be limited to research, data derived with these procedures may significantly improve our understanding of exercise, diet, and obesity. With respect to muscle activation, new research indicates that changes in the contrast of MRI images of skeletal muscle are indicative of activation of the muscle. Although the mechanisms associated with this phenomenon are still being explored, future research with MRI may reveal important new information regarding muscle activation during exercise.

In contrast to MRI, MRS does not involve imaging of the tissues under study per se, but rather it allows for the noninvasive measurement of muscle substrates and metabolites so that changes that occur during an exercise bout can be monitored. This facilitates investigations of muscle fatigue and is being used in research studies that previously would have required subjects to undergo muscle biopsy. Another potential use is for the noninvasive determination of muscle fiber type. The primary disadvantage of both MRI and MRS is the cost associated with their use. Because of the expense, the use of these technologies to study exercise physiology will likely be limited to relatively few laboratories (54).

Academic Training in Exercise Physiology

Undergraduate

Courses in exercise physiology have long been a part of the curriculum for undergraduate physical education majors. Intensive study of exercise physiology at the undergraduate level is a more recent phenomenon. Most undergraduate degrees related to exercise physiology are not exercise physiology degrees per se; rather, they are more likely to be degrees in exercise science. This more generic title allows for a broad emphasis in which exercise physiology is integrated with other areas of study, such as biomechanics and motor learning. Although an undergraduate degree may be sufficient for many purposes, it is often the case that these degrees are preparatory for more advanced training at the graduate level or in professional school.

As preparation for the core courses in the degree, mathematics and basic science courses such as chemistry, physics, and general physiology are helpful and may be required. In addition, for those individuals who wish to pursue graduate training or who will apply for professional school (such as medicine or physical therapy), these courses may often serve as requirements for application to the various programs.

Core courses in the degree program will typically include one or more courses in exercise physiology itself, with emphasis on the basic areas of study outlined in this chapter. Additional courses at the undergraduate level may include emphasis on nutrition, cardiovascular exercise physiology, exercise testing, and exercise prescription. With respect to exercise testing, these courses often provide hands-on experiences in conducting exercise tests for both fitness evaluation and clinical evaluation. Similarly, exercise prescription courses provide theoretical and practical information regarding the design and implementation of individualized exercise programs for both healthy individuals and those with conditions such as cardiovascular disease.

Graduate

Graduate programs in exercise physiology tend to be more specialized than undergraduate programs. Indeed, differences between institutions for similarly titled programs can be quite large. Outlined next are some characteristics of different types of graduate programs at both the master's and doctoral levels. For those interested in pursuing graduate training in exercise physiology, it is advisable to research the specific programs of interest carefully to make sure that the chosen program fits the specific needs and goals of the student.

Master's.   At the master's level, many programs emphasize training in clinical exercise physiology. Courses in these programs tend to focus on advanced training in exercise testing and exercise prescription. Specialized training often includes in-depth analysis of exercise electrocardiograms, study of the effect of cardiovascular medications on exercise, study of the effect of exercise on cardiovascular disease, and designing exercise programs for those with cardiovascular disease. Many clinical exercise physiology programs do not require the completion of a thesis project. At the other end of the spectrum, some master's programs focus on preparation for doctoral training and have very little emphasis on clinical training. These programs tend to have an increased emphasis on basic science and perhaps statistics and research design.

Doctoral.   Doctoral education provides advanced training with a focus on developing research skills. The two most common degrees in exercise physiology are the Doctor of Philosophy (Ph.D.) and the Doctor of Education (Ed.D.). In general, the Ph.D. degree emphasizes training in research, while the Ed.D. degree, as the title suggests, tends to place more emphasis on training in education. Traditionally, the Ed.D. degree tends to require more formal coursework than the Ph.D., while the scientific rigor of the Ph.D. dissertation is expected to be higher than that for the Ed.D. degree. It is often the case, however, that there is little difference in the two degrees, and many fine educators hold Ph.D. degrees, while a number of outstanding researchers have an Ed.D.

During the training for the doctoral degree, the coursework typically includes courses in exercise physiology, but many courses are taken outside the primary department. For example, training in statistical procedures often occurs through statistics departments or other departments with statistical specialists, such as Psychology or Educational Psychology. Advanced basic science courses such as endocrinology, immunology, and neurophysiology are taught in biology departments or through affiliated allied health and/ or medical schools.

The culminating step in the doctoral degree is the completion of a dissertation. Traditionally, the dissertation project is the first independent research project by the doctoral candidate. The process involves developing a dissertation proposal, completing the data collection and analysis, writing the document, and finally defending the dissertation before a faculty committee.

Exercise Physiology as Part of a Preprofessional School Degree

Physical Therapy.   Physical therapists are primarily involved in the rehabilitation of patients following injury and disease. As part of the treatment process, physical therapists are often involved in the design of exercise programs to increase cardiovascular fitness, muscular strength, and flexibility (7, 8). Therefore, expertise in exercise physiology can be of great benefit for many physical therapists.

Training to become a physical therapist may occur at the bachelor's degree level; however, a large percentage of physical therapy education programs are postbaccalaureate. That is, they require a bachelor's degree for admission. The postbaccalaureate programs do not typically require that an applicant receive his or her undergraduate degree in a specific major for admission; however, most require broad training in the sciences (biology, chemistry, and physics) and have specific requirements for the humanities. Many of these requirements overlap with requirements for exercise science and, combined with the overlap in content area, make training in exercise science an appealing choice for preparation for admission to physical therapy school.

Medicine.   Admission to both allopathic (grants the Medical Doctor, M.D., degree) and osteopathic (grants the Doctor of Osteopathy, D.O., degree) medical schools requires high-level performance in basic science courses at the undergraduate level. As with physical therapy, many of the courses required for admission to medical school are also prerequisites for many courses in exercise physiology. More importantly, training in exercise physiology may be very useful to practicing physicians. Therefore, an undergraduate degree with emphasis in exercise science, along with the appropriate premedical requirements, is an attractive option for those seeking admission to medical school.

Chiropractic.   In general, the admission requirements for chiropractic schools are similar to those of medical schools. Therefore, as with the M.D. and D.O. programs, undergraduate training in exercise physiology is an appealing approach for those who wish to pursue the D.C. degree.

Other Preprofessional Opportunities.   A strong background in the basic sciences as well as exercise physiology provides a foundation for other professional schools, such as dentistry, physician's assistant, and optometry.

Professional Organizations

American College of Sports Medicine

The American College of Sports Medicine (ACSM) was founded in 1954 and has grown to become the largest organization in the world dedicated to the disciplines associated with exercise science and sports medicine. Its membership has grown from an initial 11 founding members to over 16,000 today. The ACSM has 11 regional chapters that hold their own meetings and programs (96). The annual national meeting grows almost every year and attracted over 5,500 participants for the 1999 meeting. The national meeting includes lectures, tutorials, colloquia, and research presentations addressing all areas of exercise science and sports medicine. The journal *Medicine and Science in Sports and Exercise* is the official journal of the ACSM and publishes research in exercise physiology and other areas of exercise science and sports medicine. *Exercise and Sport Sciences Reviews* is an annual publication that contains timely review articles by leading researchers. In addition, a new journal, (starting in 1997) entitled *ACSM's Health and Fitness Journal,* has been published and focuses on more applied information for health and fitness professionals. The Web page for the ACSM can be found at http://www.acsm.org and includes more information regarding membership, publications, and certification.

American Society of Exercise Physiologists

The American Society of Exercise Physiologists (ASEP) is a new organization (founded in 1997) and its membership is currently relatively small. The impetus for the organization is to facilitate professionalization of exercise physiology and improve career opportunities for exercise physiologists. The ASEP Web page, which can be found at http://www.css.edu/users/tboone2/asep/toc.htm contains information regarding the charter of the organization, membership, goals and objectives, and other topics.

American Physiological Society

The American Physiological Society (APS) is an organization of scientists who specialize in the physiological sciences. The APS publishes several different journals, one of which is the *Journal of Applied Physiology,* which is a primary journal for original research in exercise physiology. In addition, the *American Journal of Physiology* also regularly publishes original research in exercise physiology. Other publications of the APS include the *Journal of Neurophysiology, Physiological Reviews, News in the Physiological Sciences, The Physiologist,* and *Advances in Physiology Education.* Regular membership is restricted to those who conduct original research in physiology; however, other membership categories, such as student membership, are available. The APS Web page is at http://www.faseb.org/aps.

American Alliance for Health, Physical Education, Recreation, and Dance

The American Alliance for Health, Physical Education, Recreation, and Dance (AAHPERD) is the primary professional organization for individuals in physical education and related disciplines. Because of the ties between exercise physiology and physical education, many exercise physiologists have AAHPERD membership and are active in the organization. Its research journal, the *Research Quarterly for Exercise and Sport,* has historically published and continues to publish research in exercise physiology. However, because of AAHPERD's primary focus on teaching at the kindergarten through twelfth grade levels and minimal emphasis on basic science and clinical exercise physiology, the activity level of exercise physiologists in this organization is less than for the ACSM. The Web page for AAHPERD can be found at http://www.aahperd.org.

National Strength and Conditioning Association

The National Strength and Conditioning Association (NSCA) was started in 1978 and was originally called the National Strength Coaches Association, which reflects its roots as an organization for individuals who work as strength and conditioning coaches, often at the collegiate or professional level. Since that time, however, the organization has grown in size (currently 13,000 or more members) and scope and attracts members from the health and fitness industry, as well as from competitive athletics. The NSCA publishes two journals, *Strength and Conditioning* and the *Journal of Strength and Conditioning Research,* which as the name suggests, is a research journal in which original investigations that have application to strength training and conditioning are published. *Strength and Conditioning* publishes reviews and opinion articles with more direct application to the strength and conditioning professionals. The Web page for the NSCA can be found at http://www. nsca-lift.org.

American Association of Cardiovascular and Pulmonary Rehabilitation

The American Association of Cardiovascular and Pulmonary Rehabilitation (AACVPR) is an organization of physicians, nurses, exercise physiologists, and other health care professionals who specialize in cardiac and pulmonary rehabilitation. The official journal of the AACVPR is the *Journal of Cardiopulmonary Rehabilitation,* which publishes research articles addressing issues of cardiac and pulmonary rehabilitation. In addition, members of AACVPR receive a quarterly newsletter. Student memberships are available. The AACVPR Web page is at http://www.aacvpr.org.

Certifications

American College of Sports Medicine

A variety of organizations have certification programs related to exercise science and exercise physiology. Of these, the largest and most prestigious is the American College of Sports Medicine (ACSM). The ACSM began certification in 1975 and has two tracks: the health/

fitness track and the clinical track. The emphasis of the health/fitness track is on work with apparently healthy individuals, whereas the clinical track has an increased emphasis on individuals with disease or who are at high risk. Both tracks have three certification levels. The certification levels of the health/fitness track are Health Fitness Director (HFD), Health Fitness Instructor (HFI), and Health Fitness Leader (HFL). Both the HFD and HFI require at least an undergraduate degree with training in exercise and fitness, as well as knowledge and experience in exercise testing and prescription, behavior modification, and exercise leadership. In addition, the HFD certification requires supervisory, administration, and management experience. The HFL certification requires practical experience in exercise instruction and leadership, but does not require formal college training.

The three certification levels of the clinical track are Program Director (PD), Exercise Specialist (ES), and Exercise Test Technologist (ETT). The PD, the highest level of the clinical track, requires formal education beyond the bachelor's degree, extensive knowledge in exercise science, and supervisory and administrative competencies. The ES also requires extensive training in clinical aspects of exercise science, but does not require graduate training or administrative expertise. The ETT certification emphasizes competencies in performing graded exercise tests in a clinical environment, but requires no formal college training.

Specific requirements and competencies are described in detail in various ACSM publications, such as *ACSM's Guidelines for Exercise Testing and Prescription* (1). Certification examinations in both tracks include written and practical components. Therefore, both formal academic training and hands-on experience are necessary prior to sitting for the examination.

National Strength and Conditioning Association

The National Strength and Conditioning Association (NSCA) began a certification in 1985 called the Certified Strength and Conditioning Specialist (CSCS). To sit for the CSCS examination, a minimum of a bachelor's degree (or senior-level standing at an accredited institution) and CPR certification are required. The focus of the examination is on the design and implementation of strength training programs for application to sports conditioning. The examination includes questions on both the scientific and practical–applied aspects of strength and conditioning training.

Recently, the NSCA instituted another certification track for those individuals who are or will be personal fitness trainers. The NSCA-certified Personal Trainer certification is the only personal trainer certification recognized by the National Commission for Certifying Agencies (13). This distinction is important because there are many personal trainer certification examinations, and it is difficult for employers and trainers alike to determine the quality of the certification examination. Indeed, many certification examinations are given by for-profit organizations and have suspect standards.

Employment Opportunities

Clinical Exercise Physiology

Exercise physiologists have been working in clinical settings for many years, and the two most common areas of clinical exercise physiology, cardiac rehabilitation and pulmonary rehabilitation, have been addressed previously in this chapter. Recently, the ACSM developed a definition and description of a clinical exercise physiologist (3); however, the impact of this work remains to be seen.

The education required for expertise in clinical exercise physiology is not standardized. At the very minimum, a bachelor's degree in Exercise Science or related discipline with specialized coursework in clinical topics of exercise physiology, such as exercise testing and electrocardiography, is important. A master's degree is often necessary. Hands-on experience, often gained from an internship as part of an academic program, is very helpful, as is ACSM certification in the clinical track.

One important task of a clinical exercise physiologist is to perform clinical exercise testing. Currently, clinical exercise testing (stress testing) is used almost exclusively for assessing individuals with suspected or diagnosed cardiovascular or pulmonary disease. The general approach is to stress the client with a progressive exercise test so that indications of disease, severity of disease, and exercise capacity can be determined; *progressive* in this context means that the exercise intensity starts at a low level and increases over time until the subject can no longer continue or signs and symptoms develop such that stopping the test is warranted. Unless an orthopedic or neurological condition prevents lower-body exercise, testing is usually performed with a treadmill or, less often, a cycle ergometer.

Clinical exercise testing always includes electrocardiographic monitoring and may, but does not always, include metabolic measurements by indirect calorimetry. ECG monitoring is important for client safety, but is also used as a diagnostic tool for assessing coronary artery disease. The diagnostic utility comes from the fact that heart size and occlusion of coronary arteries due to atherosclerosis result in specific alterations in ECG signals. These effects may not show up at rest, but because exercise places stress on the heart, coronary artery occlusion will become evident during exercise and result in these changes in the ECG. Similarly, pulmonary dysfunction may not be fully exhibited with resting pulmonary measurements, whereas ventilatory and metabolic changes during exercise testing can provide diagnostic information (52). For both cardiac and pulmonary disease, impairments in peak workload attained during exercise, low maximal oxygen consumption, abnormalities in blood pressure response, and other information from the exercise test, considered in context with other diagnostic information, can be useful in the diagnostic process.

In addition, the exercise testing data provide information regarding the severity and progression of disease and can be used to monitor the effects of interventions such as exercise training. With respect to exercise, data such as maximal oxygen consumption, heart-rate response to different exercise intensities, and ventilatory responses to the exercise test are used to design the exercise program for the client. Finally, exercise test data are used to predict outcomes and survival in patients.

A typical workday for a clinical exercise physiologist in cardiac rehabilitation is shown in Figure 6.3.

Health and Fitness

For those with training in exercise physiology, there appear to be two primary types of positions in the health and fitness industry; one is to work in a private health club, YMCA/

FIGURE 6.3   A day in the life of clinical exercise physiologist Scott Hayford

Scott Hayford, CSCS, MS is a clinical exercise physiologist at Pinecrest Rehabilitation Hospital in Delray Beach, Florida. He is the program coordinator of the Cardiac and Pulmonary Rehabilitation Programs, having taken the position in 1996 after spending 6 years as a Clinical Exercise Specialist of Boca Raton Community Hospital. Scott earned his B.S. in Physical Education from the University of Vermont and his Master of Science Degree from Pennsylvania State University.

Current duties as program coordinator include patient monitoring during exercise, intake evaluations, patient scheduling, staff scheduling, ordering of supplies, equipment maintenance, and other day-to-day administrative duties. As the program coordinator, he is also responsible for leading and directing the program (including keeping current with national organizations and guidelines), attending management meetings, and acting as a liaison between his staff and administration. Scott also performs many marketing tasks, such as promoting cardiac rehabilitation or pulmonary rehabilitation weeks, visiting physician's offices, and promoting guest lecturers on a regular basis. Scott occasionally will visit local communities to deliver presentations on exercise-related topics.

Monday–Wednesday–Friday

7:00 A.M.   Arrive at clinic to open and prepare for the arrival of the first class of cardiac rehabilitation patients, which starts at 7:30 a.m.

7:30 A.M.–
12:30 P.M.   Conduct five 1-hour exercise classes with our two registered nurses and another master's degree exercise physiologist. Each class starts at half past and runs for exactly 1 hour. During that time the patients will be monitored with continuous ECG, blood pressure pre-, during and postexercise, along with constant evaluation and assessment by our staff members. They are taught to warm up and cool down properly and to reach their appropriate peak exercise levels during the aerobic phase. Classes have up to 10 patients, with two staff members (5:1 patient:staff ratio). On Monday and Friday we conclude with dumbbell resistance exercises and flexibility and on Wednesday substitute a short educational topic before check-out with ECG and blood pressure check.

12:30–1:00 P.M.   Lunch

1:30–3:30 P.M.   Conduct last two exercise classes of the day. During peak season in South Florida, which is from December to April, we will run classes until 4:30 P.M..

Tuesday and Thursday

8:00 A.M.   Arrive and prepare for patient intake evaluation at 8:30 and 10:30, each 45–60 minutes long. This is the initial meeting with cardiac and pulmonary patients and serves as an introduction to the facility and protocol, a screening tool, and an opportunity to gather valuable medical history data and information. The patient will be given a time for attending the regular exercise sessions and instructions on proper dress, eating, etc.

8:30 A.M.   Conduct patient evaluation.

9:30 A.M.   Monitor cardiac rehabilitation class (only one on T–TH).

(continued)

FIGURE 6.3 Continued

10:30 A.M.	Conduct patient evaluation.
11:30 A.M.–12:30 P.M.	Time for monthly meetings with supervisor, marketing representative, or staff or administrative duties.
12:30–1:00 P.M.	Lunch
1:00–2:30 P.M.	Time available for assembling patient files, completing patient progress or final discharge reports, or other administrative duties.
2:30–3:30 P.M.	Monitor pulmonary rehabilitation class. These hourly classes run from 12:30–3:30 P.M. on Tuesday and Thursday and are staffed by a respiratory therapist and either an RN or exercise physiologist. The hour is designed similarly to the cardiac rehabilitation classes, with the main difference being the patient's diagnosis and consequent limitations. The pulmonary patients, with COPD, have moderate to severe shortness of breath and are taught to exercise within their limitations. Ratings of perceived exertion (RPE), dyspnea, and oxygen saturation are primary tools used to determine intensity, with heart rate and blood pressure also used for monitoring. This is a twice weekly program of up to 24 sessions.
3:30–4:30 P.M.	Perform documentation and administrative duties.

YWCA, or corporation-based center, and the other is to serve as a personal trainer. Employment in health clubs involves tasks such as providing fitness evaluations, designing exercise programs, and educating members about exercise, nutrition, and health. Personal trainers are often employed through a health club, but many are entrepreneurs who contract their services to clients on an individual basis. Regardless of the route of employment, personal trainers design exercise programs for their clients and then supervise individual exercise sessions of their clients.

Sports Conditioning

The area of sports physiology, a subdiscipline of exercise physiology, emphasizes the study and application of exercise physiology to the improvement of athletic performance. Most coaches have historically been involved in the design and implementation of exercise and conditioning programs to improve the performance of their athletes. A strong knowledge base in sports physiology is clearly helpful in this regard. More recently, the emergence of the personal trainer has led to many individuals serving as one-on-one conditioning coaches for some athletes, especially for individual sports such as distance running and cycling. As with many personal trainer situations, these types of positions are often entrepreneurial in that the trainers contract their services individually with their clients. At colleges, universities, and many large high schools, full or part-time strength and conditioning coaches develop the conditioning programs for the athletes in many different sports. These types of positions require knowledge in not only sports physiology, but also in other areas of exercise science (for example, biomechanics and sports nutrition).

List of Prominent Journals

Primary Journals
Acta Physiologica Scandinavia
American Journal of Physiology
American Journal of Sports Medicine
British Journal of Sports Medicine
Canadian Journal of Applied Physiology
European Journal of Applied Physiology
International Journal of Sports Medicine
Journal of Applied Physiology
Journal of Cardiopulmonary Rehabilitation
Journal of Physiology
Journal of Sports Medicine and Physical Fitness
Journal of Strength and Conditioning Research
Medicine and Science in Sports and Exercise
Pediatric Exercise Science
Pflugers Archives: European Journal of Physiology
Research Quarterly for Exercise and Sport
Sports Medicine

Associated Journals
American Heart Journal
American Journal of Clinical Nutrition
American Journal of Physical Medicine and Rehabilitation
American Journal of Sports Medicine
Archives of Physical Medicine and Rehabilitation
Circulation
Ergonomics
International Journal of Sports Nutrition
Journal of Orthopaedic and Sports Physical Therapy
Muscle and Nerve
Physical Therapy

Summary

Exercise physiology is the study of how the body responds, adjusts, and adapts to exercise. The knowledge base of exercise physiology is applicable to many settings, including clinics, laboratories, and health clubs. It is important for exercise science students to study the principles of exercise physiology and to be able to utilize this knowledge base to improve human performance and quality of life. For example, a track coach may use the principles of exercise physiology to design training programs for athletes which will enable them to improve their running times, whereas a fitness instructor may use the principles of exercise physiology to design exercise programs for the elderly which will make the performance of the activities of daily living easier. The area of exercise physiology has applications in a number of areas of exercise science.

STUDY QUESTIONS

1. Distinguish between a response and an adaptation to exercise. Provide examples of each.

2. Explain why the study of the cardiovascular system is of prime importance to the study of exercise physiology.

3. Define an ergogenic aid and provide examples of different ergogenic aids, including their potential uses and dangers.

4. Explain the importance of the study of exercise and the skeletal system.

5. Describe the stages of cardiac rehabilitation programs.

6. Define obesity and outline current areas of study in exercise physiology related to obesity.

7. Outline the advantages and disadvantages of treadmill versus cycle ergometer exercise modes.

8. Differentiate between the ACSM, APS, AAHPERD, NSCA, and AACVPR.

9. Outline the two ACSM certification tracks and differentiate between the different certifications.

10. Explain the difficulty in defining an exercise physiologist.

11. Describe the process of clinical exercise testing and explain its uses.

12. Describe the process of fitness testing and explain its uses.

13. Differentiate between undergraduate and graduate study in exercise physiology.

14. Explain the relationships among exercise physiology, physiology, and physical education.

GLOSSARY

Adenosine triphosphate (ATP)   A molecule in which energy (for example, a for muscle contraction) is stored in high-energy phosphate bonds.

Aerobic exercise   Exercise that primarily depends on ATP production involving the use of oxygen.

Anabolic steroids   A class of drugs derived from testosterone; used as an ergogenic aid in strength and power sports.

Atherosclerosis   A disease in which fatty deposits in artery walls lead to a reduction in blood flow through the artery; can lead to heart attack and stroke.

Autonomic nervous system   The branch of the nervous system that controls the involuntary functions of the body.

Cholesterol   A steroid molecule found in the blood that can contribute to lipid deposition and atherosclerosis of artery walls.

Concentric contraction   A muscle contraction in which shortening of fibers occurs.

Diabetes   A disease of the insulin system in which insufficient insulin is produced (Type I diabetes) or the body is insensitive to insulin (Type II diabetes).

Eccentric contraction   A muscle contraction in which the muscle actively lengthens under tension.

Electromyography   The measurement of muscle electrical activity.

Endocrine gland   A ductless gland that secretes hormones into the blood.

Ergogenic aid   A substance or device that is believed to enhance athletic performance.

Ergolytic   A substance or device that can impair performance.

Hemiparesis   A loss of motor control (including strength) on one side of the body.

Hemoglobin   A blood protein involved in the transport of oxygen and carbon dioxide.

Hormone   A chemical released from an endocrine gland into the blood that exerts its biological effect elsewhere in the body.

Indirect calorimetry   The measurement of energy expenditure by determination of oxygen consumption and carbon dioxide production.

Insulin   A hormone released from the pancreas that functions to facilitate glucose transport from the blood into cells.

Osteoporosis   A condition in which a loss of bone mineral density increases the risk for fracture.

Parasympathetic nervous system   The branch of the autonomic nervous system that is most active at rest and is involved in restorative functions.

Spasticity   A condition of excessive muscle tone and resistance to stretch.

Sympathetic nervous system   The branch of the autonomic nervous system that is most active during periods of stress and activity.

VO_2 max   The maximal rate at which an individual can take in and utilize oxygen.

SUGGESTED READINGS

Brooks, G. A., T. D. Fahey, and T. P. White. *Exercise Physiology.* Mountain View, CA: Mayfield Publishing Company, 1996

Foss, M. L. and S. J. Keteyian. *Physiological Basis for Exercise and Sport.* Dubuque, IA: WCB/McGraw-Hill Companies, 1998.

Wilmore, J. H. and D. L. Costill. *Physiology of Sport and Exercise.* Champaign, IL: Human Kinetics, 1994.

REFERENCES

1. American College of Sports Medicine. *ACSM's Guidelines for Exercise Testing and Prescription,* 5th ed. Baltimore, MD: Williams and Wilkins, 1995.

2. American College of Sports Medicine. *ACSM Membership Directory,* American College of Sports Medicine, Indianapolis, IN, pp. 113, 1995.

3. American College of Sports Medicine. Action items. ACSM Board of Trustees. *Sports Med. Bulletin* 31:6–7, 1996.

4. American College of Sports Medicine. ACSM Position Stand on Osteoporosis and Exercise. *Med. Sci. Sports Exerc.* 24:i–vii, 1995.

5. American College of Sports Medicine. Position stand on the prevention of thermal injuries during distance running. *Med. Sci. Sports Exerc.* 19:529–533, 1987.

6. American College of Sports Medicine. *Position stand. The use of blood doping as an ergogenic aid.* Med. Sci. Sports Exerc. 28:i–viii, 1996.

7. American Physical Therapy Association. *1994 Directory of Physical Therapy Education Programs,* American Physical Therapy Association, Alexandria, VA, pp. i–viii, 1994.

8. American Physical Therapy Association. A guide to physical therapist practice, volume 1: A description of patient management. *Phys. Ther.* 75:709–748, 1995.

9. American Thoracic Society. Pulmonary rehabilitation: Official American Thoracic Society position statement. *Am. Rev. Respir. Dis.* 124:663–666, 1996.

10. Arena, B., N. Maffulli, F. Maffulli, and M. A. Morleo. Reproductive hormones and menstrual changes with exercise in female athletes. *Sports Med.* 19:278–287, 1995.

11. Astrand, P.-O. Influence of Scandinavian scientists in exercise physiology. *Scan. J. Med. Sci. Sports* 1:3–9, 1991.

12. Bach, J. R., and J. R. Moldover. Cardiovascular, pulmonary, and cancer rehabilitation. 2. Pulmonary rehabilitation. *Arch. Phys. Med. Rehabil.* 77:S45–S51, 1996.

13. Baechle, T. R. NSCA Certified Personal Trainer Program measures up. *Stren. Cond.* 18:37, 1996.

14. Bailey, D. A., R. A. Faulkner, and H. A. McKay. Growth, physical activity, and bone mineral acquisition. *Exerc. Sport Sci. Rev.* 24:233–266, 1996.

15. Baldwin, K. M., T. P. White, S. B. Arnaud, V. R. Edgerton, W. J. Kraemer, R. Kram, D. Raab-Cullen, and C. M. Snow. Musculoskeletal adaptations to weightlessness and development of effective countermeasures. *Med. Sci. Sports Exerc.* 10:1247–1253, 1996.

16. Ballor, D. L., V. L. Katch, M.D. Becque, and C. R. Marks. Resistance weight training during caloric restriction enhances lean body weight maintenance. *Am. J. Clin. Nutr.* 47:19–25, 1988.

17. Balsom, P. D., K. Soderlund, and B. Ekblom. Creatine in humans with special reference to creatine supplementation. *Sports Med.* 18:268–280, 1994.

18. Barr, R. N. Pulmonary rehabilitation. In: *Essentials of Cardiopulmonary Physical Therapy,* E. A. Hillegass and H. S. Sadowsky (Eds.). Philadelphia: W. B. Saunders Company, 1994.

19. Bergstrom, J. Muscle electrolytes in man. *Scand. J. Clin. Lab. Invest.* 68(Suppl):1–110, 1962.

20. Bhasin, S., T. W. Storer, N. Berman, C. Callegari, B. Clevenger, J. Phillips, T. J. Bunell, R. Tricker, A. Shirazi, and R. Casaburi. The effects of supraphysiologic doses of testosterone on muscle size and strength in normal men. *New Eng. J. Med.* 335:1–7, 1996.

21. Berryman, J. W. *Out of Many. One. A History of the American College of Sports Medicine.* Champaign, IL: Human Kinetics, 1995.

22. Bigland-Ritchie, B., and J. J. Woods. Changes in muscle contractile properties and neural control during human muscular fatigue. *Muscle Nerve* 7:691–699, 1984.

23. Kleiger, E., and J. N. Rottman. Frequency domain measures of heart period variability and mortality after myocardial infarction. *Circulation* 85:164–171, 1992.

24. Blimkie, C. J. R. Resistance training during pre- and early puberty: Efficacy, trainability, mechanisms, and persistence. *Can. J. Sports Med.* 17:264–279, 1992.

25. Borer, K. T. The effects of exercise on growth. *Sports Med.* 20:375–397, 1995.

26. Brooks, G. A. The exercise physiology paradigm in contemporary biology: To molbiol or not to molbiol—that is the question. *Quest* 39:231–242, 1987.

27. Brooks, G. A. 40 years of progress: Basic exercise physiology. In: *40th Anniversary Lectures,* American College of Sports Medicine, Indianapolis, IN, 1994.

28. Brooks, G. A., and T. D. Fahey. *Exercise Physiology: Human Bioenergetics and Its Applications.* New York: Macmillan, Inc., 1985.

29. Buskirk, E. R. Exercise physiology. Part I. Early history in the United States. In: *History of Exercise and Sport Science,* J. D. Massengale and R. A. Swanson (Eds.). Champaign, IL: Human Kinetics, 1996, pp. 367–396.

30. Buskirk, E. R. From Harvard to Minnesota: Keys to our history. *Exerc. Sport Sci. Rev.* 20:1–26, 1992.

31. Chapman, C. B. The long reach of Harvard's Fatigue Laboratory. *Persp. Biol. Med.* 34:17–33, 1990.

32. Convertino, V. A. Exercise as a countermeasure for physiological adaptation to prolonged spaceflight. *Med. Sci. Sports Exerc.* 28:999–1014, 1996.

33. Costill, D. L. 40 years of progress: Applied exercise physiology. In: *40th Anniversary Lectures,* American College of Sports Medicine, Indianapolis, IN, 1994.

34. Curtis, C. L., and J. P. Weir. Overview of exercise responses in healthy and impaired states. *Neur. Report.* 20:13–19, 1996.

35. Davis, J. M., and S. P. Bailey. Possible mechanisms of central nervous system fatigue during exercise. *Med. Sci. Sports Exerc.* 29:45–57, 1997.

36. Dempsey, J. A., S. K. Powers, and N. Gledhill. Discussion: Cardiovascular and pulmonary adaptation to physical activity. In: *Exercise, Fitness, and Health. A Consensus of Current Knowledge,* C. Bouchard, R. J. Shephard, T. Stephens, J. R. Sutton, and B. D. McPherson (Eds.). Champaign, IL: Human Kinetics, 1990, pp. 205–215.

37. DeVries, H. A., and T. J. Housh. *Physiology of Exercise for Physical Education, Athletics, and Exercise Science,* 5th ed. Dubuque, IA: W. C. Brown, 1994.

38. Dill, D. B. Arlie V. Bock, pioneer in sports medicine. *Med. Sci. Sports Exerc.* 17:401–404, 1985.

39. Dill, D. B. Historical review of exercise physiology science. In: *Structural and Physiological Aspects of Exercise and Sport.* W. P. Johnson and E. R. Buskirk (Eds.). Princeton, NJ: Princeton Book Company, 1980, pp. 37–41.

40. Engardt, M., E. Knutsson, M. Jonsson, and M. Sternhag. Dynamic muscle strength training in stroke patients: Effects on knee extensor torque, electromyographic activity, and motor function. *Arch. Phys. Med. Rehabil.* 76:419–425, 1995.

41. Evans, W. J. What is sarcopenia? *J. Gerontol.* 50A(Special Issue):58, 1995.

42. Fox, E. L., R. W. Bowers, and M. L. Foss. *The Physiological Basis for Exercise and Sport,* 5th Ed. Dubuque, IA: W. C. Brown, 1993.

43. Gollnick, P. D., and D. King. Effects of exercise and training on mitochondria of rat skeletal muscle. *Am. J. Physiol.* 216:1502–1509, 1969.

44. Haas, F., J. Salazar-Schicchi, and R. Fain. Cardiopulmonary exercise evaluation. *Phys. Med. Rehabil. Clin. North Amer.* 7:241–251, 1996.

45. Halar, E. M. Physical inactivity. A major risk factor for coronary heart disease. *Phys. Med. Rehabil. Clin. North Amer.* 6:55–67, 1995.

46. Heyward, V. H. Evaluation of body composition. Current issues. *Sports Med.* 22:146–156, 1996.

47. Hoberman, J. M., and C. E. Yesalis. The history of synthetic testosterone. *Sci. Amer.* Feb:76–81, 1995.

48. Holloszy, J. Effects of exercise on mitochondrial oxygen uptake and respiratory enzyme activity in skeletal muscle. *J. Biol. Chem.* 242:2278–2282, 1967.

49. Hough, D. O., and K. L. Dec. Exercise-induced asthma and anaphylaxis. *Sports Med.* 18:162–172, 1994.

50. Housh, D. J., T. J. Housh, G. O. Johnson, and W. Chu. Hypertrophic response to unilateral concentric isokinetic resistance training. *J. Appl. Physiol.* 73:65–70, 1992.

51. Housh, T. J., G. O. Johnson, J. Stout, and D. J. Housh. Anthropometric growth patterns of high school wrestlers. *Med. Sci. Sports Exerc.* 25:1141–1150, 1993.

52. Jones, N. L. *Clinical Exercise Testing,* 3rd ed. Philadelphia: W. B. Saunders, 1988.

53. Kearny, J. T. Training the Olympic athlete. *Sci. Amer.* June:52–63, 1996.

54. Kent-Braun, J. A., R. G. Miller, and M. W. Weiner. Human skeletal muscle metabolism in health and disease: Utility of magnetic resonance spectroscopy. *Exerc. Sport Sci. Rev.* 23:305–347, 1995.

55. Kroll, W. P. *Perspectives in Physical Education.* New York: Academic Press, 1971.

56. Kuczmarski, R. J., K. M. Flegal, S. M. Campbell, and C. L. Johnson. Increasing prevalence of overweight among US adults. The National Health and Nutrition Examination Surveys, 1960 to 1991. *J.A.M.A.* 272:205–211, 1994.

57. Lawless, D., C. G. R. Jackson, and J. E. Greenleaf. Exercise and human immunodeficiency virus (HIV-1) infection. *Sports Med.* 19:235–239, 1995.

58. Lindermann, J. K., and K. L. Gosselink. The effects of sodium bicarbonate ingestion on exercise performance. *Sports Med.* 18:75–80, 1994.

59. Lynch, J., S. P. Helmrich, T. A. Lakka, G. A. Kaplan, R. D. Cohen, R. Salonen, and J. T. Salonen. Moderately intense physical activities and high levels of cardiorespiratory fitness reduce the risk of non-insulin-dependent diabetes mellitus in middle-aged men. *Arch. Int. Med.* 156:1307–1314, 1996.

60. MacLaren, D. P. M., H. Gibson, M. Parry-Billings, and R. H. T. Edwards. A review of metabolic and physiological factors in fatigue. *Exerc. Sport Sci. Rev.* 17:29–66, 1989.

61. Malina, R. M. Physical growth and biological maturation of young athletes. *Exerc. Sport Sci. Rev.* 22:389–433, 1994.

62. McArdle, W. D., F. I. Katch, and V. L. Katch. *Exercise Physiology. Energy, Nutrition, and Human Performance,* 4th Ed. Baltimore, MD: William and Wilkins, 1996.

63. Moritani, T. Time course of adaptations during strength and power training. In: *Strength and Power in Sport,* P. V. Komi (ed.). London: Blackwell Scientific Publications, 1992.

64. Moritani, T., and H. A. deVries. Neural factors versus hypertrophy in the time course of muscle strength gain. *Am. J. Phys. Med.* 58:115–130, 1979.

65. National Strength and Conditioning Association. Youth resistance training: Position paper and literature review. *Stren. Cond.* 18:62–75, 1996.

66. Nieman, D. C., L. M. Johanssen, J. W. Lee, et al. Infectious episodes in runners before and after the Los Angeles Marathon. *J. Sports Med. Phys. Fit.* 30:316–328, 1990.

67. Nieman, D. C. The immune response to prolonged cardiorespiratory exercise. *Am. J. Sports Med.* 24:S-98 to S-103, 1996.

68. Pate, R. R., M. Pratt, S. N. Blair, et al. Physical activity and public health. A recommendation from the Centers for Disease Control and Prevention and the American College of Sports Medicine. *J.A.M.A.* 273:402–407, 1995.

69. Pi-Sunyer, F. X. Medical hazards of obesity. *Ann. Int. Med.* 119:655–660, 1993.

70. Pivarnik, J. M. Maternal exercise during pregnancy. *Sports Med.* 18:215–217, 1994.

71. Poehlman, E. T., P. J. Arciero, and M. I. Goran. Endurance exercise in aging humans: Effects on energy metabolism. *Exerc. Sport Sci. Rev.* 22:251–284, 1994.

72. Potempa, K., L. T. Braun, T. Tinkell, and J. Popovich. Benefits of aerobic exercise after stroke. *Sports Med.* 21:337–346, 1996.

73. Potempa, K., M. Lopez, L. T. Braun, J. P. Szidon, L. Fogg, and T. Tincknell. Physiological outcomes of aerobic exercise training in hemiparetic stroke patients. *Stroke* 26:101–105, 1995.

74. Power, S. K., and E. T. Howley. *Exercise Physiology: Theory and Application to Fitness and Performance,* 2nd ed. Dubuque, IA: W. C. Brown, 1994.

75. Ragnarsson, K. T. Guest Editorial. Health maintenance and reduction of disability through physical exercise. In: *Physical Fitness: A Guide for Individuals with Spinal Cord Injury,* T. T. Sowell (ed.). Washington, D.C. Department of Veterans Affairs, 1996.

76. Regensteiner, J. G., and W. R. Hiatt. Exercise rehabilitation for patients with peripheral arterial disease. *Exerc. Sport Sci. Rev.* 23:1–24, 1996.

77. Rogers, M. A., and W. J. Evans. Changes in skeletal muscle with aging: Effects of exercise training. *Exerc. Sport Sci. Rev.* 21:65–102, 1993.

78. Ryan, A. S., R. E. Pratley, D. Elahi, and A. P. Goldberg. Resistive training increases fat-free mass and maintains RMR despite weight loss in postmenopausal women. *J. Appl. Physiol.* 79:818–823, 1995.

79. Saltin, B. Cardiovascular and pulmonary adaptation to physical activity. In: *Exercise, Fitness, and Health.*

A Consensus of Current Knowledge, C. Bouchard, R. J. Shephard, T. Stephens, J. R. Sutton, and B. D. McPherson (eds.). Champaign, IL: Human Kinetics, 1990.

80. Schneider, F. J. Traumatic spinal cord injury. In: *Neurological Rehabilitation,* 2nd Ed., D. A. Umphred (ed.). St. Louis: Mosby, 1990, pp. 423–483.

81. Shi, X., G. H. J. Stevens, B. H. Foresman, S. A. Stern, and P. B. Raven. Autonomic nervous system control of the heart: Endurance exercise training. *Med. Sci. Sports Exerc.* 27:1406–1413, 1995.

82. Siebens, H. The role of exercise in the rehabilitation of patients with chronic obstructive pulmonary disease. *Phys. Med. Rehabil. Clin. North Amer.* 7:299–313, 1996.

83. Smith, H. L., D. L. Hudson, H. M. Graitzer, and P. B. Raven. Exercise training bradycardia: The role of autonomic balance. *Med. Sci. Sports Exerc.* 21:40–44, 1989.

84. Spelsberg, A., and J. E. Manson. Physical activity in the treatment and prevention of diabetes. *Comp. Ther.* 21:559–564, 1995.

85. Stiens, S. A., M. C. Johnson II, and P. J. Lyman. Cardiac rehabilitation in patients with spinal cord injuries. *Phys. Med. Rehabil. Clin. North Amer.* 6:263–296, 1995.

86. Sulzman, F. M. Overview. *J. Appl. Physiol.* 81:3–6, 1996.

87. Sutton, J. R., J. T. Maher, and C. S. Houston. Operation Everest II. *Prog. Clin. Biol. Res.* 136:221–233, 1983.

88. Tesch, P. A., P. V. Komi, and K. Hakkinen. Enzymatic adaptations consequent to long-term strength training. *Int. J. Sports Med.* 8:66–69, 1987.

89. Thoden, J. S. Testing aerobic power. In: *Physiological Testing of the High-performance Athlete.* J. D. MacDougall, H. A. Wenger, and H. J. Green (Eds.). Champaign, IL: Human Kinetics, 1991.

90. Tipton, C. M. Exercise physiology. Part II. A contemporary historical perspective. In: *History of Exercise and Sport Science,* J. D. Massengale and R. A. Swanson (eds.). Champaign, IL: Human Kinetics, 1996.

91. Tomassoni, T. L. Introduction: The role of exercise in the diagnosis and management of chronic disease in children and youth. *Med. Sci. Sports Exerc.* 28:403–405, 1996.

92. Tsuji, H., F. J. Venditti, E. S. Manders, J. C. Evans, M. G. Larson, C. L. Feldman, and D. Levy. Reduced heart rate variability and mortality risk in an elderly cohort. The Framingham Heart Study. *Circulation* 90:878–883, 1994.

93. Urban, R. J., Y. H. Bodenburg, C. Gilkison, J. Foxworth, A. R. Coggan, R. R. Wolfe, and A. Ferrando. Testosterone administration to elderly men increases skeletal muscle strength and protein synthesis. *Am. J. Physiol.* 269:E820–E826, 1995.

94. Wasserman, D. H., and B. Zinman. Exercise in individuals with IDDM. *Diabetes Care* 17:924–937, 1994.

95. Wenger, N. K., E. S. Froelicher, L. K. Smith, et al. *Cardiac Rehabilitation as Secondary Prevention. Clinical Practice Guideline.* Quick Reference Guide for Clinicians, No. 17. Rockville, MD: U.S. Department of Health and Human Services, Public Health Service, Agency for Health Care Policy and Research and National Heart, Lung, and Blood Institute. AHCPR Pub. No. 96–0673, October 1995.

96. Whitehead, J. R. The largest sports medicine and exercise science conference in the world. *Sports Med. Bull.* 31:5, 1996.

97. Williams, J. H. Caffeine, neuromuscular function and high-intensity exercise performance. *J. Sports Med. Phys. Fit.* 31:481–489, 1991.

98. Williams, M. H. Ergogenic and ergolytic substances. *Med. Sci. Sports Exerc.* 24:S344–S348, 1992.

99. Wilmore, J. H. Increasing physical activity: Alterations in body mass and composition. *Am. J. Clin. Nutr.* 63(Supplement):456S–460S, 1996.

100. Wilmore, J. H., P. R. Stanforth, J. Gagnon, A. S. Leon, D. C. Rao, J. S. Skinner, and C. Bouchard. Endurance exercise training has a minimal effect on resting heart rate: The HERITAGE study. *Med. Sci. Sports Exerc.* 28:829–835, 1996.

101. Yesalis, C. E., and M. S. Bahrke. Anabolic–androgenic steroids. Current issues. *Sports Med.* 19:326–340, 1995.

102. Young, J. C. Exercise prescription for individuals with metabolic disorders. Practical considerations. *Sports Med.* 19:43-54, 1995.

7 Exercise and Sport Nutrition

JOAN M. ECKERSON

Related Disciplines

Areas of Study and Research in Nutrition
Sport-related Aspects
Health-related Aspects

Historical Aspects of Nutrition

**Technology Used to Study Health
and Exercise-related Aspects of Nutrition**
Muscle Biopsy Technique
Blood and Urine Analysis
Calorimetry
Metabolic Measurements
Dietary Recall and Analysis
Body Composition Assessment

Academic Training and Certifications
Dietetics

Licensure
Undergraduate Programs in Exercise
and Sport Nutrition
Graduate Programs in Exercise
and Sport Nutrition

Employment Opportunities
Dietetics
Exercise and Sport Nutrition

Professional Journals and Related Sources

Summary

Study Questions

Glossary

Suggested Readings

References

The role of nutrition in health and sports performance has gained importance primarily through increased knowledge of exercise physiology. *Nutrition* is the science of food and is generally described as the sum total of the processes involved in the intake and utilization of food, including the ingestion, digestion, absorption, and metabolism of food (35). *Exercise nutrition* is a relatively new area of study that integrates the principles of nutrition and physical activity as they relate to the enhancement of sports performance or prevention of chronic disease.

Although the interactions between nutrition and various forms of sport or exercise have been studied for more than 100 years, only recently have extensive investigations been performed regarding specific dietary recommendations for athletes and the general public. For example, research suggests that carbohydrate intake prior to and during exercise bouts of long duration at moderate to high intensities and with adequate fluid intake before and during endurance events performed under warm or hot environmental conditions are two dietary practices that have consistently resulted in enhanced performance capacity (35). In addition, a significant amount of research suggests that both diet and physical activity play important roles in the development or progression of chronic diseases, such as coronary heart disease (CHD), hypertension, osteoporosis, and a variety of cancers (4). For example, a considerable amount of evidence supports relationships between serum cholesterol and CHD, calcium and osteoporosis, fats and cancer, and diets low in fat and rich in fiber and antioxidant nutrients and both heart disease and cancer (see Figure 7.1). Several factors, including an interest in exploring relationships among food and health and performance, make exercise nutrition a viable field of study.

Related Disciplines

Biology and chemistry serve as the foundation for understanding almost every aspect of nutrition, exercise, and health. Biology is the science of life and living things. Chemistry is the science that studies the structure and composition of matter: the solids, liquids, and gases that are the basic building blocks of our universe. Biochemistry is the chemistry of living things, the science of the chemical changes associated with the vital processes of plants and animals (30).

Dietetics and food science are interrelated disciplines in that they both involve the study of food. Traditionally, however, dietetics has been associated with the study of foods in health and disease, whereas food science uses principles of biological and physical sciences to study the nature of foods, the causes of food deterioration, and the principles underlying the processing and preparation of food (that is, the application of science and technology to the provision of a safe, wholesome, and nutritious food supply). Pharmacology, which is the study of drugs, their origin, nature, properties, and effects on living things, is also an important discipline to consider, because drugs may have a significant effect on performance or health due to alterations in nutritional status. In addition, some nutrients may act as *neutraceuticals,* a term used to describe nutrients that exhibit druglike properties when taken in appropriate dosages.

Areas of Study and Research in Nutrition

Sport-related Aspects

Although genetic endowment is an important factor when considering the potential for success in an athletic event or sport, the nutritional status of the athlete may also exert a significant impact on performance. True athletic potential may not be attained if the athlete has insufficient fuel stores or lacks the nutrients that are necessary for optimal performance. In fact, many athletes spend considerable time, money, and effort striving for peak performance and fall short because of inadequate, counterproductive, and sometimes harmful nutritional practices (35). Inadequate intakes of nutrients, electrolytes, and water can hinder athletic performance. Conversely, excessive intakes of some nutrients may

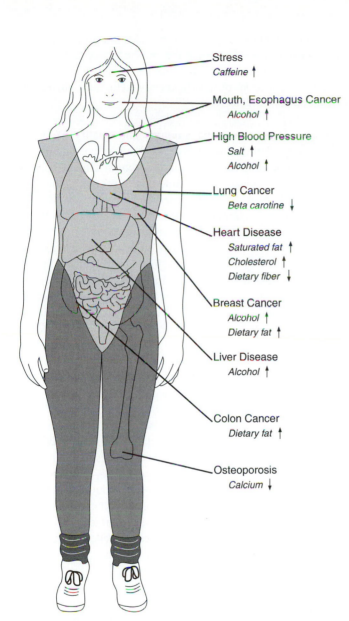

Stress
Caffeine ↑

Mouth, Esophagus Cancer
Alcohol ↑

High Blood Pressure
Salt ↑
Alcohol ↑

Lung Cancer
Beta carotine ↓

Heart Disease
Saturated fat ↑
Cholesterol ↑
Dietary fiber ↓

Breast Cancer
Alcohol ↑
Dietary fat ↑

Liver Disease
Alcohol ↑

Colon Cancer
Dietary fat ↑

Osteoporosis
Calcium ↓

FIGURE 7.1   Possible health problems associated with poor dietary habits. The upward arrow represents excessive intake, while the downward arrow represents low intake or deficiency.

Source: Williams, M. H. *Nutrition for Fitness and Sport,* 4th ed. Dubuque, IA: W. C. Brown Communications, Inc., 1995. Reproduced with permission of the McGraw-Hill Companies.

impair athletic performance by disrupting normal physiological processes or by leading to undesirable changes in body composition (35).

Carbohydrate Intake and Performance.   All biological functions require energy; therefore, the use of dietary manipulation to determine how the body uses and stores energy for biological work has been, and continues to be, a major research interest. In 1939, Christensen and Hansen first examined the effects of dietary manipulation on exercise performance, and today it is well known that the availability of carbohydrates to muscles is a limiting factor in prolonged exercise of moderate intensities (11). The use of the muscle biopsy technique has been instrumental in establishing the role of diet and exercise on muscle glycogen depletion and repletion and has led to effective applications of specific dietary techniques, such as carbohydrate loading, to enhance athletic performance (11).

Protein Intake and Performance.   Determining the amounts and quality of protein necessary to build muscle size and strength is an area of research that is of considerable interest to athletes, trainers, and coaches. Athletes, particularly strength athletes such as weight lifters and body builders, routinely consume large amounts of protein in the belief that these diets enhance performance. In addition, a wide variety of commercially available protein supplements claim to enhance muscle strength and size by stimulating protein synthesis through enhanced absorption and/or inhibition of protein breakdown.

Compared to the study of carbohydrates and athletic performance, the study of protein nutrition and its effects on muscular strength and hypertrophy is insufficient to provide definite conclusions and guidelines. The question of whether increased dietary protein improves nitrogen metabolism through a relatively simple caloric effect or by specific effects unique to amino acids warrants further study (7). There is an emerging consensus among researchers, however, that initiation of increased exercise workloads (endurance or strength training) most likely increases protein requirements, at least for a relatively short time period of 4 to 8 weeks (7).

Athletes view protein powders as a cost-effective and convenient source of additional dietary protein, and the demand for these products equates to millions of dollars for commercial suppliers of protein supplements. Some companies claim improved or faster absorption over dietary proteins and decreased protein catabolism using their "secret formula" of amino acid mixtures. Many of these manufacturers' claims are indirectly based on peer-reviewed clinical studies, which show that specific combinations of amino acids can enhance the healing of body tissues and, therefore, speed recovery (5, 28). Therefore, theoretically, similar combinations of amino acids taken by athletes should enhance protein synthesis and lead to improved performance. However, very few well controlled laboratory studies have been performed to support or contradict these manufacturers' claims. Much more research regarding the effects of amino acid mixtures is needed to determine whether protein supplementation is effective and/or warranted by athletes.

Fat Intake and Performance.   Fat represents a major source of energy for working muscles, particularly at low intensities, and training enhances the muscle's ability to utilize free-fatty acids (FFA) as an energy source during exercise. The use of dietary fat as a means to enhance athletic performance has largely been ignored because even individuals with low body fat store huge amounts of energy as triglycerides in adipose tissue and within the muscles. Furthermore, research has shown that high fat consumption (60% to 80% of caloric intake) has limited beneficial effects on muscular exercise performance and may actually decrease performance relative to high-carbohydrate diets (7). Recent evidence, however, suggests that two types of dietary fats, omega-3 fatty acids and medium-chain triglycerides (MCTs), possess interesting properties that may benefit athletic performance if manipulated correctly (7).

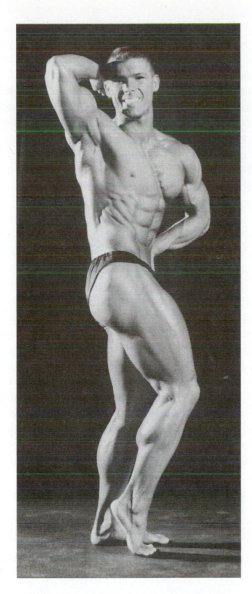

FIGURE 7.2   Bodybuilders typically consume large amounts of protein to increase muscle strength and size.

Courtesy of Dan Reeves, Mr. Natural Universe, 1996; Lifetime Professional Natural Bodybuilder.

Omega-3 FFAs are polyunsaturated fatty acids found in fish oils that have a double bond between the third and fourth carbon from the terminal, or omega, carbon. It has been theorized that the natural physiological effects of these fatty acids, including increased tissue perfusion, stimulation of regulatory hormones such as growth hormone, and conversion to antiinflammatory compounds, produce ergogenic benefits for both aerobic and strength performance (7).

Medium-chain triglycerides are saturated FFAs with chain lengths of 6 to 12 carbons and are found in human milk, coconut oil, and palm oil. Unlike other fats, MCTs possess unique physiological properties that strongly indicate a need for further study as an ergogenic aid. These triglycerides are water soluble and can be rapidly absorbed by the portal circulation, where they are readily taken up by the liver and oxidized to produce ketone bodies (substances involved in acidosis) and cellular energy. Metabolism of MCTs resembles that of carbohydrate oxidation rather than fat oxidation, in that they do not rely on carnitine to enter the mitochondria. It has been shown that MCTs are not easily stored as body fat, but rather mobilize body fat stores, increase metabolic rate, and spare lean muscle mass. Furthermore, MCTs appear to be nonatherogenic; that is, they do not promote the formation of fatty plaques on the arterial walls. Potential applications of MCTs include their use in preexercise meals to improve endurance performance, to prevent muscle mass loss from strenuous exercise, to recover from immobilizing injuries with less lean tissue loss, and to aid in body fat loss without lean body weight loss (7).

Although not a fat, glycerol supplementation has also been studied for its ergogenic (work-enhancing) effects because it is one of the by-products of triglyceride breakdown. Other supplements, such as lecithin and carnitine and the drug caffeine, have been used in an attempt to facilitate the metabolism or mobilization of FFAs (7).

Vitamin and Mineral Intake and Performance.   Although vitamins and minerals do not provide a direct source of energy, they do serve as essential links and regulators in the chain of metabolic reactions within cells and, therefore, help to release the energy trapped inside carbohydrates, fats, and proteins. Most athletes, as well as the general population, receive the *Recommended Dietary Allowances* for vitamins in their daily diets and, therefore, there is little need for concern regarding vitamin deficiency, even for athletes in sports that require low body weights (35). Although vitamin supplementation is not usually necessary, many athletes believe it is essential for athletic success and, therefore, consume vitamins with the hope of improving performance. Manufacturers of vitamin supplements are aware of athlete's perceptions regarding vitamins and suggest through their advertising that their products do, indeed, enhance performance. Although the general consensus is that vitamin supplementation does not significantly enhance either anaerobic or aerobic exercise performance, research is incomplete, especially with regard to the dosages that would be necessary for enhanced performance, effects of megadoses, time of administration, and use of different forms of vitamins (7).

Antioxidant vitamins such as vitamins E, C, and beta-carotene have received a great deal of attention in recent years because of their ability to protect the body from oxidative, free-radical-mediated damage. Free radicals are oxygen molecules with an unpaired electron, making them highly reactive, and are naturally produced through cellular metabolism (21). Free radicals destroy cells by attacking the cellular membrane and have been linked to aging, cancer, coronary heart disease, and other chronic diseases. Fortunately, a considerable amount of protection exists in the body in the form of antioxidants (such as vitamins E and C) and certain enzymes (such as glutathione peroxidase, catalase, and superoxide dismutase), which react directly with free radicals to reduce their reactivity and thus help to protect cells (34). Recently, considerable research has focused on the effect of various antioxidant supplements to reduce exercise-induced muscle damage and soreness, thereby enhancing performance. Results from preliminary studies appear promising; however, further investigations are necessary to determine the utility of antioxidant supplementation in preventing exercise-induced muscle damage (35).

Minerals are essential to human body structure and function. Most research has been devoted to the role of mineral nutrition in health and disease, including both epidemiological and laboratory research. For example, large surveys among the general population have shown that either an inadequate dietary intake of some minerals or excessive intake of others may contribute to several health problems and disease states (35).

An increasing number of studies have utilized athletes to determine the effect of mineral nutrition on performance, as well as the effect of exercise on mineral metabolism. Several major dietary concerns of the female athlete are linked to mineral deficiencies, particularly calcium and iron. Osteoporosis is commonly associated with old age; however, there is a growing concern among investigators regarding disordered calcium metabolism in young, female athletes involved in endurance and weight-control sports such as long distance running, dance, and gymnastics (35). The female athlete triad comprises three entities that are interrelated: disordered eating, amenorrhea, and osteoporosis. Many female athletes have unhealthy or inadequate dietary practices that can lead to amenorrhea (absence of menstrual cycles) and increase their risk for premature osteoporosis.

The importance of iron for oxygen transport via hemoglobin and endurance exercise has been well documented (13, 16). Female endurance athletes, in particular, frequently

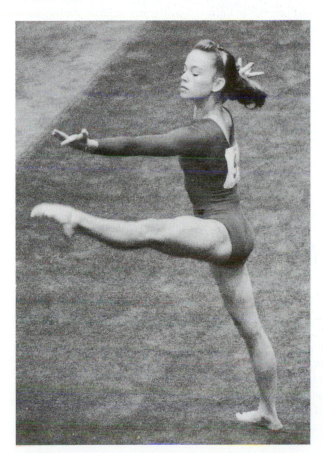

FIGURE 7.3 Gymnasts on very low calorie diets may be at risk for mineral deficiencies, such as calcium and iron. Pictured is Kelli More.

Photo courtesy of Mr. Tom Koll, TNT Gymnastics, Omaha, NE.

exhibit low levels of hemoglobin and sports anemia. Iron supplementation to anemic persons (including athletes) has been shown to improve hemoglobin concentration, red blood cell count, maximal oxygen consumption, maximal work times to exhaustion, heart-rate responses, and performance time (7). The effects of iron supplementation on athletic performance need to be explored; however, a few studies have shown that iron supplementation improves the iron status of athletes (25, 36). Much more research is needed to fully determine the effects of iron supplementation, as well as the effects of other micro- and macrominerals for both athletes and the general population.

Water, Electrolytes, and Physical Performance.   Normal body function depends on a balance between water and electrolytes. Electrolytes are substances that, when in solution, conduct a current. Some electrolytes important for normal biological function include sodium, potassium, chloride, and calcium. Of all the nutrients, water is the most important to physically active individuals and is one of the few that may have beneficial effects on performance when used in supplemental amounts before or during exercise (35). The effects of exercise on normal fluid balance and the role of water in body temperature regulation have been major areas of research focus. For example, researchers have identified how environmental heat and cold and dehydration and hypohydration effect physical performance and have established guidelines regarding the maintenance of water balance during exercise. Research has also provided guidelines for fluid and electrolyte replacement after different types of exercise and under different types of environmental conditions (35).

Ergogenic Aids.   Although the dietary intake of nutrients such as water and carbohydrates can be manipulated to enhance performance, most exercise and health professionals consider *ergogenic aids* to be artificial pharmacological agents or practices that improve performance. During the past century, a considerable number of substances have been studied for their potential ergogenic effect. Few, however, have been shown to delay the onset of fatigue and/or to be of practical value for improving performance. Although there has been a great deal of controversy regarding the effectiveness of a large number of ergogenic aids, those receiving the most attention include amphetamines, caffeine, bicarbonate, anabolic steroids, creatine, and blood doping (11).

Nutrition and Its Application to Injury Rehabilitation and Sports Medicine.   An extensive amount of laboratory research and clinical work has been performed regarding the therapeutic use of nutrients for healing. The applications of this research have resulted in recommended combinations of nutrients that enhance the healing of sports injuries and other musculoskeletal conditions. Research has shown that specific nutrients, proteases in particular, can accelerate healing rates and shorten recovery to full function for sports injuries such as bruises, strains, sprains, lacerations, and fractures (8). Nutrient combinations for these types of injuries include multiple vitamins and minerals, multiple antioxidants, and multiple proteases (enzymes that break down proteins). Although nutrients should not necessarily be used as replacements for drugs or medical care, they may have the potential to significantly affect healing and return the athlete to competition sooner when compared to traditional rehabilitation programs (8).

Health-related Aspects

Epidemiological, animal, clinical, and metabolic research has established that diet and physical activity play important roles in health promotion and disease prevention. Clinical studies, in particular, show a possible synergistic effect of diet and exercise in the prevention and treatment of *hyperlipidemia,* hypertension, diabetes, and *osteoporosis* (4). However, the mechanisms of action and optimal diet and exercise prescription needed for benefit have not been clearly illustrated. Current evidence suggests that, rather than being randomly distributed throughout the body, nutrients are directed to specific tissues and cells by physiologic processes that require more intensive study (4).

Figure 7.4 is an abstract of a health-related research study of antioxidants.

Coronary Heart Disease. *Coronary heart disease* (CHD) remains the leading cause of death in the United States and is a major contributor to disability, lost productivity, and medical costs (2, 4). This disease begins in childhood and progresses over time, resulting in atherosclerotic plaques on the walls of the coronary arteries and thus reduced blood flow to the heart. Risk factors include elevated levels of total and low-density lipoprotein (LDL) *cholesterol* and reduced levels of high-density lipoprotein cholesterol, hypertension, smoking,

FIGURE 7.4 Abstract of a research study involving dietary antioxidants and bone mineral density.

Leveille, S. G., A. Z. Lacroix, T. D. Koepsell, S. Beresford, G. Van Belle, and D. M. Buchner.
Do Dietary Antioxidants Prevent Postmenopausal Bone Loss?
Nutrition Research, Vol.17, No. 8, pp. 1261–1269, 1997.

The role of dietary antioxidants in osteoporosis has not been well explored. The objective of this study was to examine the relationship between the dietary antioxidants, vitamin E and beta-carotene, and hip bone mineral density (BMD) in postmenopausal women. Subjects were 1892 screenees, aged 55–80 years, who were volunteers for a clinical trial. Bone densitometry and osteoporosis risk factor information was obtained during screening. Dietary and supplement information was obtained by mailed food frequency and vitamin supplement questionnaires. We found no evidence of an association between dietary and/or supplemental vitamin E and bone density of the femoral neck. Dietary beta-carotene, adjusted for age and weight, was positively associated with hip BMD ($\beta = 1.5 \times 10^{-6}$ g/cm^2, $p = 0.05$). Further adjustment for osteoporosis risk factors diminished the association ($\beta = 0.7 \times 10^{-6}$ g/cm^2, $p = 0.38$). Neither total nor supplemental beta-carotene intake was found to be associated with BMD. We did not find that vitamin E or beta-carotene was associated with femoral neck bone density in postmenopausal women; however, the potential role of antioxidants and other nutrients in postmenopausal bone loss warrants further study, including research of other bone sites.

Source: Reprinted from Leveille, S. G., A. Z. Lacroix, T. D. Koepsell, S. Beresford, G. Van Belle, and D. M. Buchner. Do Dietary Antioxidants Prevent Postmenopausal Bone Loss? *Nutrition Research,* 17(8): 1261–1269, 1997, with permission from Elsevier Science.

physical inactivity, diabetes, and obesity, particularly when characterized by excessive abdominal fat (android-type obesity) (4). Although the mechanisms underlying their preventive effect are not fully understood, both diet and exercise affect several risk factors and are believed to influence both atherogenic (plaque forming) and thrombotic (blood clotting) processes (4).

Research strongly relates dietary saturated fat and serum cholesterol to the development of CHD, showing that the formation of atherosclerotic lesions in coronary arteries increases proportionately with levels of total and LDL cholesterol. Clinical trials that involve altering diet composition, especially the type and amount of fat and total intake of cholesterol, have favorably changed lipoprotein levels and considerably reduced CHD risk (4). Other dietary factors may reduce CHD risk through a variety of mechanisms. Reduced sodium chloride (salt) and alcohol intake are associated with decreased blood pressure. Conversely, moderate alcohol consumption may raise HDL levels and decrease platelet aggregation. Certain types of fiber, when consumed in adequate amounts, may reduce total and LDL cholesterol by decreasing cholesterol synthesis in the gut and facilitating its excretion. Recent studies also suggest that antioxidants (vitamins E, C, and beta-carotene) may prevent the oxidation of LDL cholesterol, which is believed to initiate an immune response that, in turn, leads to the formation of cells responsible for atherosclerotic plaques (4).

Clinical research has also shown a relationship between calcium and osteoporosis and dietary fat and certain types of cancers. Future research will continue to examine the relationships among nutrition, health, and disease to better understand their interaction. In addition, ethnic and cultural factors are now being recognized for their importance in influencing diet quality and metabolic responses to diet. The roles of nonnutrients in foods, such as estrogenic compounds, and of the overall variety in the diet are also being examined for effects on health (33).

Genetic Engineering and Transgene Technology.   The development of transgene technologies, the transfer of a gene from one species to another species, has accompanied advances in genetic engineering. The first transgenic animal was a mouse, which was produced by inserting a foreign gene into an embryo; thereafter this foreign gene became an integral part of the host animal's genetic material (31).

Transgenic animals hold significant promise for developing new animal models for human disease. Presently, there are several models for studying metabolic diseases, including diabetes, hypertension, cancer, obesity, and hyperlipidemia and for developing gene therapy technologies. The origin and development of these diseases (pathogenesis) may be discovered using these genetically engineered animals. Thus, transgenic animals will continue to play an important role in nutritional research in the next decade (31).

Obesity.   Obesity is a major health concern in the United States and other industrialized nations. Data from the most recent National Health and Nutrition Examination Survey (NHANES III) estimated that 33% of adults in the United States aged 20 to 74 years were overweight (body mass index ≥ 27.8 for men, ≥ 27.3 for women) (4). Therefore, studies regarding the development of fat substitutes, weight-loss drugs, fat patterning, and nutrients that offer health benefits will continue to be a focal point for research.

Historical Aspects of Nutrition

To provide a comprehensive historical perspective of the many facets of nutrition as it relates to athletic performance and health and disease is beyond the scope of this chapter. Therefore, this section primarily reflects on those aspects of nutrition that have made a significant contribution to the knowledge base in exercise physiology.

Nutrition science developed in this century with its roots in medicine, physiology, and the biological sciences (32). However, dietetics and interest in diet may be traced back to the ancient Egyptians, Greeks, and Romans, with the term *nutrition* in its various forms in the English language originating sometime between the fifteenth and sixteenth centuries (32). More than 2300 years ago, Egyptian physicians perceived that some of their patients were suffering from a lack of proper nutrition and prescribed enemas and nutritional clysters (injection of fluids into tissue spaces, the rectum, or abdominal cavity). Greek physicians adopted these same practices and administered rectal clysters, which included wine, whey, and milk (6).

Although the importance of nutrition was first realized over 2000 years ago, it was not officially recognized as an independent discipline until April 11, 1933, with the founding of the American Institute of Nutrition (AIN). Until the formation of the AIN, there was no organization specifically devoted to the study of nutrition science (32). Today, this organization is known as the American Society for Nutrition Science.

Early nutrition research focused on identifying all the essential nutrients and the dietary requirements for each nutrient. In addition, it was necessary to determine the distribution of each nutrient in various foods to define a nutritionally adequate diet or analyze a diet and determine whether it was nutritionally balanced (18).

Although the Nutrition Laboratory at the Carnegie Institute in Washington, D.C., had been created in 1904 to study nutrition and energy metabolism, the real impact of laboratory research in exercise physiology and exercise and sport nutrition occurred in 1927 with the creation of the Harvard Fatigue Laboratory under the direction of David Bruce Dill. Although the laboratory closed in 1947, the research conducted there in the areas of metabolism, environmental physiology, physical fitness, and nutrition formed the foundation for research in modern laboratories of exercise physiology (24).

Ancel Keys, a biochemist and physiologist associated with the Harvard Fatigue Laboratory, conducted what is now considered classical research in nutrition and semistarvation at the Laboratory of Physical Hygiene at the University of Minnesota in the late 1930s. Based on requests from the U.S. Army, Keys and his colleagues conducted experiments to develop high-calorie, nonperishable foods that could be used in the field by soldiers. Their research resulted in the Keys or K-rations, which were widely used in World War II and continue to be used today (10). Keys also envisioned the impact that the war would have on worldwide starvation and realized that experimental data on the effects of starvation were needed. His concern led to the classic Minnesota Starvation Study, which was a comprehensive evaluation of the physiological effects of starvation and the recovery that followed. The results of this study were published in the two-volume work, *The Biology of Human Starvation,* in 1950 (22). Research on starvation continued into the 1950s and contributed to a better understanding of moderate periods of semistarvation; however, none were as comprehensive as the classic Minnesota Starvation Study (10).

One of the most important developments in nutrition has been *epidemiology,* particularly the epidemiology of chronic diseases (18). Following World War II, the United States was faced with an aging population whose infatuation with the "good life" led to life-style practices that predisposed many to the deleterious effects of chronic diseases, particularly CHD (10). This disturbing state of affairs led to the recruitment of 250 middle-aged (45 to 55 years) professional men from the Twin Cities area for a longitudinal study of initially healthy men as they aged and developed evidence of cardiovascular degeneration. Over time, this study acquired the acronym CVD for (cardiovascular degeneration) (10). The study has continued for over 40 years and has had an important influence on epidemiological research in that other well-known longitudinal studies, such as the Public Health Service's Framingham Heart Study (20) and the Harvard Alumni Study (26), were able to take advantage of the protocol, design, and related administrative and scientific approaches used in the CVD study (10). The outcome of these and related studies has led to the identification of the risk-factor concept, with serum cholesterol levels, smoking, physical inactivity, and hypertension playing early and continuing roles in the development of CHD.

An association between diet and sports performance has been made as far back as descriptions of athletes exist. Early interest in sports nutrition developed from an ambiguous and indistinct search for an ergogenic food or nutrient. However, in the last 30 years a true science has developed, to parallel the increase in interest and understanding of the physiology of exercise (9). Credit is commonly given to Christensen and Hansen (as reported by Costill 11) as the first to examine the effects of dietary manipulation on exercise performance. Previous studies, however, had demonstrated the role of carbohydrates in long-term exercise and the maintenance of muscle and liver glycogen (12, 23).

The reintroduction of the muscle biopsy technique in 1962 led to studies that examined the role of diet and exercise on muscle glycogen depletion and resynthesis. Several prominent investigators from Sweden used this technique to describe the rate of muscle glycogen use during exercise performed at different intensities and durations (11, 27). The discovery of the relationship between muscle glycogen concentration and exercise time to exhaustion led to a series of studies that examined ways to elevate muscle glycogen before exercise and to speed resynthesis following maximal effort. Based on the results of these studies performed during the 1960s, Astrand (3) proposed a 7-day dietary regimen to load the muscles with carbohydrates (classic *carbohydrate loading*). Studies performed in the 1970s, however, indicated that eating a carbohydrate-rich diet only during the final 3 days before competition was adequate to maximize muscle glycogen stores (11, 29).

The muscle biopsy technique has also been used to study the effects of muscle damage on glycogen resynthesis. It appears that the highest rate of muscle glycogen resynthesis occurs within the first 2 hours after exercise, suggesting that athletes should eat a high-carbohydrate meal soon after exhaustive exercise (11).

Fluid balance during exercise has received considerable attention over the past 40 years by a number of investigators, thanks to the commercial producers of sports drinks. Probably one of the most widely known sports drinks is Gatorade™, which was developed by a University of Florida research team to help prevent dehydration and improve performance (14). The drink was first tested on University of Florida Gator football players in 1965 and was shown to increase stamina. In 1988, the Gatorade Company created the Gatorade Sports Science Institute (GSSI) to encourage and disseminate education, service, and research in sports nutrition, as well as other aspects of exercise science. The GSSI currently serves approximately 60,000 members in more than 80 countries all over the world (15). Commercial producers of sports drinks and organizations such as the GSSI have provided research funding for studies that examine the effects of water, electrolyte, and carbohydrate balance during prolonged exercise. The results of such studies have helped to establish guidelines for fluid replacement during exercise that help to prevent fluid and electrolyte imbalances and enhance performance, determine the role of gastric emptying and intestinal absorption as potential limiting factors in maintaining fluid balance, and formulate rehydration beverages that meet the fluid, sodium, and carbohydrate needs of exercise.

The use of nutrients as ergogenic aids to improve energy production and thus athletic performance has been studied and applied for thousands of years (7). Prior to the twentieth century, efforts to enhance performance could only be made by manipulating foodstuffs. However, because of a greater understanding of exercise physiology and human metabolism, as well as technological advances, hundreds of nutrients and cellular compounds have been developed, each with specific applications for improving performance (7). Although much research has been performed to evaluate the effectiveness of these compounds and nutritional supplements, many questions remain. In the past, ergogenic aids such as blood doping, caffeine, anabolic steroids, bicarbonate, and amphetamines were widely studied (11). Ergogenic aids currently receiving attention include creatine monohydrate, chromium picolinate, DHEA (dehydroepiandrosterone), different types of amino acids and proteins including whey protein, HMB (beta-hydroxy beta methylbutyrate), ephedrine, and antioxidants.

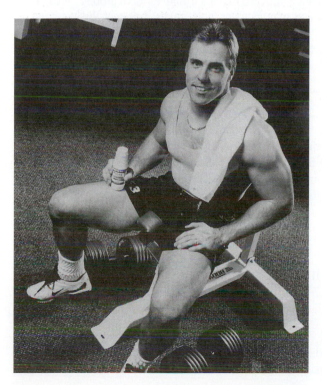

FIGURE 7.5 Many athletes consume dietary supplements to enhance performance and assure adequate nutrition. Pictured is Dennis Lane.

Photo courtesy of Experimental and Applied Sciences, Golden, CO.

FIGURE 7.6 Abstract of a research study involving creatine supplementation.

Volek, J. S., M. Boetes, J. A. Bush, M. Putukian, W. J. Sebastianelli, and W. J. Kraemer.
Response of Testosterone and Cortisol Concentrations to High-intensity Resistance Exercise Following Creatine Supplementation.
J. Strength Cond. Res., Vol. 11, No. 3, pp. 182–187, 1997.

This study investigated the influence of oral creatine monohydrate supplementation on hormone responses to high-intensity resistance exercise in 13 healthy, normally active men. Subjects were randomly assigned in double-blind fashion to either a creatine or placebo group. Both groups performed bench press and jump squat exercise protocols before (T^1) and after (T^2), ingesting either 25 g creatine monohydrate or placebo per day for 7 days. Blood samples were obtained pre- and 5 min postexercise to determine serum lactate, testosterone, and cortisol concentrations. Creatine ingestion resulted in a significant ($\rho \leq 0.05$) increase in body mass but no changes in skinfold thickness. Serum lactate concentrations were significantly higher at 5 min postexercise in both groups compared to resting values. From T^1 to T^2 there were no significant differences in postexercise lactate concentration during both exercise protocols in the placebo group, but the creatine group had significantly higher lactate concentrations after the bench press and a trend toward lower concentrations during the jump squat at T^2. There were significant increases in testosterone concentration postexercise after the jump squat, but not the bench press, for both groups; 5-min postexercise cortisol concentrations did not differ significantly from preexercise values for both groups for either protocol. Creatine supplementation may increase body mass; however, testosterone and cortisol may not mediate this initial effect.

Many significant contributions have been made to further the science of nutrition and form a firm foundation for future research. The study of nutrition will continue to evolve as new knowledge is obtained regarding the effects of nutrients on human physiology and performance and with the discovery of nutritive agents that may play a role in health and disease.

Figure 7.6 is an abstract of a research study on the effects of creatine supplementation.

Technology Used to Study Health and Exercise-Related Aspects of Nutrition

Muscle Biopsy Technique

It is well known that the availability of carbohydrates to muscles is a limiting factor for prolonged, moderately intense exercise. The use of the muscle biopsy technique has been instrumental to researchers in establishing the role of diet and exercise on muscle glycogen depletion and repletion and has led to effective applications of specific dietary techniques to enhance both high-intensity and endurance activities. The technique involves removing a very small piece of tissue from the belly of the muscle for analysis. After the area from which the biopsy is taken is deadened with a local anesthetic, a small incision is made through the skin and subcutaneous tissue with a scalpel and a hollow needle is inserted into the muscle belly. A small plunger is pushed through the center of the needle and a tissue sample is extracted. Biochemical assays may then be performed to determine the muscle's glycogen content and other factors related to substrate utilization (37).

Blood and Urine Analyses

To evaluate the effect of nutritional or pharmacological substances on exercise-induced muscle damage and performance, researchers measure markers of protein degradation such as the amino acid 3-methylhistidine, end products of lipid peroxidation such as malondialdehyde, or serum enzymes that leak from the muscle, including creatine kinase and lactate dehydrogenase (35). In addition, the influence of different supplements, diet, and exercise on metabolic hormones such as insulin, glucagon, testosterone, cortisol, and growth hormone may also be determined through blood analyses. Blood and urine analyses may also be used to examine the effects of diet and exercise intervention programs in the development, prevention, and treatment of certain metabolic diseases, such as diabetes and hyperlipidemia.

Calorimetry

To determine the energy value of food, researchers use instruments called *bomb calorimeters*. Bomb calorimeters operate on the principle of direct calorimetry, in which food is completely burned and a measurement is taken of the heat that is released. In bomb calorimetry, food is placed inside a sealed chamber filled with oxygen. An electrical current moving through a fuse at the top of the chamber ignites the food–oxygen mixture and the food literally explodes. As the food burns, the heat (energy) released is absorbed by a layer of water surrounding the bomb (see Figure 7.7). Because the calorimeter is fully insulated from the external environment, a measured increase in water temperature directly reflects the amount of heat liberated during oxidation of the food nutrient (24).

Metabolic Measurements

Direct calorimetry may also be used in humans to measure the amount of energy that the body uses at rest and during exercise. When using direct calorimetry, a person is placed inside an insulated chamber, and the heat released is calculated by measuring the increase in the temperature of a layer of water surrounding the chamber. This method is similar to the bomb calorimeter used to measure the energy value of food. A *kilocalorie* is defined as the amount of heat necessary to raise the temperature of 1 liter of water 1° Celsius. Therefore, by measuring the temperature of the water surrounding the direct calorimeter before and after the activity, the number of kilocalories used can be determined. Older direct calorimeters

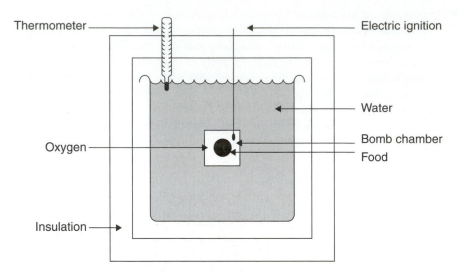

FIGURE 7.7   A bomb calorimeter.
Source: Williams, M. H., *Nutrition for Fitness and Sport,* 4th ed. Dubuque, IA: W. C. Brown Communications, Inc., 1995. Reproduced with the permission of the McGraw-Hill Companies.

were about the size of a small room and therefore were quite large. Newer calorimeters are
the size of a phone booth or the size of a space suit (34). Because of its expense and complexity, direct calorimetry is rarely used to determine energy expenditure; instead, researchers use
indirect calorimetry.

When using indirect calorimetry, a technician measures the exchange of respiratory
gases, because there is a predictable relationship between the body's use of energy and its use
of oxygen or production of carbon dioxide (CO_2). Instruments used to measure respiratory
gases (gas analyzers) are widely available and much less expensive than direct calorimeters.
These instruments can be mounted on carts (Figure 7.8) and rolled up to a hospital bed or
carried in backpacks while a person plays racquetball or rides a bicycle (34). Measurements obtained from indirect calorimetry allow for the determination of a variety of factors,
including an individual's basal metabolic rate, the amount of energy (kilocalories) used
during an activity, and the type of food (carbohydrate, fat, or protein) being used to supply
the energy.

A more recent approach to indirect calorimetry involves the use of isotopes, such as
hydrogen 2 (deuterium, or ^2H), as tracers that may be selectively followed in the body. *Isotopes* are elements with an atypical atomic weight and may be radioactive (radioisotopes)
or nonradioactive (stable isotopes). The use of isotonically (or doubly) labeled water is a
common tracer technique that is used to monitor energy expenditure. In this technique, the
subject consumes a known amount of water labeled with two isotopes ($^2H_2{}^{18}O$); thus the term
doubly labeled water. The deuterium (^2H) diffuses through the water content of the body,
while the oxygen 18 (^{18}O) diffuses through both the water and bicarbonate stores (where
much of the CO_2 from metabolism is stored). The rate at which the two isotopes leave the

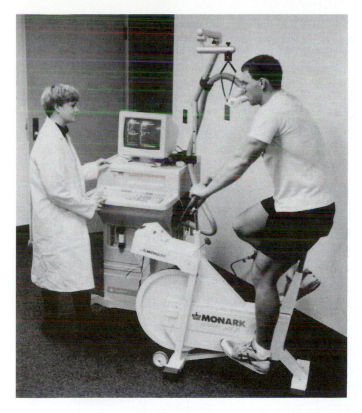

FIGURE 7.8   Metabolic measurement carts may be used to determine the metabolic rate and cost of an activity and the substrate used to supply energy.

Courtesy of the Exercise Science Department, Creighton University.

body is then measured by determining their presence in a series of blood, urine, or saliva samples. These turnover rates are then used to calculate how much CO_2 is produced, and this value is converted to energy expenditure using calorimetric equations (37).

Because isotope turnover is relatively slow, measurements of energy metabolism must be performed for several weeks. Therefore, this technique is not used for measurements of acute exercise metabolism. However, because of its accuracy and the low amount of risk involved to the subject, this technique is well suited for determining day-to-day energy expenditure. Many nutritionists consider this technique to be among one of the most significant technological advances in the field of energy metabolism this century (37).

Dietary Recall and Analysis

To determine whether an individual is meeting his or her Recommended Dietary Allowances for essential nutrients, nutritionists require individuals to keep a record of the food that they eat over several days and then use computer software programs to analyze the nutritional content of their diet. With this information, the nutritionist can determine an individual's total daily energy expenditure, discover where deficiencies or excesses are occurring, and make recommendations for changes in the individual's diet (see Figure 7.9).

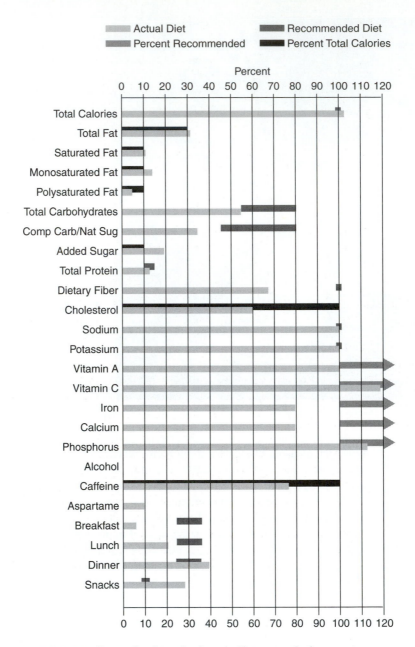

FIGURE 7.9 Example of results from a dietary analysis.
Copyright 1997, DINE Systems, Inc., Amherst, NY.

Body Composition Assessment

Assessing body composition, particularly an individual's percent body fat (% fat), is an important tool for monitoring the effects of various dietary and exercise intervention programs and for examining the distribution of fat in the body. There are many laboratory and field techniques used to estimate % fat. *Densitometry* provides a measure of body density (mass/volume) and is one of the most common laboratory techniques for assessing body composition. The mass of the body is easily determined from an accurate scale. Body volume can be obtained by several different techniques, but the most common is hydrostatic (or underwater) weighing in which the individual is weighed while totally immersed in water (Figure 7.10). The difference between the person's scale weight and underwater weight, when corrected for water density and the residual volume of the lungs, equals the body's volume. Body density is then converted to % fat using standard regression equations (37).

Other laboratory methods for assessing body composition include radiography, magnetic resonance imaging, hydrometry (for measuring total body water), photon absorptiometry, total body electrical conductivity, and dual-energy x-ray absorptiometry. Most laboratory techniques are time consuming, complex, and expensive and are therefore not well suited for mass body composition screening.

Field techniques for assessing body composition are more accessible than laboratory techniques because the equipment is less expensive, more portable, and convenient to use

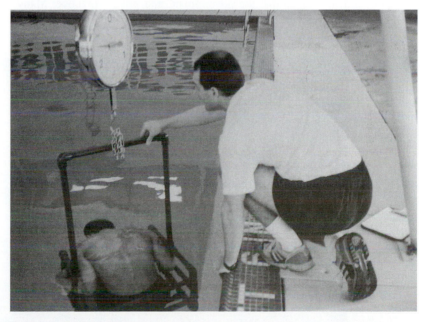

FIGURE 7.10   Underwater weighing is an accurate laboratory technique for determining body composition characteristics.
Courtesy of the Exercise Science Department, Creighton University.

for mass body composition testing. Field techniques provide reasonably accurate estimates of body composition and are based on a criterion method such as densitometry or hydrometry. The most widely applied field technique involves measuring an individual's skinfold thickness with a caliper at one or more sites on the body to obtain a sum of skinfolds (Figure 7.11). The sum of skinfolds is used, in turn, to estimate body density or % fat using regression equations. Other commonly used field techniques include bioelectrical impedance analysis, which provides an estimate of body composition from a measure of total body resistance, and near-infrared interactance (Figure 7.12) which is based on the principles of light absorption and reflection using near-infrared spectroscopy.

Academic Training and Certifications

Dietetics

Dietetics is the science of applying food and nutrition to health and disease. A dietitian is a highly qualified professional recognized as an expert on food and nutrition. A dietetic technician is trained in food and nutrition and is an integral part of health care and food service management teams. Individuals interested in dietetics can become either a registered dietitian (RD) or a dietetic technician, registered (DTR). The letters RD and DTR indicate that an individual has completed a specialized program of education and training (1). Dietetic professionals work in a variety of settings, including health care, research, fitness, food management and preparation, the government, and private practice. Many of the jobs in the field of nutrition require an RD or DTR credential (1).

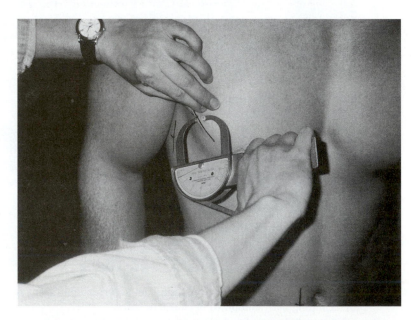

FIGURE 7.11 Body composition testing using skinfold measurements.

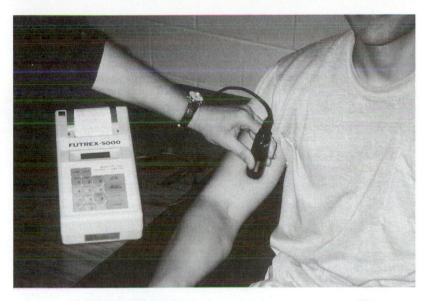

FIGURE 7.12   Body composition testing using near-infrared interactance spectrophotometry.

A registered dietitian is a legally protected professional designation. Achieving the RD credential requires at least a bachelor's degree from an accredited U.S. college or university, completion of specific coursework and a supervised practice program that has been accredited or approved by the Commission on Accreditation/Approval for Dietetics Education (CAADE) of the American Dietetic Association (ADA), and successful completion of a national credentialing examination administered in April and October of each year. The Commission on Dietetic Registration (CDR) is the credentialing agency for the ADA (1).

There are two primary avenues of academic preparation to become an RD. A Coordinated Program (CP) is a bachelor's or master's degree program that integrates classroom instruction with a minimum of 900 hours of supervised practical experience and is accredited by the CAADE. The purpose of the CAADE is to establish and enforce standards of education for the preparation of dietetics professionals and to accredit or approve those dietetics education programs that comply with the academic standards (1). Graduates of coordinated programs are eligible to take the Registration Examination for Dietitians to become certified as an RD.

A Didactic Program in Dietetics (DPD) is an academic program that has been approved by the CAADE, culminating in a minimum of a bachelor's degree. Upon graduation from a DPD, students become eligible to apply to participate in a supervised practice program by completing either a CAADE-approved preprofessional practice program (AP4) or a CAADE-accredited dietetic internship (DI). An AP4 or DI must be completed before a student can become eligible to take the registered examination to become an RD (1). By the year 2004, the AP4s will become accredited DIs to meet the supervised practice requirement. Dietetic internships provide a minimum of 900 hours of supervised practice,

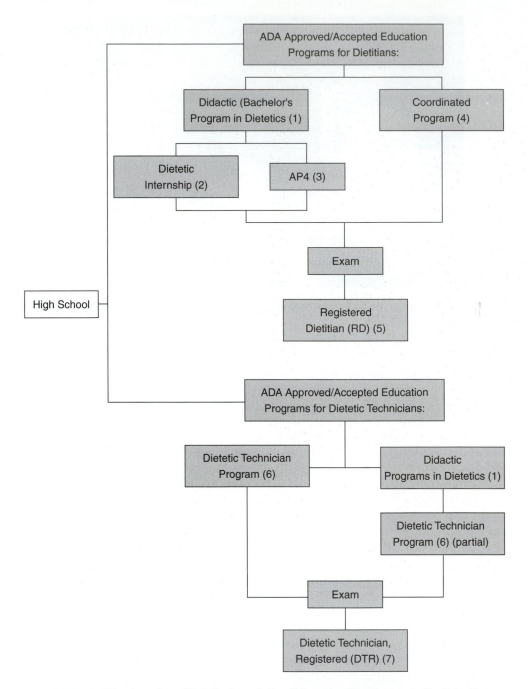

FIGURE 7.13 **The American Dietetic Association Educational pathways to Registration.**

FIGURE 7.13   Continued

Definitions:

1. *Didactic Program in Dietetics:* An academic program in a regionally accredited college or university culminating in at least a bachelors degree. The program is approved by the Council on Education Division of Education Accreditation/Approval of the American Dietetic Association to meet the minimum academic requirements for ADA membership and to apply for a supervised practice program leading to registration eligibility.

2. *Dietetic Internship:* A formalized full- or part-time postbachelor's degree educational program accredited by the Council on Education Division of Education Accreditation/Approval of the American Dietetic Association. The curriculum of the program is designed to meet the supervised practice experience requirements for registration eligibility and ADA membership. Some programs include the opportunity to complete graduate course work while enrolled in the program.

3. *AP4   Approved Preprofessional Practice Program:* A formalized full- or part-time postbachelor's degree program approved by the Council on Education Division of Education Accreditation/Approval of the American Dietetic Association. The curriculum of the program is designed to meet the supervised practice experience requirements for registration eligibility and ADA membership. Some programs include the opportunity to complete graduate course work while enrolled in the program.

4. *Coordinated Program:* A formalized bachelor's or master's degree program in dietetics accredited by the Council on Education Division of Education Accreditation/Approval of the American Dietetic Association. The curriculum is designed to coordinate academic and supervised practice experiences to meet the requirements for registration eligibility and ADA membership.

5. RD   *Registered Dietician:* A dietician who has completed the registration eligibility requirements established by the Commission on Dietetic Registration, successfully passed the Registration Examination for Dieticians, and met continuing education requirements.

6. *Dietetic Technician Program:* A two-year program in a regionally-accredited college or university combining academic and supervised practice experiences, leading to an associate degree. Dietetic Technician Programs are approved by the Council on Education Division of Education Accreditation/Approval of the American Dietetic Association. The curriculum is designed to coordinate academic and supervised practice experiences to meet the requirements for registration eligibility and ADA membership.

7. *DTR   Dietetic Technician, Registered:* A technician who has completed registration eligibility requirements established by the Commission on Dietetic Registration, successfully passed the Registration Examination for Dietetic Technicians, and met continuing education requirements.

and most appointments are awarded on a competitive basis through a computer matching process. The DI is typically completed in 6 to 24 months, depending on the availability of a part-time schedule or requirement for graduate credit, with longer internships associated with master's programs (1).

Although the two pathways sound very similar, the primary difference is that a CP is an accredited bachelor's or master's degree program that *combines* both classroom instruction and 900 hours of a supervised practice program, whereas an approved DPD requires that specific coursework and a minimum of a bachelor's degree (that is, the didactic portion) be completed first, followed by the completion of an AP4 (until the year 2004) or DI. Whether a program is approved or accredited depends on its evaluation by the CAADE. Accredited programs have been evaluated from an on-site visit by a team of professionals from the CAADE. Approved programs have been evaluated based on the submission of a program description and an educational curriculum to the CAADE (that is, approved on paper).

The Dietetic Technican Program (DTP) is a 2-year program, approved or accredited by the CAADE, that combines didactic instruction with a minimum of 450 hours of supervised practice experience and culminates in an Associate's degree. Graduates of a DTP are eligible to take the Registration Examination for Dietetic Technicians to become certified as DTR (1). In 1994, the CAADE initiated a plan that requires all DT programs to be accredited by the year 2004. Figure 7.13 shows the educational pathways to become eligible to take the registration exam for RD or DTR.

Once an individual becomes an RD or DTR, he or she must maintain registration status through participation and reporting of continuing education activities to the CDR (1). Examples of activities that meet these requirements include attending local or national meetings related to dietetics, publishing articles in peer-reviewed journals, and participating in educational workshops.

The ADA publishes a comprehensive list of colleges and universities that offer CP, DPD, DT, and accredited internship programs, which is updated annually. Visit their website for more information (www.eatright.org/caade.html). The following figure and tables provide examples of undergraduate curriculum from different schools that meet the didactic requirements set forth by the CAADE/ADA for the programs previously discussed. Figure 7.14 presents the Coordinated Program in Dietetics offered at Kansas State University by the Department of Hotel, Restaurant, Institution Management and Dietetics. Table 7.1 provides the suggested sequence of courses for meeting the requirements of the Didactic Program in Dietetics offered through the Department of Nutritional Science and Dietetics at the University of Nebraska–Lincoln. Table 7.2 includes the course requirements for the Dietetic Technician Program at the Community College of Philadelphia in Philadelphia, Pennsylvania. Keep in mind that some of these suggested sequences of courses include requirements for graduation in addition to those set forth by the CAADE/ADA.

Licensure

The ADA also encourages dietitians to pursue licensure in their state of residence. The purpose of licensure is to ensure that only qualified, trained professionals provide nutrition counseling to individuals seeking nutrition care or advice. Nonlicensed dietetics professionals who practice nutrition counseling or therapy may be subject to prosecution. States with

FIGURE 7.14   Coordinated Program in Dietetics at Kansas State University.

This program is accredited by the CAADE of the American Dietetic Association and meets academic and practice requirements that qualify graduates to take the Registration Examination for Dietitians administered by the Commission on Dietetic Registration.

Application for admission in the program should occur during the first semester of the junior year or upon completion of the general education courses required by the University. Criteria for admission are:

- An overall minimum grade-point average of 2.75 (on a 4.0 scale), with no grade lower than a C in the natural sciences and professional courses in foods, nutrition, and food service management.
- Four hundred hours of dietetic-related work experience.
- One completed recommendation form, preferably from an employer.
- Interview with the dietetics admission committee.

Criteria for progression to the senior year are a minimum grade-point average of 2.75, with no grade lower than a C in professional and supporting courses, and a recommendation of the student by faculty teaching the junior-level professional courses.

Professional Courses (55 hours)	Credit Hours
Human Nutrition	3
Science of Food	4
Nutritional Assessment	2
Public Health Nutrition	3
Nutrient Metabolism	4
Life-span Nutrition	3
Clinical Nutrition	5
Introduction to Professional Dietetic Practice	1
Principles of Food Production Management	3
Food Production Management	3
Hospitality Service Systems	3
Counseling Strategies in Dietetic Practice	3
Management in Dietetics	3
Management in Dietetics Practicum	6
Applied Clinical Dietetics	3
Clinical Dietetics Practicum	6

Source: Kansas State Undergraduate Catalog, 1996–1998.

certification laws restrict the use of titles such as dietitian or nutritionist to persons meeting specific requirements. Eligibility to take a licensing exam varies from state to state. Some states require an RD credential, while others allow individuals with a bachelor's, master's, or doctoral degree in Human Nutrition or a related field to sit for the licensing exam. As of May 1997, 40 states presently confer some form of licensure under titles such as licensed medical nutrition therapist (LMNT), certified nutritionist (CN), and licensed dietitian (LD),

TABLE 7.1   Recommended Course Sequence for the Dietetics Option at the University of Nebraska–Lincoln.

First Year

Semester 1	Credits	Semester 2	Credits
Introduction to Nutrition	3	General Biology	4
English Composition or Literature Course	3	Orientation to the Human Resources and Food Science Profession	2
Mathematics Course	3	Introduction to Dietetics	1
Introductory Psychology or Sociology Course	3–4	Introductory Political Science Course	3
Introduction to Library Research	1	Individuals and Families as Consumers	3
Clothing and Human Behavior	3	Humanities Course	3
	16–17		16

Second Year

Semester 1	Credits	Semester 2	Credits
Principles of Food Preparation	3	General Chemistry III	4
General Chemistry I	4	Introductory Anthropology Course	3
Family Science	3	Nutrition in the Life Span	3
Ethics Course	3	Computers in Restaurants/Food Service and Dietetics	3
Communications Course	3	Technical Communications I	3
		Elective	3
	16		17

Third Year

Semester 1	Credits	Semester 2	Credits
Organic Chemistry with Laboratory	4	Biochemistry	4
Quantity Food Production and Purchasing with Laboratory	4	Advanced Foods	3
Introduction to Economics	5–6	Marketing	3
History Course	3	Statistics Course	3
		Race, Ethnicity, and Gender Course	3
	16–17		15–16

Fourth Year

Semester 1	Credits	Semester 2	Credits
Advanced Nutrition	3	Clinical Nutrition	3
Applied Clinical Dietetics	3	Community Nutrition	3
Organization and Administration of Food Service	3	Senior Seminar	1
Professional Preparation for Careers in Dietetics	1	Microbiology	4
Research Experiences	1	Electives	6
Human Physiology or Comparative Anatomy and Physiology	4		
	15		17

Source: The 1996–1997 University of Nebraska–Lincoln Undergraduate Bulletin.

TABLE 7.2   Dietetic Technician Program at the Community College of Philadelphia.

First Year	Credits
Fall	
Health Field	1
Introduction to Nutrition	3
Anatomy and Physiology I	4
Food Science	4
English Composition I	3
	15
Spring	
Management Systems I	3
Supervised Experience I	1
Anatomy and Physiology II	4
Quantity Food Preparation	4
Community Health	2
English Composition II	3
	17
Summer	
Supervised Experience II	2
Nutritional Care I	3
	5

- Completion of this 10-month program (37 credits) with a 2.0 GPA qualifies individuals to sit for the certifying exam of the Certifying Board for Dietary Managers.

- Candidates for the Dietetic Technician Program must complete these courses and 29 additional credits as follows:

Second Year	Credits
Computer Assisted Management	3
Supervised Experience III	3
Supervised Experience IV	4
Dietetic Seminar	1
Personnel	3
Introduction to Psychology	3
Introduction to Sociology	3
Nutritional Care II	3
Nutritional Care III	3
Elective	3
	66 credits total

Students completing this 2-year program with a minimum 2.0 GPA receive the Associate in Applied Science degree and are eligible to take the Registration Examination for Dietetic Technicians.

Source: Dietetics Department, Community College of Philadelphia, 1997, 1700 Spring Garden Street, Philadelphia, PA 19130.

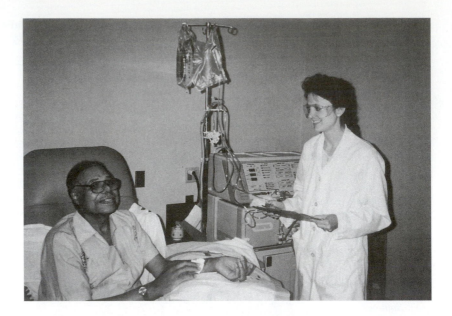

FIGURE 7.15   Clinical dietitians are important members of medical teams in hospitals, nursing homes, and other healthcare facilities.

Courtesy of the American Dietetic Association.

depending on the state in which licensure is obtained (L. Young, personal communication, November 1997). Because each state's licensure program is different, interested individuals should contact the licensure division affiliated with their State Department of Health.

Undergraduate Programs in Exercise and Sport Nutrition

Becoming a well-qualified sport nutritionist requires an extensive background in nutrition, particularly as it relates to athletic performance, experience with athletes, and the ability to effectively communicate with both coaches and athletes. Although there is currently no specific training or professional exam to take to become a certified sport nutritionist, several options exist to become qualified in the area. The best strategy depends on how many degrees a person wants to obtain. If a person is interested in obtaining a bachelor's or master's degree, he or she may want to consider becoming an RD. If a person is considering a doctoral degree in the future, a college or university with a strong human nutrition department should be selected. Science courses (such as biology, physiology, and chemistry) provide the core of the academic studies for a person interested in exercise and sport nutrition. Math, English, sociology, psychology, and business courses are also important (1). Many people combine nutrition courses with those in exercise science to broaden their educational base.

Because it is difficult to gain direct experience from every sport, it is important to read scientific literature, popular sport magazines, and newsletters to be aware of current issues in sport nutrition, better learn the specifics of the sport, understand the demands of training, and appreciate the stress of competition. Experience with physically active people and athletes may be achieved by volunteering nutrition services to high school or university sports teams, youth sports leagues, or club sports (19).

If a person is interested in searching for colleges and universities that offer degrees in nutrition and/or exercise physiology, a good place to start is the reference collection at a university library. The *College Blue Book* and *Index of Majors* are two resources commonly used to locate programs of interest at different universities. The Internet is also a good place to search for degree programs that meet an individual's personal needs. For example, the website www.collegenet.com allows one to input variables (such as cost, geographical location, and degree) that are important to a particular person and then provides a list of schools that meet these parameters. At several universities this site can be linked from the library's home page. Once the list of schools has been narrowed down, the next step is to contact the admissions office at the universities and ask the staff to send materials and a university bulletin. The following are examples of curricula associated with undergraduate and graduate programs of study in exercise and sport nutrition.

In addition to offering an ADA-approved undergraduate Didactic Program in Dietetics, the Department of Exercise and Nutritional Sciences at San Diego State University also offers a Fitness, Nutrition, and Health Specialization, which culminates in a Bachelor of Science (B. S.) degree in kinesiology (see Table 7.3).

The Nutrition and Exercise Science dual-degree program at Kansas State University is a unique program that allows an individual to receive two degrees upon graduation, a B.S. in foods and nutrition and a B.S. in kinesiology (see Table 7.4). The degrees are offered through a collaborative effort between faculty in both departments and were developed to provide depth in both nutrition and exercise science. The 145-152-credit program takes approximately 4 years to complete, but the precise length depends on the course load per semester and summer school enrollment. Students enrolled in this program also have the option of completing the necessary coursework to take the national registration exam (RD). It is important to note that this program is different from the Coordinated Program in Dietetics offered through the Department of Hotel, Restaurant, Institution Management and Dietetics at Kansas State presented in Figure 7.14.

Exercise Science majors interested in nutrition should also explore the opportunity of obtaining a minor in nutrition at their university. Some departments offer minors that generally require at least 15 credit hours, but usually no more than 19 hours. For example, at Iowa State University an individual majoring in Exercise Science may receive a minor in Food Science (15–18 hours) or Nutrition (17–18 hours). See Table 7.5. It is important to mention that entrance into a minor program in nutrition typically requires prerequisite courses in the basic sciences.

Graduate Programs in Exercise and Sport Nutrition

A large number of colleges and universities offer graduate programs in exercise science and/or nutrition. Most programs require certain prerequisites before acceptance is granted; therefore, it is important to have established some professional goals before graduating with a bachelor's degree. Admission requirements for graduate school at most universities

TABLE 7.3   Fitness, Nutrition, and Health Specialization at San Diego State University

First Year

Semester 1		*Semester 2*	
General Biology with Lab	4	Human Anatomy	4
Composition	3	Intro to. General Chem.	4
Weight Training	1	Intermediate Composition	3
Intro. to Sport and Physical Ed.	2	Activity Course	1
Introduction to Psychology	3	Introductory Sociology	3
Oral Communication	3		
	16		15

Second Year

Semester 1		*Semester 2*	
Humanities Course	3	Human Physiology	3
Introduction to Human Aging	3	Activity Course	1
Statistics Course	3	American Institution I	3
American Institution II	3	Humanities Course	3
Techniques of Athletic Training		Concepts of Health Education	3
with Laboratory	2	Nutrition for Athletes	3
Humanities Course	3		
	17		16

Third Year

Semester 1		*Semester 2*	
Growth and Development	3	Humanities Course	3
Applied Anatomy and Kinesiology	3	Electives	4
Physiology of Exercise and Lab	4	Motor Learning	3
Measurement and Evaluation	3	Leadership in Physical Education	
Biomechanics	3	and Activity	3
		Mechanisms of Sport Injury	3
		Eating Disorders and Weight Control	2
	16		18

Fourth Year

Semester 1		*Semester 2*	
Nutrition for Health/Fitness	3	Sociology Course	3
History/Philosophy of Phys. Ed.	3	Electives	6
Corrective and Orthopedic Phys. Ed.	3	Adapted Phys. Ed. Lab	1
Exercise, Fitness, and Health		Musculoskeletal Fitness and Activity	2
with Lab	3	Leading Group Aerobic Exercise	1
Exercise, Sport, and Aging	3	Administration of Fitness Programs	2
	15		15

Source: 1996 Undergraduate Bulletin at San Diego State University.

TABLE 7.4   Nutrition and Exercise Sciences Course Sequence at Kansas State University

First Year

Semester 1		*Semester 2*	
Dynamics of Sports and Exercise	3	Principles of Biology	4
Principles of Physical Fitness	1	Chemistry II	3
Expository Writing	3	Public Speaking	2
Chemistry I	4	Introduction to Sociology	3
College Algebra	3	Intro. to Personal Computers	3
General Psychology	3		
	17		16

Second Year

Semester 1		*Semester 2*	
Human Nutrition	3	Dimensions of Eating	3
Measurement and Research Techniques	3	Physiology of Exercise	3
Human Body	6	Contemporary Physical Act.	3
Expository Writing	3	Introductory Organic and Biochemistry	5
		Anthropology Course	3
	15		17

Third Year

Semester 1		*Semester 2*	
Personal Health	3	Nutrition Assessment	2
Science of Food	4	Biomechanics	3
Public Health Nutrition	3	Behavioral Course	3
Psychological Dynamics of		Elementary Statistics for the Social Sciences	3
Physical Activity	3	Principles of Macroeconomics	3
Descriptive Physics	4		
	17		14

During the summer of the first, second, and third year, 11 to 12 hours of Humanities Courses must be taken.

Fourth Year

Semester 1		*Semester 2*	
Nutrient Metabolism	4	Clinical Nutrition	4
Life-span Nutrition	3	Fitness Promotion	3
Exercise Testing and Prescription	3	Biological Course	3
Public Health and Safety	3	Expository Writing	3
Nutrition and Exercise	3	Elective Course in Hotel, Rest., Inst.	
		Mngt. and Diet	3
	16		16

Summer

Practicum (90–120 hours)	3		

Source: Survival Guide: Nutrition and Exercise Sciences, Kansas State University, Fall 1996.

TABLE 7.5   Minors in Nutrition Offered at Iowa State University

Food Science (15–18 credits)

Food and the Consumer *or*
  Food Processing   3
Introduction to Human Nutrition *or*
  Human Nutrition and Metabolism   3

Select two courses (6 credits) from:
    Scientific Study of Food
    Food Chemistry
    Food Analysis
    Experimental Study of Food
    Food Microbiology
    Food Microbiology Laboratory

Select additional 300- 400-level Food Science–Human Nutrition courses to total 15 to 18 credits for the Minor.

Nutrition (17–18 credits)

Scientific Study of Food   3
Nutrition in Growth and Development   3
Human Nutrition and Metabolism   3

Select two courses from:
    Foodborne Hazards   3
    Nutrition in Disease   3
    Community Nutrition   3
    Nutrition Education Methods   3

Source: Iowa State University 1995–1997 Catalog.

require an earned bachelor's degree in a related discipline, a grade-point average of 3.0 or higher, and satisfactory Graduate Record Examination (GRE) scores. The graduate school selected should offer a program that meets the individual's career goals. For example, if a person is interested in becoming an RD, it is important to find a university that offers a Co-ordinated Master's Program in dietetics that has been approved by the ADA. The curriculum for a master's or doctoral degree in nutrition generally has a strong foundation in biological sciences, chemistry, clinical nutrition, nutrition education, and nutrition research. However, if a person is interested in exercise and nutrition or sport nutrition, then a program that combines aspects of both disciplines is more appropriate. Universities offering these types of graduate programs are often interdisciplinary programs, that is, they are offered through a collaborative effort between the Department of Nutrition or Food Science and the Department of Kinesiology, Physical Education, or Exercise Science. The Master of Science degree (M.S.) in exercise and sport nutrition at Texas Woman's University and the M.S. in exercise and nutrition at Colorado State University are examples of such programs. Other departments combine the two disciplines, such as the Department of

Nutrition, Food, and Movement Sciences at Florida State University, which offers an M.S. in sport nutrition. Depending on the university, however, the degree may only be offered through one of the two disciplines. The Department of Nutrition and Food Science at Auburn University, for example, offers a M.S. in nutrition and food science with an emphasis in sports nutrition. Therefore, when searching for a graduate school, it may be important to inquire about the programs offered in each discipline and its related department. The University of New Mexico is unique in that it offers a dual master's degree in which an individual obtains an M.S. in nutrition and a M.S. in exercise physiology. Whereas most M.S. programs require anywhere from 30 to 45 credit hours, this program requires 52 hours of coursework.

Relatively few programs specifically offer a doctoral degree in exercise nutrition. Typically, a degree is obtained in either exercise physiology or nutrition. However, most doctoral programs allow a person to tailor a program through elective courses and thus meet his or her professional goals. Admission requirements generally require an earned M.S. degree with the completion of a thesis (that is, major research project). Therefore, after acceptance into a M.S. degree program that offers both a thesis and nonthesis option, a person considering pursuing a doctorate at some point in the future should complete the thesis option. A thesis is often required as a prerequisite for programs that culminate in a Doctor of Philosophy (Ph.D.) degree, because the focus of these programs is to prepare students to perform research, analyze data, and competently evaluate research conducted by their peers. Doctoral programs in both exercise physiology and nutrition typically require 40+ credit hours beyond a master's degree.

A person who does not possess a desire to attend graduate school, but would like to be more marketable following graduation, may wish to consider becoming a licensed nutrition therapist (described on page 180) or become certified through organizations such as the American College of Sports Medicine or the National Strength and Conditioning Association (See Chapter 6).

Employment Opportunities

Dietetics

According to the United States Bureau of Labor Statistics, employment for dietitians is expected to grow faster than the average profession through the year 2000, particularly in the areas of community, business, and consulting (1). The job market for dietetic technicians is also expected to grow at a rapid pace over the next several years. Dietetic professionals work in a variety of settings, including clinical health care, education, research, food management, fitness, and private practice.

Clinical dietitians have important roles as members of the medical team in hospitals, nursing homes, health maintenance organizations (HMOs), and other health care facilities. They work with doctors, nurses, and therapists to speed recovery following illness or injury and set goals for long-term health. Community dietitians are primarily employed in public and home health agencies, day-care centers, health and recreation clubs, and government-funded programs that feed and counsel families, the elderly, pregnant women, children, and disabled or underprivileged individuals (1).

Dietitians involved in the business world work in food- and nutrition-related industries. Their primary responsibilities include product development, sales, marketing, advertising, public relations, and purchasing. Management dietitians play a key role wherever food is served and mainly work in health care institutions, schools, cafeterias, and restaurants, where they are responsible for such things as personnel management, menu planning, budgeting, and purchasing (1).

Consultant dietitians may work full- or part-time in their own private practice or under contract within a health care facility. Consultant dietitians in private practice typically perform nutrition screening and counseling for their own clients and those referred to them by a physician. They offer advice on weight loss, cholesterol reduction, and a variety of other diet-related concerns (1).

Dietitians who are educators work in colleges, universities, and community or technical schools and teach future doctors, nurses, exercise physiologists, dietitians, and dietetic technicians the complex science of foods and nutrition. Research dietitians work in major universities and medical centers, government agencies, and food and pharmaceutical companies and conduct investigations to answer critical nutrition questions and find alternative foods or dietary recommendations for the public (1).

According to the ADA's 1995 membership database, of those registered dietitians who have been employed full time in dietetics for 1 to 5 years after registration, 63% report annual incomes between $25,000 and $35,000, and 24% report incomes between $35,000 and $45,000. Salary levels may vary with the geographical location, scope of responsibility, and supply of applicants (1).

A dietetic technician works independently or in partnership with an RD in many of the same settings described above. In clinical settings, technicians assist in the development,

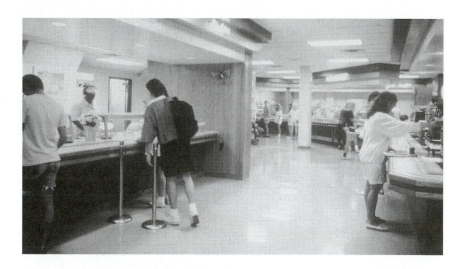

FIGURE 7.16 Management dietitians play important roles in food service.
Courtesy of Creighton University Public Relations.

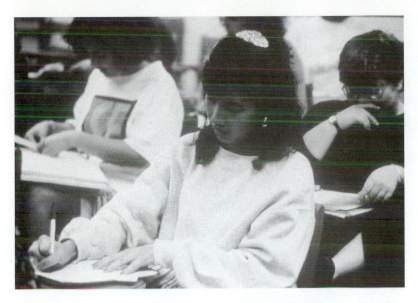

FIGURE 7.17   Educator dietitians teach nutrition-related courses in colleges and universities.
Courtesy Creighton University Public Relations.

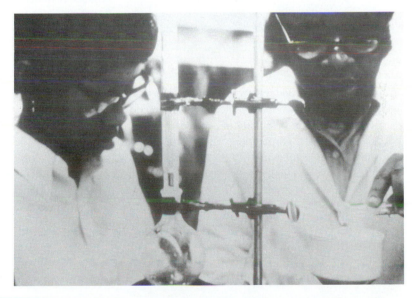

FIGURE 7.18   Research dietitians conduct studies to answer important nutrition questions and provide dietary recommendations for the public.
Courtesy of the American Dietetic Association.

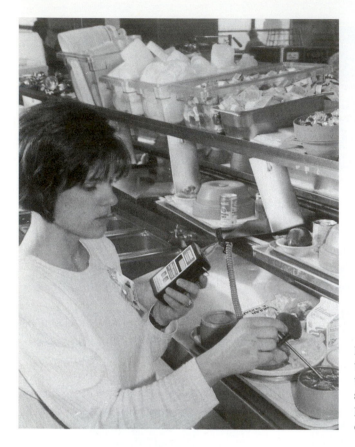

FIGURE 7.19   One of the responsibilities of a dietetic technician is to monitor the quality of food and food service in schools, restaurants, hospitals, and corporations.

Courtesy of the American Dietetic Association.

implementation, and review of nutrition care plans, and assess clients' nutritional statuses. As part of food service management teams, dietetic technicians help to supervise food production and monitor the quality of food service in schools, day-care centers, correctional facilities, restaurants, corporations, nursing homes, and hospitals. Dietetic technicians who are interested in health and wellness teach nutrition classes at health clubs, weight-management clinics, and community wellness centers (1).

The salary levels for DTRs vary with geographical location and the range of responsibilities for the position. Twenty-three percent of DTRs report annual incomes of less than $20,000, 62% report incomes between $20,000 and $30,000, and 12% report incomes between $30,000 and $40,000 (1).

Exercise and Sport Nutrition

Exercise nutrition, as an independent discipline, is still in the formative stage. It is practiced in many different settings by individuals with a wide variety of educational backgrounds and a subspecialization in nutrition. Thus, there is no definitive job description

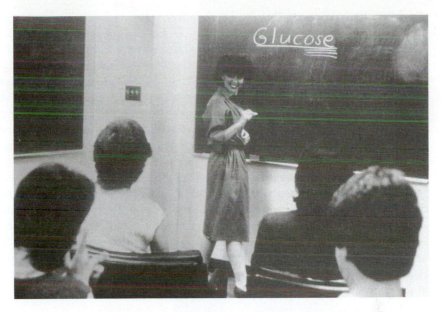

FIGURE 7.20   Teaching and performing research at a college or university typically requires a minimum of a master's degree.
Courtesy of the American Dietetic Association.

for an exercise nutritionist, nor is there a code of ethics (17). Primary employment is usually teaching and/or performing research at a college or university, acting as sport nutritionist for athletic teams, consulting within a private practice, working in cardiac rehabilitation in a hospital, or working in a corporate wellness or fitness center or health club.

Teaching and Research.   A teaching position within a college or university typically requires at least a master's degree; however, a terminal degree such as a doctorate is often preferred, especially at large institutions. Certification as an RD may or may not be a requirement depending on the department in which you are employed. For example, teaching a nutrition course as a faculty member in a Department of Exercise Science or Department of Kinesiology does not necessarily require certification. It does, however, require a strong background in nutrition principles as they relate to health and human performance. In contrast, certification may be a requirement for individuals teaching courses in a Department of Food Science or Department of Dietetics, which offers curricula approved by the CAADE of the ADA and prepares students to take the exam to become an RD.

In addition to teaching and advising students, full-time faculty members at colleges and universities are expected to be active in research and/or other scholarly activity and perform university and community service. Appointments typically range from 9 to 12 months, and salary is often commensurate with experience, ranging anywhere from $25,000 to $42,000.

Exercise and Sport Nutrition Specialists.   Only recently have athletic departments in colleges and universities begun to realize the value of the sport nutrition professional in providing both clinical nutrition services to athletes and nutrition education programs to teams, coaches, and trainers. Most positions for sport nutritionists at colleges and universities are part-time positions or may be part of the job description of the head strength coach. However, some large, NCAA Division I universities, which have several athletic programs and are self-supportive with large operating budgets, have full-time sport nutritionists. For example, the University of Nebraska–Lincoln and Pennsylvania State University each have a full-time sports nutritionist who is responsible for such things as training, meal planning, and nutrition education.

Full-time sport nutritionists typically work long hours, 6 days out of the week for 12 months. With the possible exception of the summer months, it is not uncommon for a sport nutritionist to work a minimum of 12 hrs per day. Although at any given time during an academic year at least one sport is in season, the responsibilities of the sport nutritionist may vary, depending on whether a team is in-season or off-season. During the off-season, athletes generally participate in intensive training to elicit desirable changes in body composition and engage in activities that enhance strength, speed, and power. The sport nutritionist's roles include monitoring the athletes' exercise programs, diets, and life-styles to ensure that the

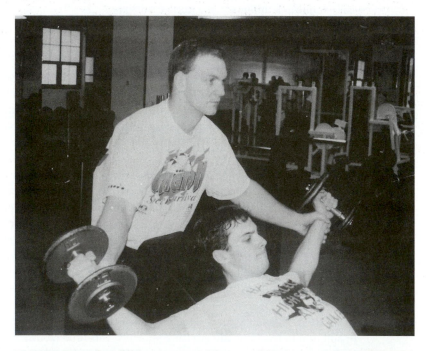

FIGURE 7.21   In addition to supervising an athlete's strength training program, many head strength coaches at colleges and universities must also provide nutrition counseling.
Pictured is Charlie Oborny, head strength coach at Creighton University.

athletes reach their off-season performance goals. It is at this time that education is stressed and goals and objectives from a dietary standpoint, including fueling tactics, are made. Body composition testing, as well as analyses of the athletes' diets, may be performed to determine where nutrient deficiencies or excesses are occurring. Workshops and/or presentations on eating disorders, proper weight gain, or weight loss are examples of educational programs provided by the sport nutritionist. During the summer months, when athletes are no longer dining at the training table, it is not uncommon for the sport nutritionist to take an athlete to the supermarket to teach him or her how to shop nutritiously or to provide counseling regarding food preparation and proper food storage.

During the in-season, the primary goal of the athlete is to maintain any changes that he or she made during the off-season with regard to performance, eating behaviors, and body composition. Sport nutritionists work closely with personnel from the campus dining facilities, both in- and off-season, to review and plan menus for the training table and to determine whether dining hours can be expanded to meet the athletes' busy schedules. To ensure that athletes eat healthily on road trips and have foods available that are familiar to them, the sport nutritionist often contacts the hotels where the athletes will be staying and dining halls and restaurants at which the team will be stopping to request in advance that meals be prepared a certain way and that foods high in carbohydrates and protein be served.

The minimum amount of education needed for employment as a sport nutritionist at a major university is a bachelor's degree in dietetics or a related discipline. Becoming certified as an RD, DTR, or obtaining licensure may also improve marketability. Because the sport nutritionist works closely with coaches, trainers, and athletes, it is important that they have strong oral and written communication skills. Sport nutritionists who are not certified often consult with a registered dietitian at the university when reviewing menus, planning meals, and preparing educational programs. Experience with athletes is also valuable. Many undergraduate students gain experience volunteering nutrition services to high school or university sport teams, a local running club, Little Leagues, or sports clubs. With an advanced degree, such as a master's or doctorate, experience with athletes can be gained through research. Although many universities cannot afford a full-time sport nutritionist, those finding a position could expect a starting salary ranging from $30,000 to $35,000, which is roughly equivalent to an assistant athletic trainer's salary (D. Ellis, personal communication, October 1996).

Nutrition Consultants.   Because many university, amateur, and professional athletic teams do not employ a full-time nutritionist, many hire an individual on a part-time basis or as a consultant. Professional teams such as the New England Patriots, Boston Bruins, New York Giants, New York Nets, and the Minnesota Vikings each employ a nutritionist on a part-time basis. Although the nutritionists employed by these teams have similar responsibilities, the job description for these individuals varies with the team's goals and needs during particular times of the season. For example, the nutritionist for the Patriots comes in 1 day per week for 6 to 8 hours during the off- season to provide educational programs on topics such as ergogenic aids, protein, fat, and meal planning for the athletes as part of their training regimen. Players are encouraged to ask questions, and the nutritionist often works one-on-one with the athletes, performing dietary recall and analysis, counseling them on proper weight-gain and weight-loss techniques, accompanying athletes to the supermarket to teach them how to shop and read labels, and providing cooking demonstrations and sample menus that are nutritious and low in fat.

At training camp, the nutritionist works with the food service facilities at the local college where the Patriots practice to review and design menus that provide plenty of carbohydrates, lean proteins, and foods low in fat. Millions of dollars are spent by the Patriots on food, so it is important to the management that the members of the team eat at the training table, rather than run to a fast-food restaurant after practice. To make sure that players do, in fact, take advantage of the training table, a wide variety of foods is available, including regional favorites, because players come from all parts of the country. During the in-season, the nutritionist works with the caterers who provide lunches at the stadium during practice to make sure that training table food is served. The nutritionist also works with airlines and hotels to provide a training table menu and proper pregame meals to the players when they travel (J. Bouchbinder, personal communication, October 1996).

Most of the consultants who work with these teams are registered dietitians who charge anywhere from $50 to $150 per hour for their services. In addition to working with their respective teams, many also work with individuals as private consultants; lecture at area high schools, universities, and business corporations; and provide nutrition counseling at cardiac rehabilitation facilities.

Cardiac Rehabilitation.   The primary responsibility of an exercise specialist working in a cardiac rehabilitation facility is to supervise Phase II and Phase III exercise programs. However, additional responsibilities may include educating patients about the synergistic effect of exercise and nutrition as it relates to primary and secondary prevention of cardiovascular disease. Therefore, a strong background in exercise nutrition is essential. Activities conducted may include developing individualized exercise prescriptions, one-on-one nutrition counseling, lipid management, cooking demonstrations using low-fat and low-sodium foods, recipe modification, and teaching patient education classes. Patient education topics include risk factor modification, weight management, and home exercise programs. Depending on the facility, research may be part of the job description, particularly as it relates to current exercise and eating habits, behavioral changes, and prevention of chronic disease. Although some cardiac rehabilitation facilities with large operating budgets hire a registered dietitian to provide clinical nutritional counseling and education, many must rely on the knowledge base of the exercise specialist. Therefore, certification as an RD may not be necessary. Salary depends on credentials earned, whether the position is full or part time, and geographical location. Salary for entry-level positions typically ranges from $26,000 to the low $30,000s and increases with experience. A registered dietitian who is a clinical nutrition manager or director of a cardiovascular disease prevention program typically earns a salary between $45,000 to $50,000 (M. Watson, personal communication, October 1996).

Corporate Fitness and Health Clubs.   Employment in a corporate or community fitness or wellness facility or commercial health club typically requires a bachelor's degree in exercise science with a strong emphasis in nutrition. Job responsibilities include personal training, teaching exercise classes, health promotion, nutrition education, fitness testing, and health screening for the risk of developing CHD. In addition to nutrition education,

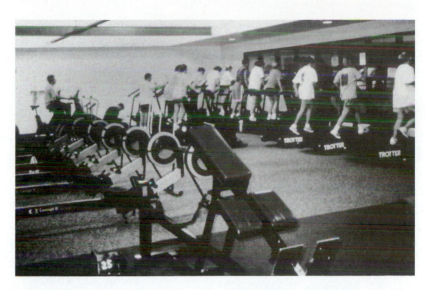

FIGURE 7.22 **Personal training and nutritional counseling are typical job responsibilities for individuals employed at corporate or community fitness facilities and health clubs.**
Courtesy of the Exercise Science Department at Creighton University.

professionals in the corporate fitness setting may assist in the planning and implementation of meals served in the company cafeteria. Entry-level, full-time salaries typically range from $18,000 to $25,000 depending on the geographical location (J. Leutzinger, personal communication, October 1996). Certifications through the American College of Sports Medicine (health fitness instructor), National Strength and Conditioning Association (certified personal trainer; certified strength and conditioning specialist), or the ADA (RD, DTR) may increase marketability and result in a higher starting salary.

Professional Journals and Related Resources

Prominent Journals in Nutrition and Exercise Nutrition

American Journal of Clinical Nutrition
Food Technology
International Journal of Obesity
International Journal of Sports Nutrition
Journal of Clinical Nutrition
Journal of Food Science
Journal of Nutrition
Journal of Nutrition Education

Journal of Strength and Conditioning Research
Journal of the American College of Nutrition
Journal of the American Dietetic Association
Journal of the American Medical Association
Medicine and Science in Sports and Exercise
Nutrition and Metabolism
Nutrition Reviews

Prominent Newsletters

Contemporary Nutrition
General Mills, Inc.
P.O. Box 1112, Dept. 65
Minneapolis, MN 55440

Diary Council Digest
National Dairy Council
6300 N. River Rd.
Rosemont, IL 60018-4233

Food and Nutrition News
National Livestock and
   Meat Board
444 N. Michigan Ave.
Chicago, IL 60611

Harvard Medical School
   Health Letter
Dept. of Continuing Education
25 Shattuck St.
Boston, MA 02115

Sports Science Exchange
Gatorade Sports Science institute
P.O. Box 049005
Chicago, IL 60604

Tufts University Diet and
   Nutrition Letter
P.O. Box 10948
Des Mones, IA 50940

University of California at Berkeley
   Wellness Letter
Wellness Letter Subscription Dept.
P.O. Box 420148
Palm Coast, FL 32142

United States Government Agencies

Center for Nutrition Policy and Promotion
1120 20th St. NW
North Lobby, Suite 200
Washington, DC 20036
(202) 418-2417

Consumer Information Center
P.O. Box 100
Pueblo, CO 81002
(719) 948-3334

Food and Drug Administration
Office of Consumer Affairs
Dept. of Health and Human Services
5600 Fishers Ln. (HFE-88)
Room 1685
Rockville, MD 20857
(301) 443-3170

Food and Nutrition Information Center
National Agricultural Library/USDA
10301 Baltimore Blvd.
Room 304
Beltsville, MD 20705
(301) 504-5719

Human Nutrition Information Service
Department of Agriculture
6505 Belcrest Road
Room 328A
Hyattsville, MD 20782

Office of Disease Prevention & Health
   Promotion
330 C St. SW
Room 2132
Suitzer Bldg.
Washington, DC 20201
(202) 205-8611

Professional and Service Organizations

American College of Sports
   Medicine
P.O. Box 1440
Indianapolis, IN 46206-1440

American Heart Association,
   National Center
7272 Greenville Ave.
Dallas, TX 75231
(214) 373-6300
1-800-242-8721

American Institute of Nutrition
9650 Rockville Pike
Bethesda, MD 20814
(301) 530-7050

Gatorade Sports Science Institute
617 W. Main St.
Barrington, IL 60010
1-800-616-4774

International Center for
   Sports Nutrition
502 South 44th St.
Suite 3012
Omaha, NE 68105
(402) 559-5505

National Center for Nutrition
   and Dietetics
The American Dietetic Association
216 W. Jackson Blvd., Suite 800
Chicago, IL 60606
(312) 899-0040
Consumer Hotline:1-800-366-1655 for referral to a local RD; 1-900-225-5267 for
   customized answers to food and nutrition questions from an RD

National Dairy Council
Dairy Center
6300 North River Road
Rosemont, IL 60018-4233
(708) 696-1033

National Strength and
   Conditioning Association
P.O. Box 38909
Colorado Springs, CO 80937
(719) 632-6722

Sports and Cardiovascular Nutritionists
   (SCAN)
A Practice Group of the American Dietetic
   Association
216 W. Jackson Blvd., Suite 800
Chicago, IL 60606-6995

Sources of Nutrition Information on the Internet

American Dietetic Association   http://www.eatright.org/
American Institute of Nutrition   http://www.faseb.org/asns
American Society for Nutrition Science   http://www.nutrition.org/nutrition
Arbor Nutrition Guide   http://www.arborcom.com
Institute of Food Technologists   http://www.ift.org

Summary

Exercise and sport nutrition is an area of study that integrates the principles of nutrition and physical activity as they relate to performance or the prevention of disease. Exercise and sport nutritionists spend a great deal of time studying the effects of carbohydrate, protein, fat, vitamins, minerals, water, electrolytes and ergogenic aids on performance. They also study the effects of diet on such health-related issues as coronary heart disease and obesity. A number of employment opportunities are available for the exercise and sport nutritionist. These include: teaching and research positions in colleges and universities as well as specialist or consultant positions for colleges, universities, amateur and professional teams, corporate fitness facilities and community health clubs. Because of the recent growing interest in nutritional agents to enhance general health as well as supplements to enhance athletic performance, the area of exercise and sport nutrition is a rapidly expanding subdiscipline of exercise science.

STUDY QUESTIONS

1. Nutrition was recognized as an independent discipline in 1933 with the founding of the:
   a. American College of Sports Nutrition.
   b. American Dietetic Association.
   c. American Institute of Nutrition.
   d. Harvard Fatigue Laboratory.
   e. Nutrition Laboratory at the Carnegie Institute.

2. Ancel Keys conducted a classic comprehensive study to evaluate the physiological effects of starvation and recovery from starvation known as the:
   a. CVD Study.
   b. Minnesota Starvation Study.
   c. Framingham Heart Study.
   d. Harvard Alumni Study.
   e. Multiple Risk Factor Intervention Trial.

3. The leading cause of death in the United States is:
   a. Obesity.
   b. High blood pressure.
   c. Accidents.
   d. Coronary heart disease.
   e. Diabetes.

4. Describe three research tools used to study health- and exercise-related aspects of nutrition and explain what types of studies could be performed using each technology.

5. Describe the two primary avenues of academic preparation to become a registered dietitian.

6. Explain the differences between dietetics, food science, and exercise nutrition and describe what types of jobs are available in each discipline.

7. Determine your professional goals for a career in exercise nutrition and develop a course of study designed to meet these goals [that is, desired degree(s), courses needed, certifications, and the like].

GLOSSARY

Antioxidants Naturally occurring or synthetic substances that help protect cells from the damaging effects of oxygen free radicals, highly reactive compounds created during normal cell metabolism.

Basal metabolic rate (BMR) The minimal amount of energy required for maintenance of life. The BMR is typically measured under strict laboratory conditions: 12 hr after eating, after a restful sleep, no exercise or activity preceding the test, elimination of emotional excitement, and in a comfortable temperature.

Bomb calorimeter Instrument used to determine the energy value of foods and nutrients.

Calorimetry The determination of heat loss or gain. A calorimeter is used to measure the amount of heat exchanged in a chemical reaction or by the body under certain conditions.

Carbohydrate loading A dietary method used by endurance athletes to increase the carbohydrate (glycogen) stores in the muscles and liver.

Cholesterol A sterol synthesized in the liver, widely distributed in animal tissues, occurring in bile, gallstones, the nerve tissue of the brain and spinal cord, blood cells, egg yolks, and oils. In most individuals, elevated levels of blood cholesterol result in an increased risk for developing coronary heart disease (CHD).

Chronic disease A disease of slow progression such as coronary heart disease, hypertension, and osteoporosis.

Coronary heart disease Narrowing of the coronary arteries, usually caused by atherosclerosis (the build-up of fatty plaques on the artery walls), that prevents adequate blood and oxygen supply to the heart.

Densitometry The determination of the density (mass/volume) of the body. Body mass may be measured using an accurate physician's scale, while body volume is commonly measured using the hydrostatic (underwater) weighing technique.

Dietetics The science of applying food and nutrition to health and disease.

Epidemiology The study of the occurrence and prevalence of disease among the population.

Ergogenic aids Agents used in an attempt to enhance athletic or physical performance.

Exercise nutrition The application of nutrition and physical activity to enhance athletic performance or prevent the development of chronic disease.

Food science Science which applies principles of the biological and physical sciences to study the nature of foods, the causes of food deterioration, and the principles underlying the processing and preparation of food.

Glycogen The storage form of carbohydrate found in the liver and in the muscles.

Hyperlipidemia An elevated level of lipids (fats) in the blood.

Kilocalories The amount of heat necessary to raise the temperature of 1 liter of water 1 degree celsius. The value of the energy of food; also known as "Calorie."

Metabolism The sum total of all physical and chemical changes that occur in the body. Metabolism involves two processes: anabolism (the building-up or synthesizing processes) and catabolism (the tearing-down or degrading processes).

Nutrition The science of food usually described as the sum total of the processes involved in the intake and utilization of food substances by living organisms, including ingestion, digestion, absorption, and metabolism of food.

Osteoporosis A disease process that results in a reduction of bone density and interferes with the mechanical support function of bone.

Recommended Dietary Allowances (RDA) The Recommended Dietary Allowances are established by the Food and Nutrition Board and represent the levels of intake of essential nutrients considered to be adequate to meet the known nutritional needs of practically all healthy people of similar age and gender.

SUGGESTED READINGS

Shils, M., et al. (Eds.). *Modern Nutrition in Health and Disease.* Philadelphia: Lea and Febiger, 1994.

Simopoulous, A., and K. Pavlou (Eds.). *Nutrition and Fitness for Athletes.* Basel, Switzerland: Karger, 1993.

Snyder, A. *Exercise, Nutrition, and Health.* Carmel, IN: Cooper Publishing Group, 1997.

Wolinsky, I., and J. Hickson (Eds.). *Nutrition in Exercise and Sport.* Boca Raton, FL: CRC Press, 1994.

Ziegler, E. E., and L. J. Filer, Jr. (Eds.). *Present Knowledge in Nutrition,* 7th ed. Washington, DC: ILSI Press, 1996.

REFERENCES

1. American Dietetics Association Home Page, http://www.eatright.org/

2. American Heart Association: Fact Sheet on Heart Attack, Stroke and Risk Factors. Dallas, TX, 1996.

3. Astrand, P. O. Diet and athletic performance. *Fed. Proc.* 26:1772–1777, 1967.

4. Blair, S. N., E. Horton, A. S. Leon, I.-M. Lee, B. L. Drinkwater, R. K. Dishman, M. Mackey, and M. L. Kienholz. Physical activity, nutrition, and chronic disease. *Med. Sci. Sports Exerc.* 28:335–349, 1996.

5. Bounous, G., G. Batist, and P. Gold. Whey proteins in cancer prevention. *Cancer Letters* 57:91–94, 1991.

6. Brooks, S., and P. Kearns. Enteral and parental nutrition. In: *Present Knowledge in Nutrition,* 7th ed., E. E. Ziegler and L. J. Filer, Jr. (Eds.). Washington, DC, ILSI Press, 1996, p. 530.

7. Bucci, L. R. *Nutrients as Ergogenic Aids for Sports and Exercise.* Boca Raton, FL: CRC Press, 1993.

8. Bucci, L. R. *Nutrition Applied to Injury Rehabilitation and Sports Medicine.* Boca Raton, FL: CRC Press, 1995.

9. Burke, L. M., and R. S. D. Read. Sports nutrition: Approaching the nineties. *Sports Med* 8:80–100, 1989.

10. Buskirk, E. R. *From Harvard to Minnesota: Keys to our history. In: Exercise and Sports Science Reviews,* Vol. 20, J. O. Holloszy (Ed.), 1992, pp. 1–26.

11. Costill, D. L. Applied exercise physiology. In: *American College of Sports Medicine—40th Anniversary Lectures.* Indianapolis, IN: American College of Sports Medicine, 1994, pp. 69–79.

12. Courtice, F. C., and C. G. Douglas. The effect of prolonged muscular exercise on the metabolism. *Pro. Roy. Soc., London* 119:381–383, 1935.

13. Gardner, G. W., et al. Cardiorespiratory hematological, and physical performance responses of anemic subjects to iron treatment. *Am. J. Clin. Nutr.* 28:982, 1975.

14. Gatorade Home Page: The Cooler Site, http://www.gator.com/

15. Gatorade Sports Science Institute Home Page, http:/;/www.gssiweb.com/.

16. Gledhill, N. The influence of altered blood volume and oxygen transport capacity on aerobic performance. In: *Exercise and Sports Science Reviews,* Vol. 13, R. L. Terjung (Ed.), 1985, pp. 75–93.

17. Grandjean, A. C. Practices and recommendations of sports nutritionists. *Intl. J. Sports Nutr.* 3:232–242, 1993.

18. Hegsted, D. M. Nutrition: The changing scene. *Nutr. Rev.* 43:357–367, 1985.

19. International Center for Sports Nutrition, Fact Sheet on the Field of Sports Nutrition, Omaha, NE.

20. Kannel, W. B., P. Sorlie, and P. McNamara. The relation of physical activity to risk of coronary heart disease: The Framingham Study. *Coronary Heart Disease and Physical Fitness.* O. A. Larson and R. O. Malmborg (Eds.), Baltimore, MD: University Park Press, 1971, p. 256.

21. Kanter, M. Free radicals and exercise: Effects of nutritional anti-oxidant supplementation. In: *Exercise and Sports Science Reviews,* Vol. 23, J. O. Holloszy (Ed.), 1995, pp. 375–397.

22. Keys, A., J. Brozek, A. Henschel, O. Mickelsen, and H. Taylor. *The Biology of Human Starvation,* Vols. I and II. Minneapolis: University of Minnesota Press, 1950.

23. Krogh, A., and J. Lindhard. The relative value of fats and carbohydrates as sources of muscular energy. *Biochem. J.* 14:290–294, 1919.

24. McCardle, W. D., F. I. Katch, and V. L. Katch. *Exercise Physiology: Energy, Nutrition, and Human Performance,* 4th ed. Baltimore, MD: Williams & Wilkins, 1996.

25. Nilson, K., R. B. Schoene, H. T. Robertson, P. Escourrou, and N.J. Smith. The effect of iron repletion on exercise-induced lactate production in minimally iron-deficient subjects. *Med. Sci. Sports Exerc.* 13:92, 1981.

26. Paffenbarger, R. S., A. L. Wing, and R. T. Hyde. Physical activity as an index of heart attack risk in college alumni. *Am. J. Epidemiol.* 108:161–175, 1978.

27. Ryan, A. J. Medical approach to care of the injured athlete. In: *American College of Sports Medicine—40th Anniversary Lectures.* Indianapolis, IN: American College of Sports Medicine, 1994, pp. 55–67.

28. Sadler, R. The benefits of dietary whey protein concentrate on the immune response and health. *S. Afr. J. Dairy Sci.* 24:53–58, 1992.

29. Sherman, W. M., et al. Effects of exercise-diet manipulation on muscle glycogen and its subsequent utilization during performance. *Intl. J. Sports Med.* 2:1–15, 1981.

30. *Stedman's Concise Medical Dictionary for the Health Professions,* 3rd ed., J. H. Dirckx, (Ed.). Baltimore, MD: Williams & Wilkins, 1997.

31. Thomas, J. A. Transgene technology. In: *Nutrition in the 90's: Current Controversies and Analysis,* Vol. 2. F. N. Kotsonis and M. A. Mackey (Eds.). New York: Marcel Dekker, 1994, pp. 133–142.

32. Todhunter, E. N. Reflections on nutrition history. *J. Nutr.* 113:1681–1685, 1983.

33. Wahlquist, M. L. New directions in food. In: *Nutrition in the 90's: Current Controversies and Analysis,* Vol. 2, F. N. Kotsonis and M. A. Mackey (Eds.). New York: Marcel Dekker, Inc., 1994, pp. 117–132.

34. Wardlaw, G. M., and P. M. Insel. *Perspectives in Nutrition,* 2nd ed. St. Louis, MO: Mosby–Year Book, 1993.

35. Williams, M. H. *Nutrition for Fitness and Sport,* 4th ed. Dubuque, IA: Brown & Benchmark Publishers, 1995.

36. Williams, M. H. The role of minerals in physical activity. In: *Nutritional Aspects of Human Performance,* 2nd ed. Springfield, IL: Charles C Thomas, 1985, p. 186.

37. Wilmore, J. H., and D. L. Costill. *Physiology of Sports and Exercise.* Champaign, IL: Human Kinetics, 1994.

CHAPTER

8

Exercise and Sport Psychology

RICHARD J. SCHMIDT

What Is Exercise and Sport Psychology?

Parent Disciplines of Exercise and Sport Psychology

Activities of Exercise and Sport Psychologists

Educational Preparation and Career Opportunities

History of Exercise and Sport Psychology

Areas of Study
  Exercise Psychology
  Sport Psychology

Theoretical Orientations and Research Methodologies
  Theoretical Orientations

Research Methodologies

Future Directions and Issues

Professional Associations

Certifications

Employment Opportunities

Prominent Journals

Summary

Study Questions

Glossary

Suggested Readings

References

What Is Exercise and Sport Psychology?

Have you ever wondered how anxiety affects a surgeon's performance in the operating room or a football team's performance on the day of the state championship game? Is it possible that a sports team's cohesion is affected by a coach's reinforcement and punishment strategies? Perhaps you have pondered the questions of whether aerobic exercise reduces anxiety and depression or whether participation in daily physical education classes increases the self-esteem of elementary school children? Do athletes possess different personality profiles and mood states than nonathletes? Are specific psychological states and traits conducive to superior athletic performance. What are the most effective ways to reduce inappropriate aggression in sport? What are the psychobiological indicators of overtraining and staleness and how can they be used to improve exercise and sport performance or speed the process of recovery and rehabilitation following injury? What are the best strategies to help athletes overcome drug abuse in sports? These are but a few examples of the types of questions asked by exercise and sport psychologists.

Exercise and sport psychology involves the study of human behavior, both in individual and group contexts, in exercise- and sport-related environments. Fundamentally, exercise and sport psychology addresses two primary questions: (1) how do exercise and sport affect one's psychological makeup and, (2) how can the principles of psychology be used to improve exercise and sport performance (1)?

Exercise psychology has been defined as the

application of psychology to the promoting, explaining, maintaining, and enhancing of the parameters of physical fitness.... It is concerned with cognitions, emotions, and behaviors that are related to the perception of and/or objective changes in muscular strength and endurance, range of motion, cardiopulmonary endurance, and body composition." (39).

Sport psychology, on the other hand, is concerned with the application of psychological principles to the various areas of sport.

The study of exercise and sport psychology focuses not only on healthy individuals involved in exercise and athletics, but also on individuals in special populations, such as the disabled (Special Olympics participants, as well as orthopedic, cardiopulmonary, diabetic patients, and others), children, athletes or patients recovering from injury, and those afflicted with mental illnesses, including chronic depression.

Basic research in exercise and sport psychology involves studying the fundamental relationships among human behavior, exercise, and sport. Applied research in exercise and sport psychology addresses practical problems or questions in exercise and sport. Information obtained from such studies is used to understand how psychological factors affect exercise and sport performance and how participation in exercise and sport affects one's psychological development, health, and well-being.

Parent Disciplines of Exercise and Sport Psychology

Exercise and sport psychology has two primary parent disciplines: *psychology* and physical education. Academic training in exercise and sport psychology crosses the boundaries of both disciplines. Psychology involves the study of human behavior and includes developmental, abnormal, counseling, clinical, experimental, personality, and physiological psychology, as well as learning and motivation.

The second parent discipline is physical education. Undergraduate training in physical education normally includes courses such as anatomy, biomechanics, exercise physiology, exercise testing and prescription, and motor learning. For physical educators, the knowledge from the study of psychology can be used to improve health and enhance human performance during physical activity, exercise, and athletic participation.

Activities of Exercise and Sport Psychologists

Exercise and sport psychologists work with the academic, applied, or clinical aspects of exercise and sport. An *academic exercise and sport psychologist* strives to expand the knowledge base of the discipline through critical research. An *applied exercise and sport psychologist* applies the knowledge base in real-world situations. A *clinical exercise and sport psychologist* specializes in helping athletes solve issues related to mental health, anxiety, and drug dependency. These three areas (academic, applied, and clinical) can be further subdivided into teaching, research, and consulting.

Teaching. Those who teach in exercise and sport psychology are usually employed as professors at colleges or universities and teach general or specific courses (such as exercise psychology and applied sport psychology) in exercise science and/or physical education programs. Professors of exercise and sport psychology may hold dual appointments in a physical education or exercise science department, as well as in a department of psychology.

Research. The goals of research are to develop new knowledge, modify present knowledge, and correct old knowledge (21). Much research in exercise and sport psychology is conducted at colleges and universities in conjunction with professional preparation programs. Some research, however, is conducted by nonuniversity-based professionals who work with individual athletes or medical or professional athletic organizations. Such research may address issues such as how mental imagery affects performance, the role of exercise in anxiety reduction and depression in cardiac rehabilitation patients, or the relationship between exercise and/or sport programs in the development of children's self-concept and self-esteem. Much of the research conducted in higher education is shared with other professionals through publication of their findings in scientific research journals or at the presentation of research findings at professional meetings.

Consulting. A consultant in exercise and sport psychology generally works with athletes for the purpose of improving athletic performance. This type of consulting may involve developing cognitive behavioral strategies or imagery training schema to enhance performance. It may also involve working with sports medicine groups to develop strategies to control pain in injured athletes or to reduce the severity and incidence of athletic injuries. Consultation may take the form of working with athletes who have eating disorders, such as anorexia nervosa, bulimia nervosa, or anorexia athletica. In contrast to working with athletic programs, consultants in exercise and sport psychology also work with K–12 physical education programs to design them in such a way as to instill in students life-long habits toward regular physical activity and proper nutrition.

Educational Preparation and Career Opportunities

Students interested in academic study in exercise and sport psychology usually begin their preparation at the graduate level. The American Psychological Association's (APA) Division 47 (Exercise and Sport), the Association for the Advancement of Applied and Sport Psychology, and the North American Society for the Psychology of Sport and Physical Activity (NASPSPA) have information available for prospective students, which they disseminate in a pamphlet called "Graduate Training and Career Possibilities in Exercise and Sport Psychology" (2). Graduate programs of study are normally housed in physical education or exercise science departments, where students usually major in a specialty area of human performance and take related coursework offered by departments of psychology.

Currently, about 50 universities provide doctoral programs and about 100 schools provide master's programs in areas related to study and research in sport psychology (2). Doctoral students complete coursework in areas such as clinical psychology, personality theory, clinical assessment, psychometric theory, group processes, psychotherapy, motivation and emotion, learning processes, education, and human development. Master's students take most of their coursework in physical education, sport, or exercise science and elective coursework in psychology and/or sociology. Typical courses in a master's program address areas such as the psychological bases of human movement or, perhaps, psychological kinesiology.

Typically, three academic tracks are available in exercise and sport psychology at the doctoral level. Track I is targeted toward those who want to teach and conduct research into the use of cognitive strategies for improving the performance of athletes. A doctoral degree (Ph.D.) in sport sciences with a specialization in sport psychology and a significant proportion of coursework in psychology or counseling are required. Professionals may find employment in academic positions in colleges or universities, as researchers in sport research institutes or medical research laboratories, or as coaching educators within college or university physical education departments or sport organizations. Work in this track may include employment as a scientist scholar–educator or as a performance-enhancement specialist working in the areas of youth sport (motivational factors, ideal experiences, or optimal learning periods), learning and expertise (learning processes, expert systems, and the like), or performance enhancement (mental preparation strategies, motivation, intervention techniques) (2, 49).

Track II focuses on teaching and research in psychology, as well as working with athletes. A doctoral degree in psychology with a significant proportion of coursework in exercise and sport sciences is required for this track. Individuals may find employment in academic positions within colleges or universities or as researchers in sport research institutes or medical research laboratories. Opportunities in Tracks I and II may include part-time consulting with amateur and professional athletes and teams and, on rare occasions, full-time consulting. As in Track I, work in Track II may include employment as a scientist, scholar–educator, or performance-enhancement specialist working in the areas of psychometrics (sport-specific psychological test construction, diagnosis, and prediction of success) and performance enhancement (2, 49).

Track III focuses on those who have an interest and aptitude in providing clinical or counseling services to various populations, including athletes. A doctoral degree from an APA-accredited clinical or counseling psychology program with a significant proportion of coursework in sports psychology and related sport sciences is required to work in this track. Primary employment may be found in private psychology practice, clinical or counseling psychology programs in a university counseling center, sports medicine clinics as a psychological consultant, or as a university-based substance-abuse specialist. Individuals in this track may opt to do part-time consulting for either amateur or professional sports teams (2, 49).

If you are interested in obtaining more specific information concerning academic programs and/or employment possibilities in exercise and sport psychology, you may wish to obtain the following materials: *Directory of Graduate Programs in Applied Sport Psy-*

chology (42), *The World Sport Psychology Sourcebook* (43), and *Graduate Training and Career Possibilities in Exercise and Sport Psychology* (2).

History of Exercise and Sport Psychology

The ancient Greeks, well noted for the primacy that they placed on love of wisdom and athletics, were among the first to recognize and write about the inseparable dichotomy of the mind and body (62). This is noted in a commonly quoted phrase found in most introductory texts in the profession of physical education: "*mens sana in corpore sano*" or "a sound mind in a sound body." Despite this early acknowledgment of the inseparability of the mind–body dyad, exercise and sport psychology is a relatively new area of academic study and research exercise science. In the United States, exercise and sport psychology had its beginnings in the late nineteenth and early twentieth centuries.

In 1884, *C. Rieger* published what is considered by some to be the first article related to psychology and exercise when he investigated the effects of hypnotic catalepsy on muscular endurance (30). Shortly thereafter, in 1897, *Norman Triplett* published the first true experimental study in exercise psychology (53). While a professor of psychology at Indiana University, Triplett was intrigued by the observation that the performance of some competitive cyclists appeared to be enhanced by the "wheel-to-wheel rival" competition of other cyclists, while the performance of others seem to be impaired. Based on these observations, Triplett designed a study (53) that compared the performance scores between two competitive groups. Employing a self-designed hand-cranked cycle ergometer, the subjects of one group cycled alone, while the other worked in competition with one another. As a result of this study, Triplett concluded that "we infer that the bodily presence of another individual contestant participating simultaneously in the race serves to liberate latent energy not ordinarily available" (p. 523). Rejeski and Thompson (38) indicated that Triplett's study was the first to observe the adverse effects of *anxiety* on competition. This study is also noted as being the first experiment in social psychology (56).

Other scholars in the late 1800s and early 1900s, such as *George W. Fitz* (16), *William G. Anderson* (3), *E. W. Scripture* (44), *G. T. W. Patrick* (35), and *Robert. A. Cummins* (12), researched the areas of reaction time, the effects of physical training, cross education, the psychology of football, and the effects of basketball practice on motor reaction attention and suggestibility, respectively, as they pertained to sport. Except for Triplett's research, the majority of the studies conducted up until the early 1920s focused on the relationship between psychology and motor learning. It is noteworthy that during this time period the American Psychological Association president, G. Stanley Hall, issued a 1908 report highlighting the psychological benefits resulting from participation in physical education.

The first person to conduct systematic sport psychology research was *Coleman R. Griffith*, who began to study the psychological factors in basketball and football in 1918 as a doctoral student at the University of Illinois. Through his work and with the assistance of the athletic director of the University of Illinois at that time, Griffith was appointed as the director of the newly developed Athletic Research Laboratory in 1925. In this new position, Griffith established himself as the pioneer researcher in the United States in the field of exercise and sport psychology. His research interests were in the areas of learning, psychomotor, and personality research. He taught sport psychology classes, published numerous research articles, and published two classic texts, *Psychology of Coaching* (18) in 1926 and *Psychology of Athletics* (19) in 1928. During his years at Illinois, Griffith was able to do collaborative research on such notables as Red Grange, Knute Rockne, and Dizzy Dean in investigating topics related to motor learning, athletic motivation, and personality. Unfortunately, financial issues caused the Athletic Research Laboratory to close in 1932. Griffith, however, continued at the University of Illinois as a professor in the department of educational psychology. He also maintained his close ties with sport psychology when he was hired by Philip Wrigley in 1938 as a team sport psychologist for the Chicago Cubs. As a result of the influence and impact of Coleman Griffith's work, he is often recognized as the Father of American Sport Psychology (27).

In 1938, *Franklin Henry* assumed a faculty position in the Department of Physical Education at the University of California–Berkeley and established the psychology of physical activity graduate program. His primary areas of research and teaching were motor learning and sport psychology. He is noted for being the leading proponent for the scientific development of the field of exercise and sport psychology (57).

Celeste Ulrich was one of the pioneer women researchers in exercise and sport psychology. Enjoying a long, prolific career in physical education, much of her research involved studying the influence of stress on athletic performance.

The 1960s and 1970s saw the maturation of exercise and sport psychology as a true discipline. This is evidenced by the establishment of the majority of professional exercise and sport psychology organizations in the United States and other countries and the development and publication of numerous texts and scholarly journals devoted to sport psychology (59, 60). Research studies during this time period focused on aggression, causal attributions, personality, arousal and anxiety, team cohesion, imagery, and achievement motivation (8, 9, 40). *Arthur T. Slater-Hammel* of the University of Indiana and *John Lawther* of Penn State University began to offer coursework in sport psychology at their respective universities. Also during this time, *Bruce Ogilvie* and *Thomas Tutko* wrote their historic book entitled *Problem Athletes and How to Handle Them* (33). As a result of his work, Ogilvie has been referred to as the Father of Applied Sport Psychology in the United States (60). It was Henry's, Lawther's, and Slater-Hammel's programs that produced graduates who were to become some of the most prolific researchers and teachers in exercise and sport psychology.

The 1980s saw the development and expansion of more critical research in exercise and sport psychology. Major emphases in research were on the psychological aspects of exercise (7, 39) and on maximizing athletic performance through psychological intervention (7). Rejeski and Thompson (39) have noted that studies in this area are historically categorized into one of the following 10 areas: (1) fitness and mental health, (2) body image and esteem, (3) stress reactivity, (4) fatigue and exertion, (5) motivation, (6) exercise performance and metabolic responses, (7) sleep, (8) cognition, (9) the corporate–industrial environment, or (10) exercise addiction (39, 46).

In 1983, the U.S. Olympic Committee established an official sport psychology committee and a registry with three categories of clinical, educational, and research sport psychology. Eleven prominent sport psychologists were assigned to U.S. Olympic teams as part of the Elite Athlete Project. The sport psychologists along with their assigned teams included John Adderson (boxing), Herbert Fensterheim (fencing), Andrew Jacobs (cycling), Dan Landers (archery and shooting), Michael Mahoney (weight lifting), Rainer Martens (Nordic skiing), Jerry May (alpine skiing), Robert Nideffer (men's track and field), Bruce Ogilvie (volleyball), Richard Suinn (women's track and field), and Betty Wenz (synchronized swimming) (47).

In 1987, exercise and sport psychology was first recognized by mainstream psychology with the formation of Division 47 (Exercise and Sport Psychology) of the American Psychological Association (60).

The 1990s have seen the continued growth and development of research and practice in exercise and sport psychology. In exercise psychology, researchers are continuing to investigate such topics as exercise adherence, motivation, mental health, body image, eating disorders, stress, and fatigue as they relate to exercise and sport. In sport psychology, investigators are continuing their efforts to better understand the relationships between psychology and athletic performance, skill development and acquisition, motivation, goal setting, sport socialization, group dynamics, and psychometrics. The future promises additional emphasis on the applied aspects of exercise and sport psychology. Although applied sport and exercise psychology must be driven by basic research, it appears that most employment opportunities will be working as professionals in school and university settings, sport and health clubs, sports medicine clinics, and counseling centers, and as independent consultants.

It has been estimated that there are over 2700 individuals working in the field today in over 61 countries (43). Most exercise and sport psychologists live in Europe and North America, but major increases in activity have occurred in Latin America, Asia, Africa, and the Middle East in the last decade.

Table 8.1 provides a chronological history of the development of exercise and sport psychology.

Areas of Study

Following are examples of several current areas of study, research, and practice in exercise and sport psychology. These overviews will serve to give you a general orientation to each topic, importance to the field, current status, examples, current research findings, and implications for practice. It is important to remember that, although exercise psychology and sport psychology are often viewed as two separately distinct domains in terms of teaching, research, and actual practice, they do share some commonality between and within specific areas (motivation, emotion, goal-setting, anxiety, overtraining, and others).

Exercise Psychology

Exercise psychology addresses a number of areas, such as psychological effects of exercise, exercise adherence, exercise and motivation, and theoretical models of exercise behaviors. A brief overview of two of these areas, exercise and mood state and exercise adherence, are presented next.

TABLE 8.1   Chronology of the Development of Exercise and Sport Psychology

Year	Event
1884	C. Regier conducts a study on the effects of hypnotic catalepsy on muscular endurance (30).
1895	George W. Fitz publishes a study on reaction time in the journal *Psychological Review* (16).
1898	Frances A. Kellor publishes *A Psychological Basis for Physical Culture* (26).
1897	Norman Triplett conducts an experiment examining the social influence (competition) on motor performance (53).
1899	E. W. Scripture of Yale University conducts a study regarding desirable personality traits that could be fostered through athletics (44).
1899	William G. Anderson publishes work on mental practice and transfer of training and muscular strength (3).
1903	G. T. W. Patrick discusses the relationship between play and psychology.
1908	American Psychological Association president, G. Stanley Hall, issues report highlighting the psychological benefits resulting from participation in physical education.
1909	In Russia, Peter F. Lesgaft notes the importance for developing the motor learning capabilities of children through special physical activity programs. The USSR Sports Psychology Federation was formed sometime after the revolution.
1914	Robert A. Cummins investigates motor reactions, attention, and abilities as they relate to sport (12).
1918	Coleman Griffith conducts studies on basketball and football players at the University of Illinois (between 1919 and 1931, Griffith publishes 25 sport psychology research articles).
1920	The world's first sport psychology laboratory (Deutsche Hochschule für Leibesubungen) is established in Berlin, Germany, under the direction of Carl Diem.
1924	The National Institute of Physical Education is established in Tokyo. Matsui Mitsuo, majoring in aviation psychology, began sports research at this time. He is known as the Father of Sports Psychology in Japan.
1925	A. Z. Puni establishes sport psychology within the Institute of Physical Culture in Leningrad.
1925	The Athletic Research Laboratory is established at the University of Illinois with Coleman R. Griffith as director.
1926	Coleman Griffith writes *Psychology of Coaching* (18).
1928	Coleman Griffith writes *Psychology of Athletics* (19).
1928	Augustin Pechlat of Charles University (Czechoslovakia) completes his doctoral dissertation, which suggests a link between physical exercise and the psychological development of individuals participating in sports.
1932	Coleman Griffith's Athletics Laboratory at the University of Illinois closes as a result of the Depression.
1933	C. O. Jackson publishes an article entitled "An Experimental Study of the Effect of Fear on Muscular Coordination" (22).

Year	Event
1935	Franklin M. Henry initiates a course at the University of California–Berkeley entitled Psychological Basis of Physical Activity.
1938	Philip Wrigley hires Coleman Griffith to be the Chicago Cubs sports psychologist.
1938	Franklin Henry establishes the Psychology of Physical Activity graduate program at University of California–Berkeley.
1949	Warren R. Johnson's study of pregame emotion in football is a precursor to later competitive anxiety studies.
1951	John Lawther (Pennsylvania State University) writes *Psychology of Coaching.*
1952	John M. Harmon and Warren R. Johnson publish a study on the emotional reactions of college athletes (20).
1953	Czechoslovakia, under the leadership of Miroslav Vanek, forms a special section of the Czechoslovakian Union of Physical Education and Sport in the area of sport psychology.
1957	Celeste Ulrich publishes a study in the *Research Quarterly* on stress, women, and competition (54).
1962	Bulgaria establishes the Committee for Sport Psychology of the Bulgarian Union for Sport and Physical Culture.
1965	First International Society of Sport Psychology (ISSP) Congress is held in Rome (Ferruccio Antonelli of Italy is elected the first president).
1966	North American Society for the Psychology of Sport and Physical Activity (NASPSPA) is officially recognized by the International Society of Sport Psychology.
1966	Bruce Ogilvie and Thomas Tutko publish their famous book entitled *Problem Athletes and How to Handle Them.*
1967	Bryant Cratty of UCLA publishes *Psychology of Physical Activity.*
1967	The British Society of Sports Psychology is established under the leadership of Bill Steele of the University of Manchester. This group later merged with the British Association of Sports Sciences in 1985.
1968	The Sports Psychology Committee within the Romanian National Committee for Physical Culture and Sport is formed.
1968	The second ISSP Congress is held in Washington, DC.
1968	Switzerland establishes the Association Suisse de Psychologie du Sport (SASP) under the direction of Guido Schilling.
1969	Bob Wilberg and his graduate students organize the first Canadian sport psychology meeting under the title Psychomotor Learning and Sport Psychology Committee of the Canadian Association of Health, Physical Education and Recreation (CAHPER).
1969	The Federation Europeenne de Psychologie des Sports et des Activites Corporelles—FEPSAC (European Federation of Sport Psychology) is founded in Vittel, France.

(continued)

TABLE 8.1 **Continued**

Year	Event
1969	The Arbeitsgemeinschaft fur Sportpsychologie (ASP) (The Working Group for Sport Psychology) is established under the leadership of Willi Essing and Erwin Hahn.
1970	*International Journal of Sport Psychology* begins publication.
1973	The Japanese Society of Sport Psychology (JSSP) headed by Matsuda Iwao as president and Fujita Atsushi as secretary general is formed.
1973	La Societe Francaise de Psychologie du Sport (SFPS) is established in France (reorganized in 1988).
1973	NASPSPA holds its first independent conference in Monticello, IL.
1974	The Israeli Association of Sport Psychology is established under the leadership of Ema Geron.
1974	The proceedings of the NASPSPA conference are published for the first time.
1974	The Associazone Italiana di Psicologia dello Sport (AIPS) in Rome is established.
1975	The Swedish Association for Behavioral Sport Science in Orebro is formed.
1976	The Finnish Society of Sport Psychology is established under the leadership of Frieedrich Blanz.
1977	The Indian (India) Association of Sport Psychology (IASP) founded.
1977	The Canadian Society for Psychomotor Learning and Sport Psychology (CSPLSP) is organized (now independent of CAHPER's Psychomotor Learning and Sport Psychology Committee).
1978	The Hellenic Society of Sport Psychology and Applied Neurophysiology (HESPAN) is formed by Pantelis Kranidiotis.
1979	*Journal of Sport Psychology* begins publication.
1979	The Oesterreiche Arbeitsgemeinschaft fur Sport Psychologie (Austrian Work Group in Sport Psychology) is established under the direction of its first president Giselher Guttman.
1979	The Brazilian Society of Sport Psychology, Physical Activity and Recreation (SOBRAPE) is formed at the University of Feevale in Novo Hamburgo.
1980	The U.S. Olympic Committee develops the Sport Psychology Advisory Board.
1980	The Federacion Espanola de Asociaciones de Psicologia de la Actividad Fiscia y el Depote is formed in Spain.
1980	The Danish Society of Sport Psychology is founded by Arno Norske.
1980	The China Society of Sport Psychology is established.
1982	Jeffrey Bond is appointed the first applied sport psychologist at the Australian Institute of Sport.
1983	The U.S. Olympic Committee establishes an official Sport Psychology Committee and a registry with the three categories of clinical, educational, and research sport psychology.
1984	American television coverage of the Olympic Games emphasizes sport psychology.
1984	The Sports Psychology Association of Nigeria is formed.
1984	The New Zealand Sport Psychology Interest Group is formed.
1985	The Sport Psychology Association of India replaces the IASP.

Year	Event
1985	U.S. Olympic Committee hires the first full-time sport psychologist.
1985	The Association for the Advancement of Applied Sport Psychology AAASP) is formed.
1986	The AAASP holds its first conference in Jekyll, GA.
1986	The Australian Applied Sport Psychology Association (AASPA) is formed.
1986	The *Sport Psychologist* begins publication.
1986	Division 47 (Exercise and Sport Psychology) becomes an official division of the American Psychological Association.
1987	The Canadian Registry for Sport Behavioral Professionals (CRSBP) is instituted under the leadership of Murray Smith.
1987	The Dutch Psychological Association forms a working group in sport psychology. This results in the formation of the Dutch Society for Sport Psychology in 1989.
1988	The *Journal of Sport Psychology* becomes the *Journal of Sport and Exercise Psychology.*
1988	The Societa Italiana di Psicologia (SIPs) inaugurates a special section in sport psychology under the guidance of Alessandro Salvini of Padova University.
1988	The U.S. Olympic team is accompanied by an officially recognized sport psychologist for the first time.
1988	The Danish Sport Federation, in funding an institution for the elite sport called Team Danmark, consolidates a sport psychology study group.
1988	The Sociedad Colombiana de Ciencias Aplicadas al deporte (Colombian Society of Applied Sport Sciences) is formed (includes a sport psychologist on the executive committee).
1988	The Mexican Society of Sport Psychology is established in Guadalajara under Guillermo Dellamary.
1989	*Journal of Applied Sport Psychology* begins publication.
1989	AAASP approves certification criteria for title Certified Consultant, AAASP.
1989	The Sport Psychology Association of Australia and New Zealand (SPAANZ) is formed.
1991	AAASP establishes the Certified Consultant, AAASP designation
1992	*Contemporary Thought on Performance Enhancement* begins.
1993	ISSP publishes the landmark *Handbook of Research on Sport Psychology.*
1994	The Canadian Mental Training Registry (CMTR) replaces the CRSBP.
1995	Stuart Biddle, editor (University of Exeter, England), along with co-authors from England, France, Switzerland, Israel, Germany, Greece, Scotland, Norway, and Czechoslovakia publish *European Perspectives on Exercise and Sport Psychology,* which emphasizes the critical need for employing multiple cross-cultural perspectives to address and solve issues related to exercise–sport psychology.
1996	Andrew Ostrow publishes the second edition of the *Directory of Psychological Tests in the Sport and Exercise Sciences.*

Additional sources for Table 8.1 from 17, 43, 47, 50, 57).

Exercise and Mood State.   One of the most researched areas in exercise psychology is the effect of acute and chronic exercise on mood states. Although almost everyone who exercises on a regular basis reports feelings of well-being, or positive affect, either as a result of an acute bout of exercise or through participation in a regular program of physical activity, researchers are as yet unclear as to the mechanism(s) underlying these perceptions. Several mechanisms have been hypothesized to account for the increases in positive affect following an acute bout of exercise (6, 13, 38, 51): an increase in circulating endorphins resulting in feelings of euphoria; the monoamine hypothesis, which holds that increased levels of central monoamine neurotransmitters give rise to feelings of positive affect; the thermogenic hypothesis, which holds that elevation in body temperature accompanying exercise contributes to the perception of positive affect; the distraction hypothesis, which holds that it is not the exercise itself, but rather the psychological distraction or break that an exercise bout gives from the trials and tribulations of daily life that is responsible for bringing about changes in affect; and the mastery hypothesis, which holds that exercise may increase one's sense of self-mastery or accomplishment, thereby lead to improved affect.

One of the most popular instruments used by researchers to assess changes in mood states following exercise is the Profiles of Mood States (POMS) questionnaire (29) developed by McNair, Lorr, and Droppelman. The POMS measures the mood states of tension/ anxiety, depression/dejection, anger/hostility, vigor/activity, fatigue/inertia, and confusion/ bewilderment. In using this instrument, researchers have generally found that exercisers and athletes tend to have a more favorable mental health mood state profile than nonexercisers and nonathletes. A more favorable mental health profile is represented by low scores on tension, depression, anger, fatigue, and confusion and a high score on vigor.

In the area of athletics, Morgan et al. (32) have used the POMS to develop a mental health model useful in predicting athletic success. The model suggests that positive mental health is directly related to athletic success and high levels of performance. Elite athletes in a variety of sports (swimmers, wrestlers, oarsmen, runners) are characterized by what Morgan calls the *iceberg profile.* The iceberg profile of a successful elite athlete is formed by scoring high on the variable of vigor and low on the variables of tension, depression, anger, fatigue, and confusion (compared to the population 50th percentile). Less successful athletes have a flatter profile, scoring at or below the 50th percentile on all six psychological factors.

Exercise Adherence.   An area of great concern for exercise professionals is the high rate of attrition commonly seen in exercise programs. Specifically, *exercise adherence* refers to the degree to which an individual follows the recommended frequency, intensity, and duration. More generally, adherence to exercise has most often been defined for research purposes as a percentage of attendance. Lack of exercise adherence affects asymptomatic children and adults, as well as individuals in cardiac, pulmonary, and other chronic disease rehabilitation programs. Research has shown that approximately 50% of those who begin exercise programs drop out within the first six months (55). The dropout rate is similar for cardiac patients (34). Exercise psychologists are concerned with why there is a discrepancy between wanting to exercise and the ability to adhere to an exercise program. Although research in this area is new, some answers are available.

Research has shown that there are a multitude of psychological, physiological, cultural, socioeconomic, and program factors that contribute to exercise adherence. Some of these factors are prior exercise history, recent exercise behaviors, active versus inactive leisure time, current level of fitness, and smokers versus nonsmokers. Physiological factors include body weight, body fat, angina pectoris, and left ventricular ejection fraction (34). Psychological factors include aspects of personality such as self-motivation, attitudes toward exercise, and health knowledge and beliefs (61). Social factors include marital status, spousal and family social support, peer social support, and work demands (61). Program factors include enjoyment, convenience, quality of the exercise facility and equipment, program social support, group versus individual programs, program leadership, and program intensity (61).

Sport Psychology

Sport psychology addresses a number of areas, such as psychological characteristics and high-level performance, skill acquisition, group dynamics, motivation, overtraining, staleness, and burnout, and psychological techniques for individual performance. A brief overview of two of these areas, personality and sport and overtraining, staleness, and burnout are provided next.

Personality and Sport.   Coaches and sport psychologists have long been interested in the relationship between personality and sports performance. Early research posited a relationship between certain aspects of one's personality and level of athletic success (15). Several theories have emerged to attempt to explain this relationship.

Weinberg and Gould (57) described three theories in this regard: (1) trait theory, (2) the situational approach, and (3) the interactional approach. Basically, the *trait theory* contends that one's personality consists of identifiable and measurable stable psychological characteristics and that the assessment of these traits will allow investigators to predict athletic performance in a variety of settings. The *situational approach,* which is based on social learning theory (4), suggests that an athlete's behavior in a given setting is shaped or molded by the specific situation or environment. The *interactional approach* states that an athlete's behavior is a function of the interaction between the environmental situation and psychological traits.

Overtraining, Staleness, and Burnout.   All forms of stimuli act as a stressor on the body. Whether it be exercise, injury, or a very emotionally charged reaction, the body responds to all these forms of stimuli in a general way. Selye (45) first defined this response to such stressors as the *general adaptation syndrome.* He characterized the body as responding in three general stages depending on the duration that the stressor was applied. These three stages are the *alarm stage* (the body mobilizes its mechanisms to meet the demands of the stress), the *resistance stage* (stress syndrome disappears with the body being more resistant to the stressor), and the *exhaustion stage* (stress syndrome reappears and the body enters a state of decline). These three stages are characterized by a syndrome consisting of

(1) adrenal enlargement, (2) thymus and lymphatic shrinkage, and (3) bleeding ulcers in the digestive tract.

Athletes and exercisers of all ages and at all levels of involvement have the potential to incur staleness and/or burnout should a chronic imbalance (inordinate amount of stress) develop in their training or conditioning program. We know that principles of conditioning specify that one's systems must be overloaded on a systematic and progressive basis to make improvements in physiological adaptations and therefore performance. Scientific application of the variables of frequency, intensity, duration, mode, and progression must be followed to bring about desired outcomes in training and/or performance. At the same time, a fine balance must be struck between adequate rest and nutrition.

Overtraining has been defined as (50) "a stimulus consisting of a systematic schedule of progressively intense physical training of a high absolute and relative intensity" (50, p. 842). Overtraining, in effect, describes the application of an incorrect dose of frequency, intensity, duration, and mode in a training and conditioning program. When a chronic imbalance exists in these variables, inappropriate responses such as staleness or in more severe cases burnout may become manifest (52).

Staleness is an undesirable outcome of overtraining. Although individuals experiencing staleness may still be highly motivated in training, they tend to suffer decrements in physiological adaptations with resultant decreases in performance. Although an athlete or exerciser experiencing staleness generally exhibits a variety of behavioral disturbances, the primary disturbance is depression (31). Burnout, while sharing some of the same symptoms as staleness, "possesses the central features of loss of interest and motivation" (50, p. 842).

Although staleness and burnout are caused by a complex interaction of physiological and psychological factors, Raglin and Morgan (37) have ranked the following causes as being primarily responsible for the development of these syndromes: (1) too much stress and pressure, (2) too much practice and physical training, (3) physical exhaustion and all-over soreness, (4) boredom because of too much repetition, and (5) poor rest or lack of proper sleep.

Mild staleness may be treated by reducing training intensity and/or volume, but more severe cases of staleness and burnout usually require qualified medical and psychological intervention (5).

Theoretical Orientations and Research Methodologies

The study of exercise and sport psychology employs specific theoretical orientations and research methodologies. The specific theoretical orientations are generally classified as behavioral, psychophysiological, and cognitive–behavioral (57). Research methodologies for exercise and sport psychology include both qualitative and quantitative approaches. Qualitative research involves using any one of the five main traditions, that is, the biographical, phenomenological, grounded theory, ethnographic, or case study approach (11, 23). Quantitative research involves employing strict experimental control procedures to study the effect of the manipulation of an independent variable (for example, various intensities of exercise training) on a dependent variable (for example, changes in cardiorespiratory fitness) (21).

Theoretical Orientations

Behavioral.   The behavioral orientation views the primary determinants of an athlete's or exerciser's behavior as coming from the environment. In this view, participants are viewed as being primarily motivated by factors external to themselves (57).

Psychophysiological.   The psychophysiological orientation suggests that the best way to study exercise and sport is to examine the physiological processes of the brain and their influences on the physical activity (57). This approach is heavily involved with measuring physiological variables such as heart rate, electromyography, electroencephalography, blood lactate levels, galvanic skin response, and eye movement response patterns and then correlating these measures with exercise and sport behavior.

Cognitive–Behavioral.   The cognitive–behavioral orientation assumes that the behavior of individuals is determined by their cognitive mental (or "thinking") processes (57). Specific cognitive variables, such as self-confidence, self-efficacy, self-esteem, anxiety, fear, motivation, need for success, and fear of failure, are thought to be the determinants of the behavior that an exerciser or athlete may exhibit in any given situation.

Research Methodologies

A variety of quantitative research methodologies are used to study exercise and sport psychology. To begin with, one may employ any of the several theories or theoretical constructs available within the disciplines of psychology, sociology, anthropology, physical education, sport, or exercise science. With appropriate training and qualifications, one may use psychological tests or questionnaires on either an individual or group basis in quasi-experimental or experimental research design settings. The use of the introspective or phenomenological approach may be of value when other approaches may seem inadequate or contraindicated. Figures 8.1 and 8.2 are abstracts from research studies that have utilized quantitative methodologies to study exercise and sport psychology.

Software technology for quantitative research (descriptive and inferential statistics) has been available for some time. However, relatively new software has appeared on the market that offers computerized assistance in helping researchers to analyze data gained in qualitative research studies. One such piece of software is QSR NUD•IST, which is an acronym for nonnumerical unstructured data indexing searching and theorizing (36). It is designed to assist researchers in managing nonnumerical and unstructured data in qualitative analysis by supporting indexing, searching, and theorizing functions. Figures 8.3 and 8.4 are abstracts from research studies that have utilized qualitative methodologies to study exercise and sport psychology.

FIGURE 8.1 Abstract of a quantitative research study in exercise psychology.

Treasure, D. C., and D. M. Newbery.
Relationship between self-efficacy, exercise intensity, and feeling states in a sedentary population during and following an acute bout of exercise.
Journal of Sport Psychology, Vol. 20, 1–11, 1998.

This study examined the relationship between self-efficacy, exercise intensity, and feeling states in a sedentary population during and following an acute bout of exercise. Sixty sedentary participants were randomly assigned to either a moderate-intensity (45–75% age predicted Heart Rate Reserve: HRR), high-intensity exercise (70–75% HRR) group, or a no-exercise attention control group. Participants in both exercise groups experienced changes in feeling states across the course of the exercise bout. The moderate-intensity group reported more positive and fewer negative feeling states both during and after exercise than the high-intensity group. Participants in both exercise conditions were significantly more positively engaged than the attention control group postexercise. Consistent with social cognitive theory (Bandura, 1986, 1997), the reciprocal determined relationship between self-efficacy and feeling states was found to be strongest in the high-intensity exercise condition.

Source: Treasure, D. C., and D. M. Newbery. Relationship between self-efficacy, exercise intensity, and feeling states in a sedentary population during and following an acute bout of exercise. *Journal of Sport Psychology,* Vol. 20, 1–11, 1998.

FIGURE 8.2 Abstract of a quantitative research study in sport psychology.

Ziegler, P., S. Hensley, J. B. Roepke, S. H. Whitaker, B. W. Craig, and A. Drewnowski.
Eating attitudes and energy intakes of female skaters.
Med. Sci. Sports Exerc., Vol. 30, No. 4, pp. 583–586, 1998.

This study examined potential links between dietary intakes, body fatness, menstrual status, and hematological and serum iron status in 21 competitive female figure skaters ages 11–16 yr. Attitudes toward dieting were assessed using the Eating Attitudes Test (EAT). Dietary intakes were based on 3-d food records. Percent body fat was calculated using triceps, subscapular, suprailiac, pectoral, axillary, abdominal, and thigh skinfold measures. Blood iron status was measured using hematocrit (Hct), hemoglobin (Hgb), total iron binding capacity (TIBC), and serum iron. Menstrual status was based on a self-report questionnaire. Body weights and estimated energy intakes were all within normal range for this age group. Higher EAT scores were associated with lower micronutrient, but not lower energy intakes. Menstrual status and iron status were normal. No significant correlations between measures of body fatness, menstrual status, and hematological or serum iron status were observed. Although the measured indices of nutritional status were normal, adolescent athletes have higher energy needs than does the general population. Depending on energy expenditure levels, energy and nutrition intakes in the low normal range may put some athletes at risk for undernutrition.

Source: Ziegler, P., S. Hensley, J. B. Roepke, S. H. Whitaker, B. W. Craig, and A. Drewnowski. Eating attitudes and energy intakes of female skaters. *Med. Sci. Sports Exerc.,* Vol. 30, No. 4, pp. 583–586, 1998.

FIGURE 8.3   Abstract of a qualitative research study in exercise psychology.

Chepyator-Thomson, J. R., and C. D. Ennis.
Reproduction and resistance to the culture of femininity and masculinity in secondary school physical education.
Research Quarterly for Exercise and Sport, Vol. 68, No. 1, pp. 89–99, 1997.

The purpose of the study was to investigate ways in which gender-related perceptions and actions influenced students' construction of realities in curriculum-in-action in secondary school physical education. The participants were junior and senior secondary school students in a midwestern city in the United States. Data collection methods included observations and interviews. Data were analyzed with inductive analytical procedures. The findings of the study revealed that a majority of the female and male students reproduced traditionally dominant forms of femininity and masculinity. Female students patterned their behavior consistent with feminine ideology in selecting and participating in class activities, and male students chose and participated in class activities along masculine conceptions. The results were interpreted with reproduction and resistance theories. While femininity and masculinity cultures were reproduced through students' choice of activities and participation patterns, these cultures were resisted through students' construction of oppositional behavior.

FIGURE 8.4   Abstract of a qualitative research study in sport psychology.

Kimiecik, J. C., and A. T. Harris.
What is enjoyment? A conceptual/definitional analysis with implications for sport and exercise psychology.
Journal of Sport and Exercise Psychology, Vol. 18, No. 18, pp. 247–263, 1996.

It has been suggested that enjoyment is a key construct for understanding and explaining the motivation and experiences of sport and exercise participants (Scanlan & Simons, 1992; Wankel, 1993). In this paper, definitions of enjoyment used by sport and exercise psychology researchers are reviewed, and the conceptual and measurement implications for the study of sport and exercise experiences are discussed. In many studies investigating enjoyment, researchers have not adequately defined the construct. Also, there are possible limitations with proposed definitions of enjoyment (e.g., Scanlan & Simons, 1992; Wankel, 1993). One possible way of addressing these limitations is to conceptualize and define enjoyment as flow (Csikszentmihalyi, 1993). To support this enjoyment-equals-flow contention, enjoyment/flow is compared with other related constructs: affect, attitude, pleasure, and intrinsic motivation. Implications of the suggested definition of enjoyment as flow for past and present enjoyment research in sport and exercise psychology are discussed.

Future Research Directions and Issues

In exercise psychology, there will be a continued need for research in the area of exercise and mental health. Additional areas for further research include exercise adherence, the therapeutic effects of exercise, exercise addiction, and exercise and cognitive functioning (25, 41, 58).

In sport psychology, future research needs to be targeted toward research in the area of psychological skills training (PST) (50). Although current research has indicated the effectiveness of PST in improving sports performance, little is known about the mechanisms for this effect. Research into youth sport and cross-cultural sport will serve to address issues related to potential sport-related child abuse (10) and to answer questions regarding the relationship between sport and culture (14), respectively. Additional areas in which further research is needed include self-confidence, children and aggression in sport, the psychology of burnout, character development through sport, and gender issues in sport and exercise.

Of equal importance to these topical areas, gains must be made in constructing proper research designs to answer critical questions relevant to exercise and sport psychology. Constructs in exercise and sport psychology need to be accurately defined. Only in this way can researchers validly compare the results of one study with another investigating the same phenomenon under similar conditions. Research designs that have real-world application must be employed so that results will have applicability to real populations (46).

Professional Associations

American Alliance for Health, Physical Education, Recreation and Dance (AAHPERD, Sport Psychology Academy). AAHPERD, 1900 Association Drive, Reston, VA 22091.

American College of Sports Medicine (ACSM). ACSM, 401 West Michigan Street, Indianapolis, IN 46202-3233.

American Psychological Association (APA)—Division 47 (Sport and Exercise Psychology) and Division 38 (Health Psychology). APA, 750 First Street, NE, Washington, DC 20002-4242.

Association for the Advancement of Applied Sport Psychology (AAASP)*

Canadian Society for Psychomotor Learning and Sport Psychology (CSPLSP)*

International Society of Sport Psychology (ISSP)*

North American Society for the Psychology of Sport and Physical Activity (NASPSPA)*

Organizations marked with an asterisk do not have permanent addresses because membership chairs periodically rotate. For current addresses, consult the *Encyclopedia of Associations,* published by Gale Research, 835 Penobscot Building, Detroit, MI, 48226-4094, or http://galenet.gale.com/admin/copyright.html.

Certifications

In 1991, the Association for the Advancement of Applied Sport Psychology (AAASP) began a Certified Consultant, AAASP program that requires advanced training in both psychology and the sport sciences to ensure that individuals have the necessary sport science and psychological training to consult in exercise and sport psychology in the United States. A doctoral degree with appropriate coursework in psychology, health, exercise physiology, performance, health, psychopathology, ethics, statistics, research design, cognitive behavior, and the biological bases of behavior is required. Additional skills in counseling and a supervised practicum are also required (28).

The U.S. Olympic Committee (USOC) maintains its own sport psychology registry. Registered professionals are qualified to work with Olympic athletes as well as national teams. To be on the registry, one must be a member of the American Psychological Association and a Certified Consultant of the Association for the Advancement of Applied Sport Psychology (CC, AAASP). Other countries, such as Australia, Britain, and Canada, have established certification criteria for those who provide services in sport psychology within their respective countries.

Employment Opportunities

Employment opportunities in exercise and sport psychology are quite variable at the present time. Most positions available are in applied exercise and sport psychology at the university level, where one works as an *educational sport psychologist*. The next most popular employment areas are consultant positions with individual athletes, sports teams, and sport–health clubs or positions as qualified clinical sport psychologists. Job announcements may be found at the major annual conventions sponsored by the American Psychological Association, the Association for the Advancement of Applied Sport Psychology, the American College of Sports Medicine, and the North American Society for the Psychology of Sport and Physical Activity.

Prominent Journals

International Journal of Sport Psychology
Journal of Applied Sport Psychology
Journal of Sport and Exercise Psychology
Journal of Sport Behavior
Medicine and Science in Sports and Exercise
Pediatric Exercise Science
The Gerontologist
The Sport Psychologist

The following journals are published by the American Psychological Association (APA)—Division 47 (Sport and Exercise Psychology) and Division 38 (Health Psychology). APA, 750 First Street NE, Washington, DC 20002-4242.

Health Psychology
Journal of Applied Psychology
Journal of Counseling and Clinical Psychology
Journal of Counseling Psychology
Journal of Personality and Social Psychology
Perceptual and Motor Skills
Psychology and Aging

Summary

Exercise and sport psychology involves the study of human behavior in exercise- and sport-related environments. Both exercise psychology and sport psychology use the principles of psychology to examine (1) how exercise or sport affects psychological makeup and (2) methods for improving exercise or sport performance. Exercise psychology applies psychology to the parameters of physical fitness, whereas sport psychology applies psychological principles to the various areas of sport. Because psychological factors affect exercise and sport performance and participation in exercise and sport affects psychological development and health it is important for exercise science students to develop a clear understanding of this aspect of the discipline.

STUDY QUESTIONS

1. What is exercise and sport psychology?

2. Identify two general objectives of exercise and sport psychology.

3. Describe three roles of exercise and sport psychology specialists.

4. What career opportunities are there in exercise and sport psychology?

5. What are current areas of research in exercise and sport psychology?

GLOSSARY

Anxiety   An acute (state) or chronic (trait) of uneasiness or uncertainty about a future event or a past experience.

Applied sport psychologists   Professionals who apply sport-specific and general psychological theories to sport settings in an attempt to increase the psychological well-being, health, and performance of athletes.

Attentional focus   Concentration based on the two dimensions of width (broad versus narrow) and direction (internal versus external).

Attribution theory   How individuals explain their successes and failures.

Clinical sport psychologists   Professionals specifically trained to address emotional problems and personality disorders experienced by athletes.

Competitiveness   A contest, match, or other trial of skill or ability against oneself or another.

Educational sport psychologists   Professionals who communicate the principles of sport psychology to athletes and coaches.

Exercise adherence   Ability to comply with the prescribed frequency, intensity, duration, mode, and progression of a physical activity until a stated outcome goal is achieved.

Exercise addiction   The psychological and/or physiological dependence on regular exercise characterized by withdrawal symptoms after 24 to 36 hours.

Goal setting   The process of setting performance (process) and outcome (product) goals to attain a desired result.

Imagery   Use of mental preparation techniques prior to competition for the purpose of improving performance.

Motivation   An incentive, motive, or inducement to act.

Personality   The collective pattern of one's psychological traits and states.

Psychology   The science of mental processes and behavior.

Self-efficacy   Confidence in one's ability to successfully perform a given behavior.

Social cohesion   Degree of interpersonal attraction among team members.

Sport   A special type of game whose outcome is determined by physical skill, strategy, or chance, employed singly or in combination.

Staleness   A condition in which an individual, although motivated, suffers from decrements in physiological adaptations and performance. One experiencing this condition generally exhibits a variety of behavioral disturbances, primarily depression.

Task cohesion   Degree to which team members work together to achieve a common goal.

SUGGESTED READINGS

American Psychological Association. *Exploring Sport and Exercise Psychology,* J. L. Van Raalte and B. W. Brewer (Eds.). Washington, DC: APA 1996.

Biddle, S. J. H. (Ed.). *European Perspectives on Exercise and Sport Psychology.* Champaign, IL: Human Kinetics, 1995.

Willis, J. D., and L. F. Campbell. *Exercise Psychology.* Champaign, IL: Human Kinetics, 1992.

REFERENCES

1. Abernethy, B., V. Kippers, L. T. Mackinnon, R. J. Neal, and S. Hanrahan. *The Biophysical Foundations of Human Movement.* Champaign, IL: Human Kinetics, 1997.

2. American Psychological Association. Graduate Training and Career Possibilities in Exercise and Sport Psycholgy. Washington, DC: 1994.

3. Anderson, W. G. Studies in the effects of physical training. *Am. Physical Educ. Rev.* 4:265–278, 1899.

4. Bandura, A. Self-efficacy: Toward a unifying theory of behavioral change. *Psychol. Rev.* 84:191–215, 1977.

5. Barron, J. L., T. D. Noakes, W. Levy, C. Smith, and R. P. Millar. Hypothlamic dysfunction in overtrained athletes. *J. Clinical Endocrinology Metabolism* 60:803–806, 1989.

6. Brown, J. D. Staying fit and staying well: Physical fitness as a moderator of life stress. *J. Personality Social Psychol.* 60:555–561, 1991.

7. Browne, M. A., and M. J. Mahoney. Sport psychology. *Annual Rev. Psychol.* 35:605–625, 1984.

8. Callois, R. *Man, Play, and Games.* New York: Free Press, 1961.

9. Cox, P. H., Y. Qiu, and Z. Liu. Overview of sport psychology. In: *Handbook of Research in Sport Psychology,* R. N. Singer, M. Murphey, and L. K. Tenant (Eds.). New York: Macmillan, 1993, pp. 3–31.

10. Cox, R. H., and L. Noble. Preparation and attitudes of Kansas high school head coaches. *J. Teaching Physical Educa.* 8:329–241, 1989.

11. Creswell, J. W. *Qualitative Inquiry and Research Design: Choosing among the Five Traditions.* Thousand Oaks, CA: Sage Publications, 1998, pp. 7–8.

12. Cummins, R. A. A study of the effect of basketball practice on motor reaction attention and suggestibility. *Psychol. Rev.* 21:356–369, 1914.

13. DeVries, H. A., P. Beckman, H. Huber, and L. Dieckmeir. Electromyographic evaluation of of the effects of sauna on the neuromuscular system. *J. Sports Med.* 8:61–69, 1968.

14. Duda, J. Achievement motivation among Navajo students: A conceptual analysis with preliminary data. *Ethos* 8:131–155, 1980.

15. Fisher, A. C. New directions in sport personality research. In: *Psychological Foundations of Sport,* J. M.

Silva and R. S. Weinberg (Eds.). Champaign, IL: Human Kinetics, 1984, pp. 70–80.

16. Fitz, G. W. A local reaction. *Psychol. Rev.* 2:37–42, 1895.

17. Gill, D. L. Sport and exercise psychology. In: *The History of Exercise and Sport Science.* J. D. Massengale and R. A. Swanson (Eds.). Champaign, IL: Human Kinetics, 1997, pp. 293–320.

18. Griffith, C. R. *Psychology of Coaching.* New York: Scribners, 1926.

19. Griffith, C. R. *Psychology of Athletics.* New York: Scribners, 1928.

20. Harmon, J. M., and W. R. Johnson. The emotional reactions of college athletes. *Research Quart.* 23:391–397, 1952.

21. Hyllgard, R., D. P. Mood, and J. R. Morrow, Jr. *Interpreting Research in Sport and Exercise Science.* St. Louis, MO: C. V. Mosby, 1997, p. 38.

22. Jackson, C. O. An experiemntal study of the effect of fear on muscular coordination. *Research Quart.* 4:71–79, 1933.

23. Johnson, M. L. Qualitative effects of youth sport camp experience (Abstract). *J. Sport Exercise Psychol.* 20:S21,1988.

24. Johnson, W. R. A study of emotion revealed in two types of athletic sports contests. *Research Quart.* 20:72–79, 1949.

25. Katz, J. F., J. C. Adler, N. J. Mazzarella, and L. P. Ince. Psychological consequences of an exercise training program for a paraplegic man: A case study. *Rehabilitation Psychol.* 30: 53–58, 1985.

26. Kellor, F. A. A psychological basis for physical culture. *Education* 19:100–104, 1898.

27. Kroll, W., and G. Lewis. America's first sport psychologist. *Quest* 13:1–4, 1970.

28. McCullagh, P., and J. M. Noble. (1993). Education and training in sport and exercise psychology. In: *Exercise Psychology: The Influence of Physical Exercise on Psychological Processes,* P. Seraganian (Ed.). New York: John Wiley & Sons, 1993, pp. 377–394.

29. McNair, D. M., M. Lorr, and L. F. Droppelman. *Profiles of Mood States Manual.* San Diego, CA: Educational and Industrial Testing Service, 1971.

30. Morgan, W. P. Hypnosis and muscular performance. In: *Ergogenic Aids and Muscular Performance,* W. P. Morgan (Ed.). New York: Academic Press, 1972, pp. 193–231.

31. Morgan, W. P., D. R. Brown, J. S. Raglin, P. J. O'Connor, and K. A. Ellickson. Psychological monitoring of overtraining and staleness. *British Journal of Sports Medicine* 21:107–114, 1987.

32. Morgan, W. P., P. J. O'Connor, P. B. Sparling, and R. R. Pate. Psychological characterization of the elite female distance runner. *International Journal of Sports Medicine* 8(supplement):124–131, 1987.

33. Ogilvie, B. C., and T. A. Tutko. *Problem Athletes and How to Handle Them.* London: Pelham Books, 1966.

34. Olderidge, N. G., A. Donner, C. W. Buck, N. L. Jones, G. A. Anderson, J. O. Parker, D. A. Cunningham, T. Kavanaugh, P. A. Rechnitzer, and J. R. Sutton. Predictive indices for dropout: The Ontario exercise heart collaborative study experience. *Amer. J. Cardiology* 51:70–74, 1983.

35. Patrick, G. T. W. The psychology of football. *Amer. J. Psychol.* 14:104–117, 1903.

36. Qualitative Solutions and Research. QSR NUD•IST User Guide. Thousand Oaks, CA: Sage Publications Software, 1996.

37. Raglin, J. S., and W. P. Morgan. Development of a scale to measure training induced distress. *Med. Sci. Sports Exercise* 21(supplement):60, 1989.

38. Ransford, C. P. A role for amines in the antidepressant effect of exercise: A review. *Med. Sci. Sports Exercise* 14:1–10, 1982.

39. Rejeski, W. J., and A. Thompson. Historical and conceptual roots of exercise psychology, In: *Exercise Psychology: The Influence of Physical Exercise on Psychological Processes,* P. Seraganian (Ed.). New York: John Wiley & Sons, 1993, pp. 3–35.

40. Roberts, J. M. Games in culture. *Amer. Anthropologist* 61:597–605, 1959.

41. Sachs, M. L. Running addiction. In: *Psychology of Running,* M. H. Sachs and M. L. Sachs (Eds.). Champaign, IL: Human Kinetics, 1981, pp. 116–121.

42. Sachs, M. L., K. L. Burke, and L. A. Butcher. *Directory of Graduate Programs in Applied Sport Psychology,* 4th ed. Morgantown, WV: FIT, 1995.

43. Salmela, J. H. *The World Sport Psychology Sourcebook.* Champaign, IL: Human Kinetics, 1992.

44. Scripture, E. W. Cross-education. *Popular Sci. Monthly* 56:589–596, 1899.

45. Selye, H. *Stress in Health and Disease.* Boston: Butterworth, 1976.

46. Seraganian, P. Current status and future directions in the field of exercise psychology. In: *Exercise Psychology: The Infuence of Physical Exercise on Psychological Processes,* P. Serganian (Ed.). New York: John Wiley & Sons, 1993, pp. 383–390.

47. Silva, J. M., and R. S. Weinberg. *Psychological Foundations of Sport.* Champaign, IL: Human Kinetics, 1984.

48. Singer, R. N. United States. In: *The World Sport Psychology Sourcebook,* 2nd ed., J. H. Salmela (Ed.). Champaign, IL: Human Kinetics, 1992, pp. 54–60.

49. Singer, R. N. Future of sport and exercise psychology. In: *Exploring Sport and Exercise Psychology,* J. L.

Van Raalte and B. W. Brewer (Eds.). Washington, DC: American Psychological Association, 1996.

50. Singer, R. N., M. Murphey, and L. K. Tenant (Eds.). *Handbook of Research in Sport Psychology.* New York: Macmillan, 1993.

51. Steinberg, H., and E. A. Sykes. Introduction to symposium on endorphins and behavioral processes: Review of literature on endorphins and exercise. *Pharmacology, Biochemistry Behavior* 23:857–862, 1985.

52. Thomson, W. C., V. K. Wayda, J. Jones, and K. Flor. Avoiding burnout: Hardiness as a stress buffer in college athletes. *Research Quart. Exercise Sport* 69(supplement): S116, 1998.

53. Triplett, N. The dynamogenic effects of pacemaking and competition. *Amer. J. Psychol.* 9:507–533, 1898.

54. Ulrich, C. Measurement of stress evidenced by college women in situations involving competition. *Research Quart.* 28:160–172, 1957.

55. Wankel, L. M. Enhancing motivation for involvement in voluntary exercise programs. In: *Recent Advances in Motivation and Achievement,* Vol. 5. Enhancing motivation, M. L. Maehr and D. A. Kleiber (Eds.). Greenwhich, CT: JAI Press, 1987.

56. West, S. G., and R. A. Wicklund. *A Primer of Social Psychology Theories.* Monterey, CA: Brooks/Cole, 1980.

57. Weinberg, R. S., and D. Gould. *Foundations of Sport and Exercise Psychology.* Champaign, IL: Human Kinetics, 1995.

58. White-Welkley, J. E., E. C. Dunn, S. Nowicki, M. Duke, and L. Price. Excessive exercise, psychopathologic symptoms and eating attitudes among female non-athletic adults. *J. Sport Exercise Psychol.* 20 (supplement):S97, 1998.

59. Wiggins, D. K. The history of sport psychology in North America. In: *Psychological Foundations of Sport,* J. M. Silva and R. S. Weinberg (Eds.). Champaign, IL: Human Kinetics, 1984, pp. 9–22.

60. Williams, J. M., and W. F. Straub. Sport psychology: Past, present, and future. In: *Applied Sport Psychology,* J. M. Williams (Ed.). Palo Alto, CA: Mayfield Company, 1986, pp. 1–13.

61. Willis, J. D., and L. F. Campbell. *Exercise Psychology.* Champaign, IL: Human Kinetics, 1992.

62. Ziegler, E. F. *Philosophical Foundation for Physical, Health and Recreation Education.* Englewood Cliffs, NJ: Prentice Hall, 1964.

CHAPTER

9

Measurement in Exercise Science

DALE P. MOOD

Uses of Measurement
Classification
Motivation
Achievement Assessment
Potential and Prediction
Diagnosis
Program Evaluation
Research

Nature of Measurement
Measurement versus Evaluation
Precision of Measurement
Levels of Measurement

Domains of Human Experience

A Brief History of Measurement in Exercise Science

Applications of Measurement
Cognitive
Psychomotor
Psychological (or Affective)

Accuracy of Measurement
Reliability
Validity

Other Venues of Interest for the Measurement Specialist

The Measurement Specialist's Opportunities and Responsibilities

Prominent Journals

Summary

Study Questions

Glossary

Suggested Readings

References

All disciplines rely on the existence of accurate assessment of variables of interest. As intuitive as this statement is, it is sometimes forgotten in the excitement of proposing new ways to accomplish goals or designing research projects. For example, if we believe that exposure to a particular exercise regime will improve some attribute of a group of individuals (say, physical fitness, or attitude toward activity, or knowledge about heart rates), how do we determine if our belief is true or not? Implicit in making such a determination is the fact that we can accurately assess the amount of the attribute that the individuals possess. There exists an entire field of study involving the procedures for developing, evaluating the accuracy of, and refining measurement practices associated with variables of interest to the exercise scientist.

As has been made clear in the introductory chapters of this book, exercise science is a relatively new discipline, emerging as a specialized focus and integration of several older disciplines. The measurement practices, techniques, and concerns of exercise science also trace their roots back to these related disciplines.

Uses of Measurement

Throughout this chapter, exercise science measurement is classified in many ways. One possible scheme is to organize measurement according to its intent or purpose. The following presentation represents one of innumerable ways that this could be done, and you should notice that there is overlap among these divisions.

Classification

Assessment of the degree to which individuals possess some attribute allows classification of these individuals into discrete groups. This might be done, for example, to facilitate instruction (ability grouping) or to place subjects into appropriate treatment groups in a research project. A complex subset of this purpose of measurement is the construction of norms. A current interest among exercise scientists is determining the *cut-off points* above which a child is considered to possess enough of various attributes (for example, strength or flexibility) to be classified as physically fit in a health-related sense.

Motivation

Comparison of achievement to norms or standards can provide interest and may foster the setting of goals. Although there is some controversy regarding the soundness of using external motivators to encourage learning, there is little doubt that you will pay more attention to the material in this book if you are aware that progress toward certain goals will be measured periodically than if it were not.

Achievement Assessment

Typically, in a program of instruction of training a set of objectives or goals is determined. Measurement is used as the participants move through the program (called formative evaluation) to assess improvement and progress toward the goals and usually at the end of the program (called summative evaluation) to assess the final level of achievement obtained by each participant. Formative and summative evaluations each have inherent assumptions and concerns that the measurement specialist needs to take into account if the results of assessment are to be accurate and meaningful.

Potential and Prediction

An exciting and very useful arena for the application of measurement techniques is in forecasting an individual's potential in a future setting (for example, making the Olympic volleyball team) or in predicting the future based on known tendencies. For example, the exercise epidemiologist may use assessment of cardiovascular endurance measures, physical activity patterns, and other factors to predict your risk of developing cardiovascular disease. The development of precise measurement tools and procedures and the use of sophisticated statistical techniques are required in this measurement area.

Diagnosis

Evaluation of test results is often used to determine weaknesses or deficiencies. For example, a cardiologist may administer a treadmill stress test to obtain exercise electrocardiograms to diagnose the possible presence of or extent of coronary heart disease. Or if a student is having difficulty in learning a particular gymnastics movement, the instructor may use tests to diagnose whether it is a lack of strength, a lack of coordination, or some other problem causing the difficulty.

Program Evaluation

At times it may become necessary to investigate successful achievement of program objectives. A physical educator may need to assess whether his or her students are receiving adequate physical fitness training. A comparison of the students' fitness test results with the district (or state or national) norms may be in order. Directors of corporate or commercial fitness programs may decide to measure client success and satisfaction through testing and surveys.

Research

A knowledge of proper measurement techniques is a requirement for anyone seeking to do research in the area of exercise science. In addition, an awareness of the complexities of research design and of statistical treatment of data are required. What may not be as apparent is that exercise science practitioners also need to be equipped with much of this same knowledge to intelligently read, evaluate, and make use of this research.

Nature of Measurement

Measurement versus Evaluation

In exercise science the typical meaning of the word *measurement* refers to the act of assigning a number to each member of a group of individuals or objects based on the amount of some attribute that each possesses (see Figure 9.1). *Evaluation,* on the other hand, is a statement of quality, goodness, value, or merit about what has been measured (see Figure 9.2). The act of evaluation involves decision making, and the decision is usually based, in part, on measurements and in part on a knowledge of normative data. For example, if you use a stopwatch to time an individual running the 50-yard dash, you are making a measurement. When you comment to the individual, "Wow, that was fast," you are making an evaluation. Notice that a time of 7.5 seconds would be considered "fast" for a ten-year-old girl but the same measurement for a 15-year-old boy would be evaluated as "slow."

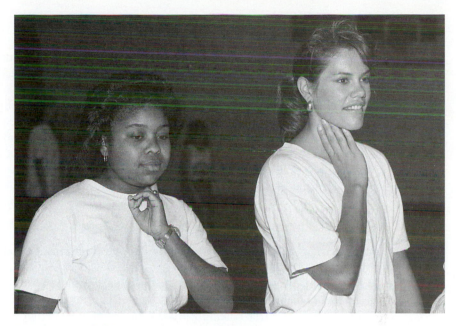

FIGURE 9.1   Subjects measuring their heart rates.

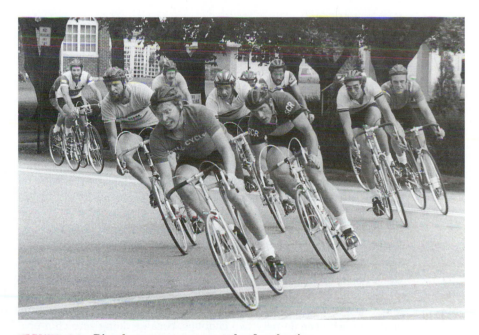

FIGURE 9.2   Bicycle racers as an example of evaluation.

Precision of Measurement

Some attributes can be measured very accurately and others cannot. Typically, the characteristics that can be measured directly (such as time to run the 50-yard dash) can be assessed with higher precision than characteristics that are measured indirectly (such as the percent of body weight comprised of fat).

Another element in the precision of measurement involves the clarity of the definition of the attributes to be assessed. For example, the measurement of response time, defined as the time elapsed between the presentation of a stimulus and the end of the required movement, is relatively unambiguous. However, even with the amount of attention it has received in recent years, there is not universal agreement among exercise scientists as to the specific elements of physical fitness.

Levels of Measurement

Measurements may be classified on the basis of the type of information that they yield. For example, it would be possible to rank a group of individuals in height by inspection, or it would be possible to assess the height of each individual using a measuring tape and recording height in inches or centimeters. The type of information resulting from the two procedures is different. In the ranking procedure, the results only permit statements such as "Sally is shorter than Betty," but use of the second procedure makes it possible to determine how much shorter Sally is than Betty. Measurements can be placed into four categories (nominal, ordinal, interval, and ratio) based on the information that they provide.

Nominal Measurement.   *Nominal measurement* conveys a minimal amount of information. It permits only the assessment of equality or difference. Nominal measurement often uses word descriptors to classify people or objects into categories. For example, a person may be classified as a letter winner, a girl, having brown hair, and so on. Occasionally, numerals are used in a nominal way. Baseball players, for example, are identified by numerals on their uniforms, but statements about the ordering or that one baseball player is greater than another based on their identification numbers are not possible.

Ordinal Measurement.   *Ordinal measurement* permits the ranking of the people or objects measured. Information regarding greater than or less than becomes relevant with ordinal measurement. Individuals' ability in handball may be ranked at the completion of a round-robin tournament, for example.

Interval Measurement.   *Interval measurement* permits the making of statements of equality of intervals. Temperature is an example of interval measurement. The same distance exists on the Fahrenheit scale between 0° and 40° as exists between 40° and 80°. However, it is not appropriate to say that 80° is twice as hot as 40°, because the zero point on the Fahrenheit scale is an arbitrary point and does not really indicate absence of heat. Likewise a fifth-grade boy who can do four chin-ups is not twice a strong as another fifth-grade boy who can do only two chin-ups, because doing zero chin-ups does not indicate the absolute lack of any upper arm strength.

Ratio Measurement. *Ratio measurement* permits statements of comparison such as twice as much or one-third as much. To achieve this level of measurement, an absolute zero point is necessary. It is possible to say, for example, that a high jump of 6 feet is twice as high as a high jump of 3 feet.

The higher the level of measurement is, the more information is gained and thus the more useful it is. Although it is true that one should always adopt procedures using the highest level of measurement possible, it is also true that there are times when only a lower level of measurement is possible. For example, if an athletic trainer is interested in evaluating various modalities for treating muscle soreness, the measurement of this condition relies on ordinal measurement. "On a scale from one to five, how sore is your muscle?" Currently, no calipers are available to assign an interval score of some sort to reflect the degree of soreness present.

Statisticians have devised many statistical tools that assume that at least interval level measures are involved. These statistical tests are categorized as parametric statistics. Another branch of statistics, called nonparametric statistics, exists also, and it consists of procedures allowing measurement at the nominal and ordinal levels. As expected nonparametric statistics are not as powerful as parametric statistics due to the reduced amount of information available from the level of measurement employed.

Domains of Human Experience

Another way to classify measurement associated with exercise science (or almost any academic discipline for that matter) is into the three domains of cognitive, affective, and psychomotor. The *cognitive domain* involves objectives in knowledge and mental achievement. The *affective domain* (sometimes called psychological) is concerned with attitudes and perceptions, and, of major interest to the exercise scientist, the *psychomotor domain* involves physiological and physical performance.

These domains have been studied over the years, and structures have been devised to explain a hierarchical nature of elements in each. These structures are called taxonomies. An example of a taxonomy (classification system) for each of the domains is presented next, but realize that others exist.

I. Taxonomy of the Cognitive Domain (1)
   1. Knowledge
      a. Knowledge of specifics
      b. Knowledge of ways and means of dealing with specifics
      c. Knowledge of the universals and abstractions in a field
   2. Comprehension
      a. Translation
      b. Interpretation
      c. Extrapolation
      d. Application

   3. Analysis
      a. Analysis of elements
      b. Analysis of relationships
      c. Analysis of organizational principles
   4. Synthesis
      a. Production of unique communications
      b. Production of a plan for operations
      c. Derivation of a set of abstract relations
   5. Evaluation
      a. Judgments in terms of internal evidence
      b. Judgments in terms of external evidence

II.   Taxonomy of the Affective Domain (4)
      a. Receiving
      b. Awareness
      c. Willingness to receive
   1. Controlled or selected attention
      a. Responding
      b. Acquiescence in responding
      c. Willingness to respond
      d. Satisfaction in response
   2. Valuing
      a. Acceptance of a value
      b. Performance of a value
      c. Commitment
   3. Organization
      a. Conceptualization of a value
      b. Organization of a value system
   4. Characterization by a value complex
      a. Generalized set
      b. Characterization

III. Taxonomy of the Psychomotor Domain (2)
   1. Reflex movements
      a. Segmental reflexes
      b. Intersegmental reflexes
      c. Suprasegmental reflexes
   2. Basic-fundamental movements
      a. Locomotor movements
      b. Nonlocomotor movements
      c. Manipulative movements
   3. Perceptual abilities
      a. Kinesthetic discrimination
      b. Visual discrimination
      c. Auditory discrimination

    d. Tactile discrimination
    e. Coordinated abilities
4. Physical abilities
    a. Endurance
    b. Strength
    c. Flexibility
    d. Agility
5. Skilled movements
    a. Simple adaptive skill
    b. Compound adaptive skill
    c. Complex adaptive skill
6. Nondiscursive movements
    a. Expressive movement
    b. Interpretive movement

These hierarchial taxonomies are of value to the measurement specialist in devising assessment procedures. The assumption is that each level of the taxonomy is based on the notion that earlier levels have been achieved.

For example, it is possible to *know* that the valence of oxygen is –2. In fact, if you just read the previous sentence (and accept it as true), you now have this knowledge. Without this type of knowledge, you cannot move to the next level (comprehension). To comprehend that valence has to do with the degree of combining power of an element based on its atomic weight requires knowledge of particular valences and much more, but it would not be possible to explain what would happen (application, the next level in this cognitive domain taxonomy) in a new situation without this comprehension. Notice how each level builds on the previous ones.

As another example, it would not be appropriate to measure complex motor skills in a young child who has not yet developed to that level of a psychomotor domain. The measurement specialist must be cognizant of these domains and taxonomies to develop measuring instruments and procedures that are appropriate for whatever situation is involved.

A Brief History of Measurement in Exercise Science

Exercise science is a very young discipline. It has developed from the field of physical education in a rather unusual way. Most disciplines move from the general to specifics. For example, physics now contains subfields such as subatomic particle physics and nuclear physics. Physical education started as a notion that there should be organized ways to teach individuals how to do certain physical skills (mostly gymnastics) and has now evolved to the study of physical activity and its impact on everything from mental well-being to the aging process. Therefore, the early history of exercise science is found in the development of physical education.

From 1776 to 1860. The United States was predominantly an agrarian society until the Industrial Revolution, which had its beginning around the turn of the century. From 1776 to 1830, education in the United States was mostly provided by and for the aristocratic segments of the population. This was the era of the Latin grammar school, with educational emphasis on classical studies. Beginning in the 1830s, a trend toward more useful education developed, and the population of the United States began to realize the necessity of universal education supported by taxes.

Physical education was very unstructured throughout this period. The basic influences on physical activity during the later stages were Johann Heinrich Pestalozzi and his disciple Joseph Neff, the German Turners, and the establishment of various religious organizations such as the YMCA. In general, the philosophy of these individuals and organizations was that physical activity (mostly in the form of gymnastic movements) should be engaged in for healthful reasons and to serve as a diversion from other aspects of life. Measurement in physical education was virtually nonexistent during this time.

From 1860 to 1900.   Some historians cite the early part of this period as the beginning of formal physical education in the United States. In 1861, Edward Hitchcock was appointed director of the department of hygiene and physical education at Amherst College. The establishment of such a department by William Stearns, the president of Amherst, gave academic status to the discipline of physical education for the first time. Like Hitchcock, many physical education leaders of this period had medical degrees and as youths had become interested in gymnastics. Dudley Sargent, professor of physical education at Harvard University, Edward M. Hartwell, director of physical education at Johns Hopkins University, and William G. Anderson, associate director of the gymnasium of Yale University, are examples of such individuals.

The medical backgrounds for many physical education leaders of this period probably explains their interest in anthropometric measurements. Students at Amherst College were periodically given a series of tests centered around anthropometric and strength measures. Cromwell investigated the growth patterns of boys and girls between the ages of 8 and 18. Statues of the typical male and female, constructed on the basis of a vast number of anthropometric measurements taken and recorded by Sargent, were displayed at the 1933 World's Fair in Chicago.

The most common form of organized physical activity during this period was gymnastics. Individuals advocated use of the German or Swedish systems or systems that they themselves had developed. The German system involved apparatus work and free exercise; the Swedish system was more scientifically and medically oriented. Dio Lewis and Francois Delsarte are two who advocated the use of their own gymnastics systems.

Although the schools of the time were heavily influenced by the proponents of these various gymnastics systems, the beginnings of two other forms of physical activity, strength development and athletics, can be traced to this period. The exercise regimens of George Winship and William Blackie are examples of programs devised during this period for the purpose of developing and maintaining strength. As previously mentioned, Hitchcock's periodic testing at Amherst involved strength measures. Sargent also expressed an interest in the measurement of strength. In fact, he devised a battery of tests that included items intended to measure the strength of the legs, back, grip, arms, and respiratory muscles. This test battery became known as the Intercollegiate Strength Test and was used as a basis for intercollegiate competition. It was later revised by Rogers and later still by McCloy. Thus, the development and consequently the measurement of various strength parameters gradually became integrated with the existing anthropometric measurement programs in this period.

Athletic programs, both intramural and intercollegiate, were common at many of the educational institutions during this period. However, athletics were primarily considered to be of recreational value, with gymnastics and physical training programs serving as the basis for physical education classes. Main events—the establishment of the United States Lawn Tennis Association in 1881, the invention of basketball in 1891, the formation of the United States Golf Association in 1894, and the participation of some athletes from the United States in the revived Olympic Games in 1896, to name a few—depict the growing interest in athletic activities. It was during the latter portion of this period that the application of measurement techniques to athletics began. For example, in 1890 Luther H. Gulick devised a pentathlon consisting of a rope climb and four track events, including the 100-yard dash, hop–skip–jump, running high jump, and shot put.

From 1900 to 1940.   Measurement in the beginning of this period continued in the trend of anthropometrics. However, several seemingly isolated events were beginning to have a cumulative effect on the educators of the time: the implications in Darwin's theories; the early development of the science of psychology as a study of the relationships between the mind and the body; and the educational theories of E. L. Thorndike, John Dewey, and G. Stanley Hall in which transfer of training, learning by doing, and identification of stages of development were integral parts.

Thomas D. Wood and Clark W. Hetherington are often cited by historians as two physical education leaders who, in the early 1900s, did much to influence the philosophy of physical education. Generally, their contention, influenced by the changing educational philosophies of the day, was that physical education should not only be education of the physical, but also education *through* the physical. Hetherington proposed that social and intellectual, as well as organic and neuromuscular objectives could be met through physical education programs.

The dramatic shift in educational philosophy during the early part of this period resulted in sweeping changes in the curricula of the schools and the methods of instruction. Along with these changes came a realization of the importance of measurement in education. The initial emphasis was the development, refinement, and administration of intelligence tests. James K. Catell, Lewis M. Terman, and Henry H. Goddard are names of some of the most prominent workers in this area.

In physical education it became important to measure many parameters besides body structure and strength. In 1902, Sargent's Universal Test for Speed, Strength, and Endurance was introduced. An interest arose in the circulatory system, as shown by Crampton's Blood Ptosis Test presented in 1905 and by the norms for blood pressure and heart rate developed by J. H. McCurdy in 1910. In 1913 the Athletic Badge Tests in baseball, basketball, tennis, and volleyball were devised. These are a few examples of the diverse areas into which the physical educators of the period were expanding.

By the middle of the period, initial tests had been developed for most of the parameters that are measured in physical education classes today. Many of these initial attempts were crude, subjective, and inexact, but they were refined as time passed. Precision, objectiveness, and test construction methods improved. Most importantly, advances made in the areas of mathematics and statistics made improved measurement techniques possible. Measurement equipment, used in some cases, improved with the increase of technological skills.

From 1940 to 1945.   World War II generated a great increase in concern for physical fitness. The main emphasis of physical education in the United States swung away from the expanded and varied program to physical training.

The elementary schools retained physical education programs in the sense that the curricula generally involved games, folk dancing, basic sports skills, and gymnastics. The secondary school physical education programs, however, were influenced more strongly by the war effort. The High School Victory Corps was organized nationally, partially to emphasize physical fitness and military drill in high school physical education classes. In colleges and universities, the physical fitness emphasis was manifested by a revival of self-defense and survival activities such as weight lifting, combatives, and swimming. Although several physical educators of the time questioned the switch in objectives by pointing out that physical education should be considered more than education of the physical, the stress on physical fitness prevailed.

Measurement in physical education followed the national trend, and measurement of physical fitness parameters became dominant. The military services established physical fitness tests during this period. Unfortunately, because of the extreme interest in and emphasis on physical fitness measurement during this time, physical education measurement became synonymous with physical fitness testing to a great segment of the population of the United States.

From 1945 to 1950.   There are abundant examples throughout history of the pendulum effect, in which emphasis swings gradually from one extreme to another. One of these examples is provided by the fluctuation of the major thrust of physical education during and after World War II.

After the war the people of the United States, tired from the strains of maintaining the war effort, became interested in peaceful pursuits. Educators began returning to the consideration of social objectives that had been becoming prevalent before the war. Physical educators shared in the movement by once again stressing the social and recreational objectives of physical education.

From 1950 to 1960.   Unfortunately, peace did not last long. The early 1950s brought the Korean conflict and the beginning of the cold war between the United States and Russia. The Minimum Muscular Fitness Test of Hans Kraus and Sonya Weber indicated a significant difference in favor of European children over U.S. children. These and other events once again stirred up a great interest in physical fitness. The return to concern for physical fitness was reflected in many events: the organization of the President's Council on Youth Fitness, development of the AAHPERD Youth Fitness Test, and President John F. Kennedy's article in *Sports Illustrated,* "The Soft American," to name only a few. The social, intellectual, and recreational objectives of physical education, although certainly not completely ignored, were once again considered of secondary importance.

From 1960 to 1970.   The period shortly after the launching of Sputnik 1 in 1957 is often cited as the beginning of the tremendous emphasis placed on the sciences in U.S. schools during the 1960s. This shift in educational philosophy resulted in critical examination of the "nonscientific" segments of school curricula and consequently a defensive attitude on the part of many physical educators. Although generalizations can be misleading, if only one word could be used to describe the greatest single concern of physical education in this decade, that word would be research. Certainly, research was done in physical education throughout the twentieth century, but during this period the volume of research quite possibly equaled all that was done previously. Three related factors lead to this occurrence.

First, the number of institutions offering undergraduate and graduate degrees in physical education had increased sharply. The ability to do research is considered important for students in these programs, so the amount of physical education research being done increased. Second, with the emphasis on the sciences, federal funding for research and research facilities was available. Third, again due to the emphasis on the sciences, nonscientific segments of the curricula were being pared, and physical educators had to have research available to argue for their retention in the curriculum. This was most likely the beginning of the change from physical education to exercise science.

The increased efforts in research had a tremendous impact on measurements in this area. During this time a great proportion of the measurement techniques and tools now in use were developed, studied, revised, and described in the literature.

From 1970 to the present.   Certainly, the most difficult time period to examine from a historical perspective is the present. It is difficult to determine whether an event is a relatively isolated occurrence or part of a developing trend. With this in mind, an examination of important recent events reveals possible directions for exercise science and consequently exercise science measurement.

One of the most important single events in this period was the Vietnam War. The sustained effort in this conflict had two major effects on exercise science. The concern for physical fitness remained a dominant influence throughout the United States. (This fact is still reflected in several current trends, including the increase in articles and books dealing primarily with physical fitness and the inclusion of physical fitness units in most physical education curricula.) Furthermore the national economic problems started during the Vietnam era have eliminated or reduced many sources of monies for research projects in many fields, including exercise science.

It appears that the type of research done in the 1970s became wider in scope. Some researchers began branching into more theoretical types of study, while others concentrated on what might be called applied research.

Perhaps we have come full circle now, because exercise science research is becoming specific rather than general. In recent history we talk about exercise physiology, motor control, biomechanics, nutrition, sports psychology, and others as areas of study within the field called exercise science (or human performance, or kinesiology, or...).

It is certainly the case that measurement since 1970 has become much more technologically oriented and that the computer has had a great influence on the measurement specialist. Highly sophisticated computer-assisted performance analyzers, magnetic resonance imaging

(Figure 3.8) tests, computer programmable treadmills, and highly complex statistical packages available on floppy disks are just a few examples of recent innovations.

Applications of Measurement

Because the exercise scientist works in such a variety of settings, the array of possible types of measurement applications is vast. No attempt will be made here to explain all that is involved in constructing valid measurement instruments or procedures. Rather, information is presented about some of the considerations around such a task and examples of some measurement instruments. Excellent textbooks (see Suggested Readings for this chapter) are available that describe the construction, validation, and use of exercise science measurement techniques. The discussion in this section is organized around the three domains described earlier: cognitive, affective, and psychomotor.

Cognitive

There are many instances when the primary objective of an exercise scientist is to determine or increase the individual's knowledge and understanding about physical activity. This typically requires measurement of cognitive processes and is usually done through the use of a written examination.

There are multiple sources of written tests. Textbook publishers, state agencies, and national corporations specializing in test construction are potential places to obtain already constructed tests. However, in the field of exercise science, outside sources of written tests are rather limited. In fact, the most common source is the exercise scientist. The upside of this situation is that the person making the assessment should be able to construct the most valid test (one that measures what it is intended to measure). The downside is that knowing what to measure is not the same as knowing how to measure it. The exercise scientist in this situation is required to learn the principles of written test construction.

The efficient written test constructor must meet five requirements. You first must be aware of the proper techniques for written test construction (more about this later). Second, you must have a very thorough knowledge about the subject area to be tested. The third qualification is to be skilled at written expression. Test questions constructed by individuals lacking in this area are often ambiguous and lead to incorrect conclusions, which reduces the usefulness of the instrument. You must also have an awareness of the range and level of understanding of the individuals to be assessed. Questions that are too difficult or too easy do not efficiently discriminate among individuals. Finally, you must realize that building adequate written tests takes a considerable amount of time and trial and error. Potential test items need to be tried out and revised, sometimes many times, before they function appropriately.

If you look over these five requirements, you will notice that the last four are characteristics of a careful researcher or exercise scientist. It is really only the first requirement, knowledge of proper test construction techniques, that requires study. Again, in this chapter it is only possible to present an outline of the types of issues to be considered.

Planning the Written Test. The first issue here is to determine if the test is to be a mastery test (designed to measure whether the examinee has enough understanding to achieve a prescribed standard) or to be an achievement test (designed to discriminate among various levels of understanding).

The next (and very important) decision in planning the test is to determine *what* is to be measured. This involves building a table of specification, which is a matrix involving educational objectives on one axis and content objectives on the other. It is a blueprint for the written test.

How to Measure. Issues to consider here include (1) when to test, (2) how many questions to include, (3) the format to use, and (4) the type of questions to use.

Administering the Written Test. Such concerns as anxiety of examinees, test distribution, security, and prevention of cheating are involved in the test administration.

Analyzing the Written Test. The major concerns in analyzing the written test are determining its reliability and validity as a measuring instrument and assessing the effectiveness of each item on the test. These procedures are somewhat complex, but necessary and important to ensure that the written test accurately assesses what it is intended to measure. Additional information about the validity and reliability of measurement is presented later in this chapter.

Psychomotor

Accurate assessment of physical characteristics is of utmost importance to the exercise scientist. Because there has been a relatively recent increase (that is, last 30 years) in interest in physical fitness in the United States, this section is divided into two parts, the assessment of fitness and the assessment of sports skills and motor abilities.

Physical Fitness. The interest in physical fitness has waxed and waned over the years. Currently, it seems to be here to stay. Early measurement of physical fitness included assessing such elements as muscular strength, posture, speed, power, agility, and muscular endurance. In the 1970s a concept involving *health-related fitness* emerged, and the characteristics deemed important changed to cardiovascular endurance, body composition, and musculoskeletal function. Precisely how these elements are to be measured is still being debated among exercise scientists, but most physical fitness tests now include some of the following types of measurements:

1. Endurance runs (distance vary according to the ages of the individuals being assessed)
2. Calculation of percentage of body comprised of fat (techniques of assessment vary from a procedure involving weighing individuals underwater to measuring skinfold thickness and various body girths)
3. Musculoskeletal function (various assessment of muscular performance, such as sit-ups, pull-ups, and sit and reach)

Many exercise scientists, including measurement specialists, are currently working on many aspects of the assessment of physical fitness. Among the issues are defining the concept (that is, precisely what is physical fitness?), how to most accurately assess those elements deemed essential, the minimal amount of each characteristic that is deemed sufficient to be considered healthy, how to define and measure physical fitness for various subsets of the population (children through older adults, males versus females, individuals with physical disabilities, and so on), and many other issues.

Sports Skills and Motor Abilities.   Exercise scientists primarily involved in the area of teaching sports skills and motor abilities (that is, physical educators and coaches) are very interested in assessing these qualities prior to, during, and after engaging in activities to improve them. Although a large number of tests and procedures has been developed over the years to make such assessments, the exercise scientist is often faced with a unique situation in which the knowledge of how to construct such a measuring instrument is invaluable.

In this chapter it is not possible to list all the tests and measuring devices that already exist (several measurement books are available for this), nor is it possible to provide details on the many considerations to be taken into account when constructing your own. Hensely (3) has provided some guidelines however, to indicate the complexity involved. He states that these tests should:

1. Have at least minimally acceptable reliability and validity.
2. Be simple to take and to administer.
3. Have easily understood instructions.
4. Require neither expensive nor extensive equipment.
5. Be reasonable in terms of preparation and administration time.
6. Encourage correct form and be gamelike, but involve only one performer.
7. Be of suitable difficulty (neither too difficult nor too simple.
8. Be meaningful to the performer.
9. Exclude extraneous variables as much as possible.
10. Provide for accurate scoring.
11. Follow specific guidelines if a target is the basis for scoring.
12. Require a sufficient number of trials to obtain a reasonable measure of performance (tests that have accuracy as a principal component require more trials than tests measuring other characteristics).
13. Yield scores that provide for diagnostic interpretation whenever possible.

Although it is probably impossible to meet all these guidelines in any single test, complying with as many as possible will provide the most valuable measurements.

Psychological (or Affective)

Of general importance in this domain are assessments of attitudes, states, and traits. Of specific interest is the assessment of these characteristics as they relate to physical performance. For example, many individuals might be concerned with the assessment of anxiety or motivation, but the exercise scientist is particularly interested in how these characteristics might affect physical performance.

As with the other two domains, it is not possible here to present in detail the myriad of complex issues associated with the development of measuring instruments in the *affective domain*. Rather an attempt will be made to indicate the type and scope of concerns in this arena.

Because it is well known that the mind affects the body, the way individuals think and feel has a strong influence on physical performance. This connection is the major interest of exercise scientists concentrating in this field. Such psychological factors as anxiety, motivation, concentration, personality, confidence, and mental practice are among the most commonly investigated. Another main focus has to do with the possibility that the body can affect the mind. For example, there are many who study whether sport and physical activity might have the capacity to positively influence mental health through reduction in depression and an increase in self-worth.

Some of the most interesting areas of research for the exercise scientist interested in the psychological domain include the following:

1. State versus trait measures (state measures are more concerned with the situation at hand and trait measurements with a more stable characteristic within the individual)
2. General versus sport-specific measures (Should personality traits be assessed globally or in the context of specific sport situations?)
3. How should team members be selected with regard to assessment of psychological traits?
4. What factors affect individuals' attitudes toward physical activity and their motivation to participate in these types of experiences?

Exercise scientists working in the affective domain in the past probably relied, more than those studying the cognitive or psychomotor domains, on measuring instruments constructed by experts, rather than developing their own. This is changing today as the trend seems to be shifting toward assessment of more specific traits as opposed to relying on general tests. Thus, as with exercise scientists working in the cognitive and psychomotor domains, those working in the psychological domain must become increasingly aware of how to recognize when a measuring instrument is accurately assessing the desired characteristics. To do this, it is necessary to understand two very important constructs: validity and reliability. These are the focus of the next section.

Accuracy of Measurement

The two most fundamental questions to be answered regarding the accuracy of a measurement process are whether it actually measures what it is intended to measure (validity) and whether it does so consistently (reliability). *Validity,* then, is the degree of truthfulness in a measurement, and *reliability* is the consistency or repeatability of a measurement.

Reliability

The typical procedure in making a measurement is to use some test, device, or procedure to assign a numerical score to reflect the amount of some characteristic possessed by an individual. We can recognize by intuition that no matter how carefully this is done there exists the possibility of error entering into this process. For example, we could misread the scale, we could record an incorrect number, we could not record the individual's best effort, and so on. Only when no error is present (a condition seldom, if ever, achieved) is a measurement perfectly reliable. As the amount of error increases, the reliability of the measurement decreases.

One way to think about this is to consider an observed score (the one that you assign) to be the sum of the true score and any error that might have occurred. Then for any set of individuals measured, we would have three columns of scores: observed, true, and error. Each column would have a mean and some variability in the values listed, as shown in Table 9.1.

In theory, if the error that occurs is random (that is, is not systematic, like a scale that is off by 2 pounds for everyone, but rather is due to imprecision in our process), the sum of the error scores and thus the average (x) error score should be zero. However, as shown in Table 9.1, error of measurement did occur for all individuals except F and J. The variability of the scores in the three columns is reflected by a statistic called *variance* (s^2). Notice that the sum of the true score variance and the error score variance is equal to the observed score variance. One method of expressing the reliability of a measurement is to calculate the ratio of the true score variance to the observed score variance (in this example the ratio is 105.0/120.2 or .87. It can be seen that if no error were present the ratio would be 105.0/105.0 or 1.00, indicating perfect reliability).

Of course, this is a fictional example because the only column you actually ever know is the "observed." This example is helpful, however, because reliability can be calculated through various procedures, and it is most often expressed as a correlation coefficient (a statistic having a range of –1.0 to +1.0). Thus, if a test were reported to have a reliability of .87 (calculated by using a test–retest procedure), we could interpret what this represents

TABLE 9.1

Individual	Observed	=	True	+	Error
A	3		5		–2
B	17		15		+2
C	16		20		–4
D	23		25		–2
E	27		25		–2
F	25		25		0
G	35		25		+10
H	26		30		–4
I	33		35		–2
J	45		45		0
x	25		25		0
s^2	120.2		105.0		15.2

in terms of true and observed variance and thus have some notion of reliability of the measure in question.

Methods for assessing reliability include test–retest (actually a stability indicator), equivalence (two "equivalent" but not identical measurements of the same characteristic are compared), split halves (one-half of a measuring instrument, for example, the odd-numbered items on a written test are compared with the other half, the even-numbered items), and intraclass (used when more than two trials of a test are available; for example, 4 trials of the standing long jump are measured on a group of individuals). Each of these methods has its proper situation for use, but the net result is a reflection of the consistency of the measurement expressed as a correlation coefficient.

Another helpful way to interpret a reliability coefficient is to determine its square root. This produces a statistic called the index of reliability and is the theoretical correlation between the observed scores and the true scores. In our example (rel = .87) this value would be .93.

It should be intuitive that to be of any value a measurement process must result in a consistent score being assigned to an individual. How much confidence would you have, for example, in a scale that gave you a different weight each time that you stepped up on it? However, reliability is not the only concern regarding the accuracy and usefulness of a measurement. For example, if you had a very reliable scale, but someone told you it was a measure of your flexibility, you might raise questions about the measurement (weight in pounds) reflecting much if anything about flexibility. This is the issue of validity.

Validity

Validity deals with the truthfulness of the measurement (that is, whether the measurement reflects the amount of the characteristic that you actually are trying to measure). It is rather easy to see in the preceding example that weight in pounds is probably not a very good (valid) measure of flexibility. Sometimes the invalidity of a measurement is not so obvious. Consider a device to measure biceps strength consisting of a bar held in front of the body with both hands with a 90° angle at the elbow. Assume that the bar is attached to a dynamometer anchored in the floor and that the dynamometer records the force when the individual attempts to pull up on the bar.

At first inspection this apparatus would seem to measure biceps strength, but what if a particular individual's wrists were not able to remain extended? Perhaps this individual's biceps strength score would be lower than he or she could actually achieve if the test did not also rely on wrist strength.

As with reliability, there are various ways to examine validity and their use is situation specific. Three will be briefly described here: content-, criterion-, and construct-related evidence.

Content-related Evidence.   Evidence for *content validity* considers the degree to which the sample of tasks or items on a test represents the actual content to be assessed. For example, you might examine the questions on a written examination to determine how well they cover the material to be tested. As another example, some might question the content validity of selecting offensive linemen for a football team on the basis of their time to run a 40-yard dash, a task they seldom perform in the game.

Criterion-related Evidence.   Evidence for *criterion validity* is based on examination of how well the measurement correlates with a criterion measure believed to be a true assessment of the characteristic of interest. For example, the VO_2 max test performed on a treadmill is considered to produce an accurate measurement of cardiovascular endurance. However, this test requires a great deal of equipment, time, and personnel to administer. Because the correlations between VO_2 max tests and various distance-run tests (depending on age and gender of the participants) have been found to be quite high; the distance-run tests are thought to be valid indicators of cardiovascular fitness.

Construct-related Evidence.   Evidence for *construct validity* is collected to validate measures that are nonobservable yet are thought to exist. For example, the concept of IQ is a construct. It is not tangible. The typical procedure for collecting construct validity evidence is to conduct experiments with the hypothesis that a particular construct does exist. For example, is it possible that some individuals possess a higher degree of kinesthetic awareness than others? If so, and if a test of jumping forward while blindfolded to land at a certain spot on the floor actually measures the construct of kinesthetic awareness, it would be hypothesized that divers and gymnasts should perform better on the test than nonathletes. If this were confirmed, it would be evidence (not conclusive) that the test validity measured the construct.

The concepts of validity and reliability are critical to all scientists. Without accurate measurement, research and experimentation are impossible. This is as applicable to the exercise scientist as to the physicist or chemist. It is important to notice that a measurement does not have *a* validity or *a* reliability. The validity and reliability of a measurement are situation specific and relative. For example one individual might produce very reliable skinfold measurements and another individual might not. (This illustrates an important subset of reliability called *objectivity*.) A shuttle run test designed to validly measure the agility of 14-year-old boys may not measure this characteristic at all for 6-year-old girls. Thus, it is imperative to clearly understand the concepts of validity and reliability to evaluate the worth of any measurement process.

Other Venues of Interest for the Measurement Specialist

The measurement specialist in exercise science is primarily concerned with the accurate assessment of characteristics related to human performance from the cognitive, psychomotor, and affective domains. Closely related to this focus are expertise in the use of two tools. One is computers and the other is statistics.

Probably because the computer can efficiently and accurately manipulate numerical data and because the measurement specialist often works with numerical data sets, it is natural for the measurement specialist to become proficient in computer hardware and software use. Whether located in academia, a laboratory setting, or industry, it is very common for the measurement specialist in exercise science to also be the resident computer expert.

Statistics is a branch of mathematics, which in recent years has become very important to the researcher in exercise science. Statistical tests have a wide variety of applications, but primary among them is to determine if apparent relationships among variables are real or could possibly be due to chance. Although this is a vast oversimplification, the basic premise in using statistics is to determine the probability of an event occurring if no relationship between the variables of interest actually exists. If that probability is very small, it is taken as evidence that the relationship does exist. For example, assume that you randomly place 20 individuals into one of two groups. The 10 individuals assigned to one group are taught to ski using short skis, and the other 10 individuals assigned to the other group are taught to ski using conventional-length skis. Assume for the purposes of this illustration that all other conditions (except ski length) are identical for both groups.

Following the instructional period, a valid and reliable test of skiing ability is administered to all 20 individuals, with higher scores on the test indicating better skiing ability. Assume that the mean score for the short-ski group is 75 and the mean score for the conventional-length-ski group is 71. The question that a statistical test (called an independent t-test) could answer in this situation (if all 20 scores were available) is whether 75 is really significantly different from 71. In other words, what is the probability of this event (mean scores of 75 and 71) if there really is no connection between learning to ski with one of these two methods and the individual's skiing ability as reflected by the test? If the probability of this event is 1 in 100, we might be willing to believe that the two variables (method and skiing proficiency) are, in fact, related and thus it is better to teach people to ski using short skis. On the other hand, if the probability of this event is 50 out of 100, we probably would conclude that it was just chance that the short-ski group's score was higher than the other group's score.

As indicated, a vast number of statistical tests have been devised over the last 75 years, and each requires certain assumptions to be met if the test is to be employed. The measurement specialist, again because of the "number" connection, is often attracted to learning about statistics.

The natural connection between the computer software available for computing relatively complex statistical tests further cements the common venues of measurement, computer, and statistics often found to be of interest to the exercise science measurement specialist. It also should be apparent that knowledge in these areas often makes the measurement specialist a valuable consultant for other exercise scientists.

The Measurement Specialist's Opportunities and Responsibilities

In the past, most exercise science measurement specialists found employment in academia. They were most often located in physical education departments (now commonly called by many other names, such as human performance or kinesiology); taught measurement, statistics, and computer courses; did their own research in these areas; and served as consultants to departmental colleagues. For some, this is still the preferred avenue for using their interests and abilities. However, it is now also the case that exercise science measurement specialists are being employed elsewhere. Two of the most common areas are (1) the many venues that have sprung up with the recent increased awareness of the importance of wellness and physical fitness (for example, corporate wellness centers and exercise prescription consultants) and (2) laboratory settings dealing with the same issues, often under the direction of hospitals, corporations, and insurance companies.

It is interesting to notice that there are not many institutions of higher education producing exercise science measurement specialists, yet there are many professionals out in the field who serve in this capacity. This has come about mostly through need. Virtually all doctorate programs in exercise science have as a graduation requirement a relatively sophisticated level of exposure to statistics and research design courses, no matter what the area of specialization may be. Many times this exposure is obtained in graduate-level courses taught in education, psychology, or other disciplines.

When an exercise science department that does not have a resident measurement specialist decides to offer courses in measurement, statistics, computers, research design, and related areas, often the faculty member with the most interest in these topics is asked to teach the courses and in the process, over time, becomes the measurement specialist in the department.

For the measurement specialist located in an academic setting as a faculty member, the types of activities that he or she would be engaged in vary considerably. And the type of institution can range from a community college to a research university. Although the emphasis and amount of time devoted to each activity would vary, the main activities can be placed into the three categories of scholarship, teaching, and service.

In the scholarship area the measurement specialist's activities focus on the creation of new knowledge and/or the application of previously discovered knowledge to new and different situations. For example, a measurement specialist might work to determine a noninvasive technique for determining muscle fiber type or might devise methods of modifying a measure of muscular strength designed for one segment of the population for use with a different subset. The types of measurement issues to be studied are virtually limitless.

Part of the work in this area is often done through experimentation and the gathering of data, and part of the work is in disseminating the results through writing articles or making presentations at relevant meetings. Occasionally, the measurement specialist may even contribute to a textbook as part of his or her scholarship effort.

A large portion of the time of a measurement specialist as a faculty member involves teaching. Most curricula in departments of physical education, human performance, kinesiology, and the like, contain many courses involving content in measurement, statistics, research design, and computers in varying combinations. Of course, teaching involves much more than presenting materials to a class of students. Preparation time, meeting with students, correcting assignments, constructing exams (something for which the measurement specialist should be well prepared), and the many other duties of a teacher are involved. Depending again on the institution, teaching duties can range from undergraduate and graduate classes to running seminar and journal clubs to directing theses and dissertations. The measurement specialist typically is involved with a large number of thesis and dissertation committees because they frequently include aspects of measurement and statistics.

Service responsibilities take many forms and can include work at the institution, state, region, national, and even international levels. Serving in various capacities on committees for the institution and for professional organizations (for example, the Measurement and Evaluation Council of the American Alliance for Health, Physical Education, Recreation and Dance) are examples. Being an editor or reviewer for various journals is another service activity.

Acting as a consultant for colleagues and students is another activity for the measurement specialist. It might be in conjunction with a research project or a grant proposal or to help with a statistical question. Because the measurement specialist in exercise science usually is equipped with many "tools," he or she is often the "mechanic" of many of a department's activities.

The measurement specialist located in a corporation, hospital, or business setting generally has two major functions. The first is to act as a consultant to colleagues in the area of measurement and research design, and the second is to act as fund raiser. Depending again on the specific location, the fund raising could be in the form of being the principle investigator or a consultant on a grant application, or it could be as a negotiator in obtaining a contract for services provided by the organization. In some cases the measurement specialist may concentrate on collecting, organizing, analyzing, and interpreting data collected by himself or herself or by others. An insurance company setting and a laboratory involved with tracking health and disease issues are examples of locations where data analysis and interpretation would be the major activities for the exercise science measurement specialist.

Along with expertise in computer usage, the measurement specialist typically has two other major areas of focus: statistics and measurement. Figures 9.3, 9.4, and 9.5 provide abstracts of recent journal articles in the areas of statistics, measurement, and computer applications in exercise science.

Prominent Journals

Because the measurement specialist can deal with a very large variety of assessment issues, it is difficult to restrict the identification of professional journals containing relevant information. The following list contains two sections: List A includes those journals most likely to contain articles specifically about the measurement process, and List B includes journals containing articles whose content is focused on other areas of the discipline, but which necessarily contain measurement practices.

List A

Applied Psychological Measurement
Educational and Psychological Measurement
Educational Measurement
Journal of Physical Education, Recreation and Dance
Measurement in Physical Education and Exercise Science
Research Quarterly for Exercise and Sport

FIGURE 9.3   Abstract of a research study in the area of statistics.

Thomas, J. R., M. R. Lochbaum, D. M. Landers, and C. He.
Planning Significant and Meaningful Research in Exercise Science: Estimating Sample Size.
Research Quarterly for Exercise and Sport, 68:33–43, 1997.

Exercise science researchers are familiar with the use of parametric tests to detect significant differences among treatment groups. However, in planning research a question asked with increasing frequency is, "How many participants are needed to detect real and meaningful differences among groups?" In this paper, we provide an overview of the use of alpha, power, and effect size in planning sample sizes that allow tests of real and meaningful differences among groups. Because effect size is the parameter most often missing, we have located meta-analyses in sport and exercise psychology ($n = 26$) and motor behavior ($n = 6$). We provide examples and a discussion of how researchers can use these effect sizes along with common estimates of alpha and power to plan for the sample size needed to detect real and meaningful group differences.

FIGURE 9.4   Abstract of a research study in the area of measurement.

H. W. Marsh.
Physical Self-description Questionnaire: Stability and Discriminate Validity.
Research Quarterly for Exercise and Sport, 67: 249–264, 1996.

The Physical Self-description Questionnaire (PSDQ) is a multidimensional, physical self-concept instrument designed to measure 11 scales: Strength, Body Fat, Activity, Endurance/Fitness, Sports Competence, Coordination, Health, Appearance, Flexibility, Global Physical Self-concept, and Global Esteem. High school students completed the PSDQ on four occasions over a 14-month period. Across the 11 PSDQ scales, the internal consistency at each occasion was good (median alpha -.92) and the stability over time varied from median $r = .83$ for a 3-month period to median $r - .69$ for the 14-month period. The data were used to demonstrate the application of confirmatory factor-analysis models of multitrait–multimethod (MTMM) data (with occasions as the multiple methods), which supported the discriminant validity of the PSDQ scales. Augmented MTMM models that included two field tests of cardiovascular endurance provided additional support for the construct validity of PSDQ responses and interpretations of the MTMM models. These results contribute to the growing body of support for the construct validity of physical-self-concept responses and illustrate the application of CFA MTMM models.

FIGURE 9.5   Abstract of a journal article about computer applications in exercise science.

J. C. Wendt and J. R. Morrow.
Microcomputer Software: Practical Applications for Coaches and Teachers.
Journal of Physical Education, Recreation and Dance, 57: 54–57, 1986.

Software is available to record sport performance, evaluate physical parameters to obtain health and nutrition data, receive scouting statistics, plan strategies, and schedule tournaments. Most current software is easy to use, has appropriate documentation, and is flexible enough to meet user demands.

Reprinted with permission from *Journal of Physical Education, Recreation, and Dance,* February, 1986, 54–57. *JOPERD* is a publication of the American Alliance for Health, Physical Education, Recreation and Dance, 1900 Association Drive, Reston, VA, 20191.

List B
Adapted Physical Activity Quarterly
American Heart Journal
American Journal of Epidemiology
American Journal of Health Promotion
American Psychologist
American Journal of Public Health
Archives of Physical Medicine and Rehabilitation
Circulation
Journal of Applied Physiology
Journal of Behavior Medicine
Journal of Chronic Diseases
Journal of Clinical Investigation
Journal of Educational Physiology
Journal of Health Education
Journal of Human Movement Studies
Journal of Occupational Medicine
Journal of Pediatrics
Journal of Sport and Exercise Physiology
Journal of Sport Psychology
Journal of Sports Medicine and Physical Fitness
Journal of Teaching Physical Education
Journal of the American Medical Association
Journal of the American Physical Therapy Association
Medicine and Science in Sports and Exercise
New England Journal of Medicine
Pediatric Exercise Science
Perceptual Motor Skills
Phi Delta Kappan

Quest
Sport Psychologist
The Physical Educator

Summary

The accurate measurement of variables is critical to all disciplines. In order for exercise scientists to be producers and/or wise consumers of the available information from research, they must be well grounded in measurement practices and techniques.

Measurement practices can be organized according to their purpose (such as: classification, motivation, achievement assessment, potential and prediction, diagnosis, program evaluation, and research.) Within each category, there are differences in the precision with which a variable can be measured. The level of measurement can be placed into four categories (nominal, ordinal, interval, and ration) based on the information that they provide.

Two important aspects of measurement are reliability and validity. Reliability is the extent to which a test consistently yields the same results when repeated under the same conditions. Validity is the degree to which a test measures what it is intended to measure. Research in all disciplines including exercise science requires that variables are reliable and valid.

STUDY QUESTIONS

1. Explain and give examples of several uses of measurement in exercise science.

2. What is the differences between measurement and evaluation?

3. Name the four levels of measurement and explain the type of information associated with each.

4. Define the three primary domains of human experience.

5. Explain the importance of the concepts of reliability and validity to the measurement specialist.

6. Give examples of how one might collect evidence for the reliability and validity of measurement process.

7. What is the basic premise of statistics?

8. Opinions differ regarding the need for the exercise science measurement specialist. One view is that this is a specialized position in its own right, and highly trained individuals serve a valuable purpose. Another view is that detailed knowledge of measurement and statistical procedures should be a part of any exercise scientist's training. Select one of these positions and defend it.

GLOSSARY

Affective (or psychological) domain   Area concerned with objectives of interests, attitudes, values, and the development of appreciations.

Cognitive domain   Area concerned with objectives that deal with the recall or recognition of knowledge and the development of intellectual skills and abilities.

Construct validity   The degree to which a test measures an intangible quality or attribute (such as sportsmanship or creativity).

Content validity   The extent to which the items on a test adequately sample the subject matter and abilities that the test was designed to measure.

Criterion validity   The extent to which a test correlates with another valid measure of the same concept.

Evaluation   A judgment of merit based on a comparison of various measurements, impressions, and other evidence of some standard.

Interval measurement   A level of measurement resulting in values that permit the making of statements of equality of intervals in addition to statements of sameness or difference (nominal) or greater than or less than (ordinal).

Measurement   The process of assigning numerical or symbolic values to members of a group for the purpose of distinguishing among the members on the basis of the degree to which they possess the characteristic being assessed.

Nominal measurement   A level of measurement that permits only the making of statements of sameness or difference.

Objectivity   The aspect of test reliability that is concerned with the variability in scores resulting from different individuals administering and scoring a test.

Ordinal measurement   A level of measurement that permits the ordering of the individuals measured in addition to statements of sameness or difference (nominal).

Psychomotor domain   Area concerned with objectives that deal with movement and factors that influence movement.

Ratio measurement   A level of measurement that permits the making of statements of equality or ratios, such as one value is twice another, in addition to statements of sameness or difference (nominal), greater or lesser (ordinal), and equality of intervals (interval).

Reliability   The extent to which a test consistently yields the same results when repeated under the same conditions.

Validity   The degree to which a test measures what it is intended to measure.

SUGGESTED READINGS

Baumgartner, T. A., and A. S. Jackson. *Measurement for Evaluation in Physical Education and Exercise Science,* 5th ed. Madison WI: Brown and Benchmark, 1995.

Morrow, J. R., A. W. Jackson, J. G. Disch, and D. P. Mood. *Measurement and Evaluation in Human Performance.* Champaign IL: Human Kinetics, 1995.

Safrit, M. J., and T. M. Woods. *Introduction to Measurement in Physical Education and Exercise Science,* 3rd ed. St. Louis, MO: C. V. Mosby, 1995.

REFERENCES

1.   Bloom, B. S. *Taxonomy of Educational Objectives: Cognitive Domain.* New York: David McKay Co., 1956.

2.   Harrow, A. J. *A Taxonomy of the Psychomotor Domain.* New York: David McKay Co., 1972.

3.   Hensley, L. D. *Tennis for Boys and Girls: Skills Test Manual.* Reston, VA: American Alliance for Health, Physical Education and Dance, 1989.

4.   Krathwohl, D. R., B. S. Bloom, and B. A. Masia. *Taxonomy of Educational Objectives: Handbook II: The Affective Domain.* New York: David McKay Co., 1964.

10 Motor Control and Motor Learning

DAVID E. SHERWOOD

Motor Control and Motor Learning
History of Motor Control and Motor Learning

Theoretical Approaches
Multilevel Movement Control
Open-loop and Closed-loop Control Theories
Dynamic Pattern Theory
Theories of Motor Learning

Future Directions and Issues

**Educational Preparation
and Career Opportunities**

Professional Associations

Prominent Journals

Summary

Study Questions

Glossary

Suggested Readings

References

Motor Control and Motor Learning

Have you ever watched an elite ice skater like Michelle Kwan and been impressed with the beauty, style, grace, and power of her performance? How did she get to the point where she can give us the impression that her performance seems so effortless and smooth when deep down inside we know that her heart must be racing. How do we design practice schedules to develop these skills in elite athletes? What kind of feedback do we give novices or elite performers to maximize their performance? These questions are central to the study of the acquisition of motor skills or *motor learning*.

At the same time, have you ever wondered how our nervous system can control the elegant and complex movements of the ice skater? Or how you find yourself dropping a hot frying pan before even knowing that it was too hot to handle? How does the nervous system know what muscles to activate, in what time sequence, while minimizing activity in muscles that would interfere with the chosen activity? What specific structures in the nervous system are responsible for controlling movement? What happens when these structures are damaged by injury or disease? All these questions are asked by investigators in *motor control*.

Even though the terms motor learning and motor control have been introduced in separate paragraphs, they are very closely linked. When we talk about motor learning, we are really talking about how one learns to control the proper muscles and coordinate the limbs to produce the chosen action. So to understand how one learns motor skills one also needs to have an understanding of how actions are produced by the nervous system.

As with the other areas of exercise science described in this book, the areas of motor learning and motor control are complex and can be studied from a number of different perspectives. At the most global level, one can study motor learning and control at the behavioral level by observing the change in the actual performance as the level of skill increases. Investigations at this level might focus on how the movements of the joints and limbs (that is, biomechanics) change with practice. Or one might address questions about learning and control at a level "closer" to the nervous system itself by studying the electrical signal associated with muscle contraction (electromyography, EMG). Here one might assess changes in the timing or amplitude of the EMG signal from various muscles over practice trials. Finally, one might investigate control and learning issues by recording from structures within the nervous system itself (typically done with animal subjects) or by using positron emission tomography (PET) scans (see Chapter 3) to assess the areas of the brain that are most active during movement.

Another way to outline the characteristics of this field of study is shown in Figure 10.1. Here the learning process has been divided into three phases: Before Practice, During Practice, and After Practice. Within each of these phases the issues that would be faced by

FIGURE 10.1   Issues in Motor Learning and Motor Control across the Learning Process

Before Practice
1. How do I want to present the skill to be learned (live demonstration, videotape, verbal explanation)?
2. How do I motivate my students so that they will want to practice?
3. What kind of knowledge do I want my learners to have before they practice (rules, strategies, physical principles, biomechanics)?
4. How do I want to organize the practice session? Do I use blocked, random, or variable practice? Massed or distributed practice? How much practice time should be devoted to each task?
5. Do I break down the skill and teach it in parts or as a whole unit?
6. What kind of individual differences should I expect?

During Practice
1. How do I give feedback during practice? What should I give feedback about, how often, and how precise should the information be?
2. How do I keep motivation up during practice? How much rest should I give between trials?
3. What should the learners be paying attention to as they practice?
4. Should I have them evaluate their own errors?

After Practice
1. What kind of postperformance feedback should I give, videotape feedback or verbal feedback?
2. How do I help them remember what they learned today?
3. How much retention should I expect?

the instructor in each phase are outlined. Each issue in each phase is a research area in motor learning and motor control.

History of Motor Control and Motor Learning

The goal in this section is not to present an exhaustive history of motor control and motor learning, but to highlight the people and historical events that shaped our modern-day thoughts about how movements are controlled and learned. The focus is on the following issues. First, how did we come to understand how the nervous system causes muscle contraction? It was a question that was pondered for over 1500 years until it was resolved in the mid-1800s. Second, how did we come to know about cerebral localization, or the idea that specific mental, motor, and sensory processes are correlated with discrete regions of the brain? Finally, why did it take so long for a theory of motor learning to emerge?

Animal Spirits or Bioelectricity?   The most basic issue in motor control is to discover how the nervous system can control the contraction of the muscles. The view advanced by the Roman physician Claudius Galen (A.D. 129–199) was that the nervous system controlled muscular contraction with a hydraulic system whereby the passage of fluids (he called them "animal spirits") down the nerves caused the muscles to inflate. When the fluid was evacuated, the muscle relaxed (22). This hydraulic model was clearly in evidence as late as the mid 1600s when the French philosopher René Descartes (1596–1650) proposed his model of muscle activation (51). Figure 10.2 shows his model. According to Descartes, movement was stimulated by a sensory signal that caused the influx of animal spirits,

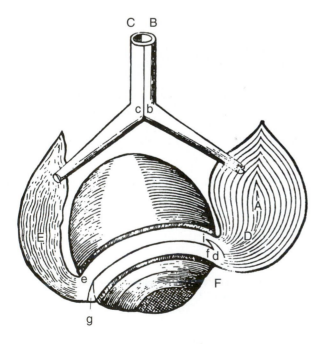

FIGURE 10.2   Representation of the command for muscular contraction according to Descartes (1664). Animal spirits by nervous tubes *B* and *C*. In the case presented here, animal spirits inflate muscle *A*, while muscle *E* relaxes. A movement (here, of the ocular globe) is produced, toward muscle *A*. To explain this reciprocal innervation mechanism by the hydraulic model, Descartes had to postulate the existence of a complicated system of valves that allowed for the evacuation or retention of animal spirits. In the case presented here, valve *H* closes, which allows muscle *A* to be filled, while muscle *E* can freely empty by evacuation canal *e*.

Source: Marc Jannerod, *The Brain Machine* (tr. David Urion). Cambridge, MA: Harvard University Press, 1985.

which were present in the heart and arteries, selectively into the muscles required for the movement. Even though scientists of the time demonstrated evidence against the hydraulic model by showing that nerves were not tubes, liquid did not run out when a nerve was severed, and muscle volume was constant before and after a contraction (22), the hydraulic model persisted until the late 1700s, when it was replaced by the notion of bioelectricity.

The shift toward a bioelectric explanation for the control of muscle was instigated by scientists who noticed that some animals, like eels, were capable of giving shocks when touched, which "sparked" the notion that animals could generate electricity in their bodies. One of the first to study animal electricity was the Italian physician Luigi Galvani (1737–1798) from Bologna. Around 1780, Galvani noted that an electric current applied to the muscle or nerve would cause a contraction of the muscle of a frog. He also noted that muscular contractions occurred when the frog preparation was connected to lighting rods during thunderstorms (Figure 10.3), as well as when a circuit was completed using other means (Figure 10.4) in the absence of thunderstorms. Galvani concluded that certain tissues were capable of generating animal electricity that caused muscle contraction. Later, working with his cousin, Giovanni Aldini (1762–1834), Galvani demonstrated a muscle contraction in one frog by touching it with a nerve from a different frog, establishing the existence of bioelectricity (35). The paradigm shift was now complete. Nerves were not

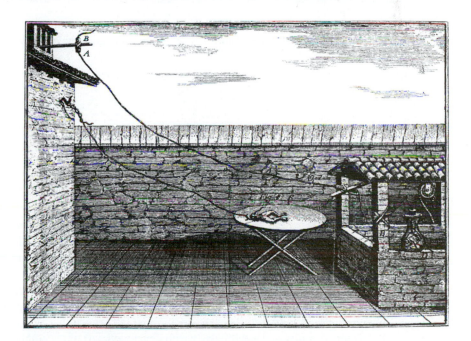

FIGURE 10.3 Figure 3.3 from *The Ambiguous Frog* shows Plate 2 from Galvani's *Commentarius* on how frog musculature was activated by lightning rods during thunderstorms.

Source: Marcello Pera, *The Ambiguous Frog* (tr. Jonathan Mandelbaum). © 1988 by Princeton University Press. Reprinted by permission.

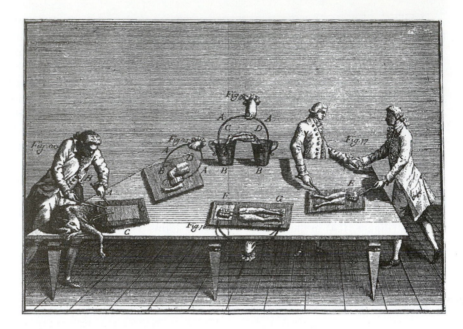

FIGURE 10.4   Figure 6.6 from *The Ambiguous Frog* shows Plate 4 from Galvani's *Commentarius* on how frog musculature was activated by circuit completion by the holding of hands and by conductive metals.

Source: Marcello Pera, *The Ambiguous Frog* (tr. Jonathan Mandelbaum). © 1988 by Princeton University Press. Reprinted by permission.

water pipes or channels as Descartes had thought, but were electrical conductors. Information within the nervous system was carried by electricity generated directly by the organic tissue (35).

Cerebral Localization.   Even though the general idea of cerebral localization had been present for many years (see the discussion of Pythagoras, Hippocrates, Plato, Erisistratus, and Galen in Chapter 3), it was not until the 1800s that the attempt to show empirical support for localization was made. The first empirical efforts came from Franz Josef Gall (1758–1828), a German neuroanatomist and physiologist, who noted apparent relationships between unusual talents and striking differences in facial and/or cranial appearance. Based on the assumptions that the size and shape of the cranium reflected the size and shape of the underlying regions of the brain and that the level of development of a given ability was a reflection of the size of the cerebrum, Gall argued that a correlation between a well developed ability and a particularly well developed part of the cranium was evidence of localization of that ability in that portion of the cerebrum (51).

The correlational methods of Gall were replaced by the neurosurgical techniques utilized by the child-prodigy Marie-Jean-Pierre Flourens (1794–1867), who earned a medical degree before he turned 20. Flourens completely uncovered the brain and then removed a specific portion of the brain (called ablation) and noted the effect on the behavior of the animal (a pigeon, in this case). He was able to localize a motor center in the medulla oblongata and stability and motor coordination in the cerebellum (51). However, when he ablated the cerebrum, many of the higher cognitive functions were damaged, leading Flourens to conclude that the functions of intelligence, perception, and drive were distributed throughout the cerebrum.

The next breakthrough was made possible by a technological development pioneered by Gustav Fritsch (1838–1927) and Eduard Hitzig (1838–1907) in the area of electrical stimulation. They developed a method whereby one could electrically stimulate one area of the cerebral cortex and note the effect on the behavior of the animal. They demonstrated that stimulation of certain areas of the cortex resulted in movements of the contralateral (opposite side) limbs and that ablation of these areas led to weakness of these limbs. In the coming years, David Ferrier (1843–1928) mapped areas of the sensory cortex and motor cortex in many species, confirming the concept of cerebral localization for sensory and motor processes.

Theoretical Developments in Motor Learning.   Motor learning and control are thought to be one of the younger areas of exercise science because theoretical developments in this subdiscipline were delayed relative to other areas. How did this come about?

One problem with the early work in motor learning and control was that researchers focused on understanding the performance of the skill, rather than on the factors that influenced long-term retention or learning of the skill. For example, in the late 1800s and early 1900s researchers investigated issues such as the contribution of visual information to accuracy of hand movements (9) and speed–accuracy trade-offs in rapid movements (19). Although motor skills were the focus of these studies, they shed little light on the processes underlying the learning of skills. The other major roadblock to the development of a motor learning theory was the research emphasis on specific skills and the solving of practical problems. For example, research on telegraphy, typing, and other vocational skills dominated this time period.

During the 1920s and 1930s, some researchers, mostly from psychology departments, began to focus on more basic research issues, rather than on the acquisition of specific skills. Studies on how to organize practice schedules appeared (21), as well as studies on the transfer of training from one skill to another (31), the retention of skills (7), and individual differences in motor skills (26). One of the most debated topics of the time was on the existence of *plateaus* in the learning curve, where gains in performance stalled for some time before gains were again noted. Although some evidence was shown for plateaus (8), many studies failed to replicate the earlier studies (26). Also, the well-known psychologist E. L. Thorndike (1874–1949) published his *law of effect,* which would guide researchers work in knowledge of results for years to come (44). The law states that responses that are rewarded will be repeated, but those actions followed by punishment will be extinguished. It would be many years until this law was replaced in the minds of many people as to how skills were learned. Even though the beginnings of theory were noted during this time, much of the research focused on industrial applications as in earlier years. Studies of time–motion and efficiency in shoveling coal or mixing mortar were common (38).

The major impact on research in motor skills during the 1940s and 1950s came from World War II. The military spent significant amounts of money on research related to pilot and military training. For example, the Air Force began a psychomotor testing program to help to identify potential pilots by correlating motor, perceptual, and intellectual abilities with flying ability. After the war, military spending in motor skill research continued, but with a broader focus that included the teaching, transfer, and retention of motor skills (3). The second factor that had a major impact on motor learning research was the emergence of general learning theories from psychologists such as C. L. Hull. Hull believed that his theory covered all kinds of behavior, both verbal and motor, so many of the experiments used to test the theory used motor skills as the learning task (20). Even though Hull's theory was later shown to be incorrect, it did stimulate research and thinking about motor skills.

The 1960s were an exciting time in motor learning because the discipline finally began to come into focus. Individuals like Franklin Henry, Alfred Hubbard, Arthur Slater-Hammel, and Jack Adams developed highly active university research laboratories dedicated to the study of motor skills. They trained graduate students like Richard A. Schmidt, George Stelmach, Ronald Marteniuk, and Walter Kroll, who had major impacts on the field themselves. The first scientific journal dedicated to research in motor control and learning (the *Journal of Motor Behavior*) was founded by Richard A. Schmidt in 1969 and has become one of the most well respected journals in the field.

During the 1970s, interest in motor skills reached a peak when Jack Adams published his paper, "The Closed-Loop Theory of Motor Learning" in 1971, outlining the first true theory specific to motor learning (2). Throughout the rest of the 1970s, a number of papers were published testing the predictions of Adams's theory, which in general held up reasonably well to scientific scrutiny. In 1975, Richard A. Schmidt published the second theory of motor learning in his paper "A Schema Theory of Discrete Motor Skill Learning," which challenged Adams's theory on several points (37). For the next 10 years or so, the battle between the two theories was fought on the pages of the *Journal of Motor Behavior* and *Research Quarterly for Exercise and Sport*. It was a intellectually challenging and thrilling time to be a graduate student in the field (more about these theories later).

Another major paradigm shift was also underway, away from the more traditional stimulus–response (SR) approach championed by Thorndike to the information-processing approach sparked by the work of people like Neisser (33). In the newer approach, the human was modeled as a active processor of information who needed to code sensory information, store it, and plan actions based on environmental information. Researchers focused on the stages of information processing (stimulus identification, response selection, and response programming) and short- and long-term memory stores. The information-processing approach continues to be a focus for many motor skill researchers today.

The field was established now, and it continues to grow today in new and exciting directions. See Table 10.1 for a timeline of important dates and contributions.

Theoretical Approaches

Now that you are familiar with how the field of motor control and learning developed, we can return to the issues presented at the beginning of the chapter. That is, how are movements controlled and learned? What are the current ideas about how the nervous system controls movement? How do we plan teaching strategies to maximize learning? As this

TABLE 10.1   Chronology of Significant Events in Motor Control and Motor Learning Since 1882.

Year	Event
1882	Bowditch and Southard publish work on visual control of hand movements (9).
1897	Bryan and Harter publish work on the learning of telegraphy and Morse code, find learning plateaus (8).
1899	Woodworth identifies fundamental principles of rapid arm movements (50).
1901	Thorndike and Woodworth propose identical elements theory for the transfer of motor skills (45).
1906	Sherrington begins work on voluntary and reflexive control of movement. Coins terms reciprocal innervation, final common path, and proprioception (40).
1909	Hollingworth studies speed–accuracy trade-offs in rapid movements (19).
1914	Thorndike's book *Educational Psychology* is published, suggesting that individual differences decrease with practice (43).
1925	Book demonstrates excellent long-term retention of typing skills (7).
1925	Kincaid publishes reanalysis of Thornkike's work on individual differences; also concludes that "Nature does not always triumph over nurture"(26).
1927	Thorndike publishes paper on the law of effect (44).
1929	McGeoch convincingly disproves the idea of learning plateaus (30).
1938	Franklin Henry establishes a graduate program in the psychology of physical activity at University of California–Berkeley.
1939	Woodrow publishes a pretheoretical paper claiming that motor learning involves restructuring of native abilities (49).
1940	Gibson proposes theory of perceptual learning (15).
1941–1945:	World War II
1943	Hull publishes *Principles of Behavior* (20).
1948	Bartlett states the importance of KR when he is quoted as saying "practice makes perfect is not true. It is practice *the results of which are known* that makes perfect" (5).
1948	Craik suggests the study of human motor control from an information-processing perspective. Gives rise to the single-channel hypothesis and the psychological refractory period (10).
1952	Hick finds reaction time a linear function of the $\log_2$ of the number of stimulus alternatives (Hick's law).
1953	*Perceptual and Motor Skills* begun by Robert Ammons and Carol Ammons.
1953	Merton publishes work on the mechanism of the muscle spindle (32).
1953	Fleishman's work on motor abilities provides the basis for the modern view of individual differences (14).
1954	Fitts presents relationship between movement, time, distance, and accuracy (Fitts's law).
1960	Henry and Rogers publish paper on the memory drum theory (18).

(continued)

TABLE 10.2   Continued

Year	Event
1964	Henry publishes a paper on the academic discipline of motor learning and motor control (17).
1964	Cratty publishes first textbook on motor learning (11).
1967	Bernstein's work on coordination translated into English (6). Neisser's book, *Cognitive Psychology,* establishes the information-processing approach (33). The North American Society for Psychology of Sport and Physical Activity (NASPSPA) is founded.
1968	Adams (1) and Keele (23) write reviews on motor learning and motor control, respectively.
1969	Richard A. Schmidt founds the *Journal of Motor Behavior.*
1971	Adams publishes his "Closed-loop Theory of Motor Learning" in the *Journal of Motor Behavior* (2).
1972	Work by Grillner (16), Evarts (12), and Matthews (28) uses neurophysiological techniques to study nervous system structures during complex movement in animals.
1975	Schmidt publishes "A Schema Theory of Discrete Motor Skill Learning" in *Psychological Review* (37).
1979	Shea and Morgan's paper on contextual interference is published (39).
1981	Kelso, Holt, Rubin, and Kugler provide theory and data on the dynamical systems approach (25).
1984	Salmoni, Schmidt, and Walter publish outstanding review of the KR literature (36).
1986	Feldman's paper on the equilibrium-point model is published in the *Journal of Motor Behavior* (13).
1987	Adams publishes paper on the historical foundations of motor learning (3).
1990	Magill and Hall's paper on contextual interference in motor learning is published (27). Van Rossum publishes major analysis of schema theory (46).
1995	Kelso publishes *Dynamic Patterns: The Self-organization of Brain and Behavior* (24).
1997	Thomas publishes book chapter on the history of motor behavior (42).

information is presented, you will understand the various theoretical approaches that are used to help to guide our investigations in the area.

Multilevel Movement Control

One approach that has been taken to help us to understand the motor control process has been to conceptualize the neuromuscular system as having a number of levels. Each level of the system involves unique physiological structures that contribute to the control of movement. The upper level is composed of the brain structures that are responsible for the planning and initiation of movement. For example, the *supplementary motor cortex* has been shown to be involved in the movement planning process, whereas movement initiation is controlled by both the *basal ganglia* and the *motor cortex* (Figure 10.5). Specifically, the basal ganglia initiates action and also controls movement amplitude or distance (22). The motor cortex is involved in determining which muscles are involved in the action and the particular level of force required for the action. Also, the motor cortex is organized *somatotopically* (Figure 10.5), which means that each region in the motor cortex is dedicated to the control of a certain part of the body. Parts of the body that require very fine muscular control (for example, the fingers and lips) are represented by more nerve cells (neurons) than muscles that are involved in gross movement (for example, trunk muscles). The somatosensory cortex, which lies just posterior to the motor cortex, is involved in processing the sensory feedback from sensory receptors for touch, vision, hearing, and proprioception. The somatosensory cortex is also somatotopically organized. The *cerebellum*, located at the base of the brain (Figure 10.6), helps to regulate coordination and the control of fine movements, like touching your finger to your nose with your eyes closed. Damage to the cerebellum can result in a loss of muscular strength and coordination.

How do these structures work together to plan and initiate an action? Suppose that you want to throw a dart to the bull's-eye. The movement plan is sent from the supplementary motor cortex to the motor cortex, where the relevant muscles are chosen for the task. The basal ganglia provides the activation for the movement and arm amplitude information. The movement commands from the motor cortex are also sent to the cerebellum, allowing for adjustments in the movement program. The pathway from the motor cortex to the cerebellum and back again is called the cerebro-cerebellar loop, and it provides for very rapid adjustments (10 milliseconds) in the original movement commands. The motor commands that move the arm are sent down to the next lowest level, the spinal level, through efferent pathways.

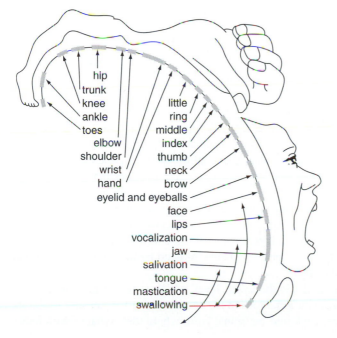

FIGURE 10.5 The motor homonculus (little man), showing the extent of representation of the various body muscles in the motor cortex.

Source: G. Sage, *Motor Learning and Control.* New York: McGraw-Hill Book Co., 1984.

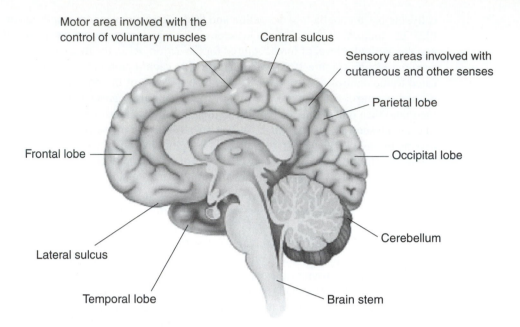

Motor area involved with the
control of voluntary muscles

Central sulcus

Sensory areas involved with
cutaneous and other senses

Parietal lobe

Frontal lobe

Occipital lobe

Cerebellum

Lateral sulcus

Temporal lobe

Brain stem

FIGURE 10.6   Motor areas of the cortex. Note that the striped area labeled "motor areas involved with the control of voluntary muscles" is the motor cortex. The supplementary motor
cortex (not labeled) is just anterior of the motor cortex toward the frontal lobe. The basal ganglia
(also not labeled) are deep within the cerebral cortex. The "sensory areas involved with cutaneous
and other senses" is the somatosensory cortex.

    Two major efferent pathways connect the upper level of the nervous system to the
spinal level, the *pyramidal tract* and the *extrapyramidal tract.* The upper motor neurons (or
first-order neurons) of the pyramidal tract descend without synapse from the motor cortex
to the spinal cord (Figure 10.7). Some nerve fibers cross over the midline of the body in the
medulla, forming the lateral corticospinal tract, while some fibers remain on the same side
of the body, forming the ventral corticospinal tract. The upper motor neurons synapse with
the lower motor neurons (second-order neurons or alpha motor neurons) that travel from
the spinal cord to the muscle. Damage to the pyramidal tract causes paralysis in the muscles. The extrapyramidal tract is a very complicated tract that involves many of the structures already discussed in the upper level. The first-order neurons originate in many areas
of the cerebral cortex, including the motor cortex, and synapse on several cortical and subcortical areas, including the basal ganglia, cerebellum, thalamus, and brainstem. Second-
order neurons descend to the spinal level from some of these structures. It is thought that
the extrapyramidal system helps to refine movements initiated by the pyramidal tract and
acts to control posture and balance.

    The middle level in the model is the spinal level, which is where the upper motor
neurons synapse with the lower motor neurons in the spinal cord. Also, sensory receptors
in the muscle send nerve fibers back into the spinal cord, where they synapse with lower

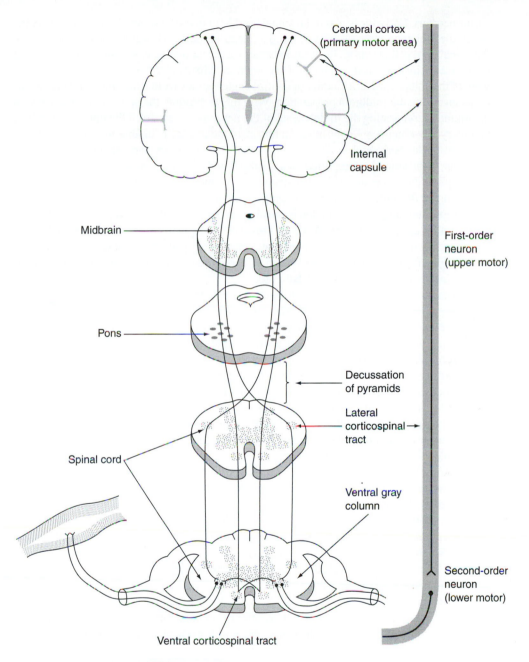

FIGURE 10.7 The pyramidal motor pathways.

Source: G. Sage, *Motor Learning and Control.* New York: McGraw-Hill Book Co., 1984.

motor neurons. Early ideas about the spinal cord held that it was merely a relay station between the brain and the muscles similar to a telephone cable. However, the current view of the spinal cord is that it is an integration center for motor and sensory information and that it plays a major role in the control of locomotion. Much of the evidence for the current view of the spinal cord as a locomotor control center comes from experimental work on animals involving the midbrain preparation. With this technique, the spinal cord is severed in the midbrain, separating the middle level of the nervous system from the upper level where voluntary movements are controlled. In this state the animal is unable to sense any stimulation from the body and is also unable to perform voluntary movements of the limbs. However, if the animal is supported on a treadmill and is stimulated by an electrical current to the spinal cord, the animal begins stepping movements similar to normal gait patterns. Interestingly, the animal continues stepping even when the electrical stimulus is turned off. In addition, stepping can be initiated by turning on the treadmill, and stepping speed can be increased by increasing treadmill speed. This work has given rise to the concept of a central pattern generator in the spinal cord that controls gait patterns without the involvement of the higher centers of the nervous system. Clearly, the spinal cord is much more complex than a simple relay station, as once believed.

The lowest level of the model includes the muscles, tendons, ligaments, and sensory receptors in the muscles involved in movement control. One way that the spinal level and the lower level interact is through the control of reflexes. For example, we have all had our reflexes tested by tapping the knee with a small mallet, which should results in a small kick of the foot. This *monosynaptic stretch reflex* (Figure 10.9) is mediated by muscle receptors called *muscle spindles* (Figure 10.8) that lie in parallel with the main skeletal muscle fibers, called *extrafusal muscle fibers.* The polar ends of the muscle spindle are composed of contractile tissue called *intrafusal muscle fibers.* From the nuclear bag and nuclear chain fibers in the central part of the muscle spindle emerges the *Ia afferent fiber,* which carries sensory information about the amount of stretch on the spindle to the spinal cord. When the patellar tendon is tapped, the quadriceps muscle is stretched, stretching both the extrafusal muscle fibers and the muscle spindles within the muscle. Since the muscle spindle is sensitive to muscle stretch, the Ia afferent fiber increases its firing rate in this situation. The signal is passed along the Ia afferent fiber to the spinal cord, where it synapses with the alpha motor neurons for the quadriceps, resulting in a small contraction and thus the kicking action. The muscle spindle is also sensitive to the velocity or speed of muscle stretch, which is signaled by the group II afferents.

As you can see, all levels of the nervous system are involved in the control of movement. Voluntary movements utilize all levels of the system, from the upper level where movements are planned and initiated, to the lower level where the alpha motor neurons for the appropriate muscles are activated. For reflexive movements, in which a stimulus leads to an involuntary response, only the spinal and lower levels may be involved.

Open-loop and Closed-loop Control Theories

Another way to conceptualize how the nervous system organizes movement is to consider whether movements are controlled with an open- or closed-loop system (Figure 10.10). In an *open-loop control* system the higher centers are responsible for the planning and initiat-

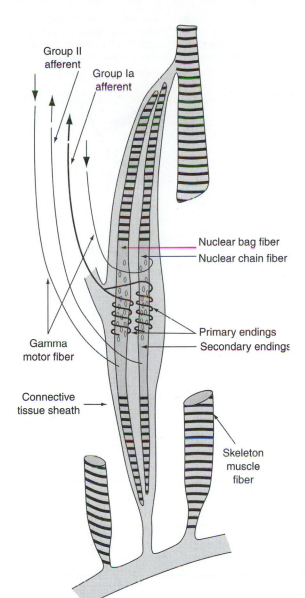

Group II
afferent

Group Ia
afferent

Nuclear bag fiber
Nuclear chain fiber

Primary endings
Secondary endings

Gamma
motor fiber

Connective
tissue sheath

Skeleton
muscle
fiber

FIGURE 10.8   Schematic representation of a muscle spindle.

Source: G. Sage, *Motor Learning and Control.* New York: McGraw-Hill Book Co., 1984.

ing of the movement, the selection of the relevant muscles, and the output of the efferent signals to the spinal and the lower levels. Some of the best evidence for open-loop control comes from animal studies showing that monkeys could climb and move about their cages even after *deafferentation* (cutting only the sensory nerves entering the spinal cord) (41). Since feedback from the limbs was not available due to deafferentation, control must have

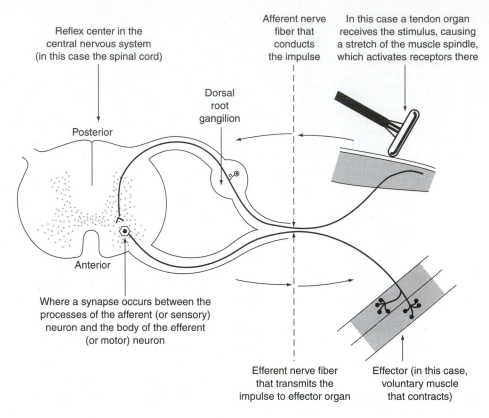

Reflex center in the
central nervous system
(in this case the spinal cord)

Afferent nerve
fiber that
conducts
the impulse

In this case a tendon organ
receives the stimulus, causing
a stretch of the muscle spindle,
which activates receptors there

Dorsal
root
gangilion

Posterior

Anterior

Where a synapse occurs between the
processes of the afferent (or sensory)
neuron and the body of the efferent
(or motor) neuron

Efferent nerve fiber
that transmits the
impulse to effector organ

Effector (in this case,
voluntary muscle
that contracts)

FIGURE 10.9   Basic nervous unit for reflex behavior.

Source: G. Sage, *Motor Learning and Control.* New York: McGraw-Hill Book Co., 1984.

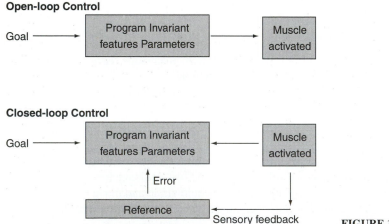

Open-loop Control

Goal ——→ | Program Invariant features Parameters | ——→ | Muscle activated |

Closed-loop Control

Goal ——→ | Program Invariant features Parameters | ←— | Muscle activated |

↑ Error

| Reference | ←— Sensory feedback

FIGURE 10.10   Closed-loop Control

been achieved by the higher centers using efferent commands exclusively. Another example of open-loop control comes from *motor program theory* championed by Schmidt (38). According to Schmidt, practicing motor skills results in the learning of stored motor programs that control the action without the influence of peripheral feedback. The motor program selects the muscles involved and controls the timing and the sequence of movements in the action, all without the need for sensory feedback. Schmidt has also suggested that the motor program is *generalized* to control a class of actions such as throwing or kicking. In this way, a separate program does not have to be stored for every possible movement that we can make, thus avoiding a storage problem for the brain. According to this idea, all movements within the general class of movements share the same invariant characteristics, those features that do not change from movement to movement. The program can be flexible by using different parameters (for example, force, time, and amplitude) to meet the goals of the task, even though the invariant features (the overall movement pattern) remain the same. Figure 10.11 is an abstract from a research study in motor control involving motor programs.

  Closed-loop control on the other hand, uses both efferent and afferent information to control the action. As with open-loop control, the higher centers plan and initiate the action, but, in addition, closed-loop control utilizes sensory feedback from the relevant muscles to make corrections in the original movement plan. For example, the spinal feedback

FIGURE 10.11   Abstract of a concept paper in motor control.

Wickens, J., Hyland, B., and Anson, G.
Cortical cell assemblies: A possible mechanism for motor programs.
Journal of Motor Behavior, Vol. 26(1), 66–82, 1994.

The concept of a motor program has been used to interpret a diverse range of empirical findings related to preparation and initiation of voluntary movement. In the absence of an underlying mechanism, its explanatory power has been limited to that of an analogy with running a stored computer program. We argue that the theory of cortical cell assemblies suggests a possible neural mechanism for motor programming. According to this view, a motor program may be conceptualized as a cell assembly, which is stored in the form of strengthened synaptic connections between cortical pyramidal neurons. These connections determine which combinations of corticospinal neurons are activated when the cell assembly is ignited. The dynamics of cell assembly ignition are considered in relation to the problem of serial order. These considerations lead to a plausible neural mechanism for the programming of movement and movement sequences that is compatible with the effects of precue information and sequence length on reaction times. Anatomical and physiological guidelines for future quantitative models of cortical cell assemblies are suggested. By taking into account the parallel, reentrant loops between the cerebral cortex and basal ganglia, the theory of cortical cell assemblies suggests a mechanism for motor plans that involves longer sequences. The suggested model is compared with other existing neural network models for motor programming.

Source: Wickens, J., Hyland, B., and Anson, G. Cortical cell assemblies: A possible mechanism for motor programs. *Journal of Motor Behavior,* Vol. 26(1), 66–82, 1994.

loop involving the muscle spindles requires 30 to 60 milliseconds and provides rapid, small-amplitude corrections to the movement. Feedback loops involving higher centers require 60 to 120 milliseconds, depending on the type of correction involved. The other major difference between the open- and closed-loop system is the need for a reference mechanism in the closed-loop system. The reference mechanism is a perceptual–motor template of the desired action that is stored in the higher centers. For the motor system to detect errors, feedback from the limbs must be compared to the reference. If there is a mismatch between the incoming feedback and the reference, an error is detected, and the higher centers can correct the error with additional efferent signals.

One model that utilizes closed-loop control is the equilibrium point model (EP) (13). Unlike the motor programming theory in which the level of force is part of the program commands, the EP model claims that the relative tension between the agonist and antagonist muscles is what is controlled by the higher centers. Suppose that you want to move a limb from a stationary position to another position. According to the EP model, a limb is stationary because the tensions created by the agonists and antagonists muscles are equal. To move to another position, the relative tensions between the agonist and the antagonists must be changed. For example, the force in the biceps could be increased relative to the triceps, resulting in forearm flexion. To stabilize the limb at a new position, the triceps force would have to increase so that the forces could be brought into equilibrium. Sensory feedback from the muscles and joints is used to help to keep the limb at the equilibrium point, so the EP model can be classified as a closed-loop model. Figure 10.12 is an abstract from research study in motor control.

Dynamic Pattern Theory

A relatively recent theory of motor control is the dynamic pattern theory introduced by Kelso and others in the last 15 years (25). This theory focuses on the coordination between

FIGURE 10.12   Abstract of a research study in motor control.

Lyons, J., Fontaine, R., and Elliott, D.
I lost it in the lights: The effects of predictable and variable intermittent vision on unimanual catching.
Journal of Motor Behavior, Vol. 29(2), 113–118, 1997.

In this study, two competing views of interceptive action were examined by assessing the influence of variability in the interval between visual samples in a unimanual ball-catching task. Subjects were required to catch tennis balls projected over a distance of 14 m, under conditions of intermittent vision in which the between-sample intervals were either predictable or unpredictable. Results indicated that, although performance was best with shorter between-sample intervals, the temporal predictability of samples did not reliably affect catching performance. This suggests that between-sample retinal expansion provides sufficient information for the timing of the interceptive act.

Source: Lyons, J., Fontaine, R., and Elliott, D. I lost it in the lights: The effects of predictable and variable intermittent vision on unimanual catching. *Journal of Motor Behavior,* Vol. 29(2), 113–118, 1997.

components within the nervous system, using the principles of nonlinear dynamics and chaos theory (47). Even though the details of nonlinear dynamics are far beyond the scope of this chapter, some examples of how these ideas have been applied to motor control are presented. The paper by Wallace (47) is an excellent introduction into this area.

One major focus of dynamic pattern theory is how patterns of coordination change as a function of some outside variable called a control parameter. Suppose that you are walking on a treadmill and the treadmill speed is gradually increased (the control parameter). At some critical speed, you will change from a walking pattern to a running pattern. The change in patterns seems to happen automatically, without thinking about it. One idea is that as the treadmill speed is increased the walking pattern becomes unstable or more variable, and the switch is made to the more stable, less variable running pattern. In dynamic pattern theory, the motor output is not simply a function of what was programmed by higher centers, as in the motor programming theory, but the control of the movement and the shift from one pattern to another are complicated functions of afferent input, efferent commands, and many other factors (anatomical, psychological, biomechanical, and biochemical). The coming years should be quite exciting as researchers use the motor programming, the EP model, and dynamic systems approaches to investigate how our nervous system controls actions.

Theories of Motor Learning

Turning now to the issue of how we learn motor skills, we will briefly discuss two theories of motor learning, Adams's closed-loop theory (2) and Schmidt's schema theory (37). Adams's closed loop theory arrived in 1971 and sparked a renewed interest in research in motor learning. Adams's theory assumed a closed-loop approach to motor control and focused on how we acquire slow positioning movements. Adams states that we form a reference of the correct movement, called a perceptual trace, over repeated practice trials. Early in practice the perceptual trace is weak because the learner has not achieved many correct responses. But as performers receive verbal feedback from the instructor termed *knowledge of results* (KR), the learner is able to correct his or her movement errors. KR provides error information about the result of the event like "Your serve was 2 feet long" or "Your golf ball sliced 35 yards." Once the learner corrects major errors and begins to repeat the correct response on a regular basis, the perceptual trace gains strength. After a great deal of practice, the perceptual trace is strong and can be used as a reference mechanism in a closed-loop control system. For example, during an action like a tennis serve, the sensory feedback from the moving limbs (called intrinsic feedback) is compared to the perceptual trace. If there is a mismatch, then an error is registered, and the higher centers can issue a correction. Once the perceptual trace is strong, Adams claimed that the learner could continue to improve without KR, since learners could detect and correct their own movement errors with the perceptual trace. Adams also proposed a mechanism called the memory trace that was responsible for movement initiation. According to Adams theory, the best way to strengthen the perceptual trace and the memory trace was to use constant practice, that is, to attempt to repeat the correct movement time and time again, with KR on every practice trial. Figure 10.13 is an abstract of a research study in motor learning that involves practice.

FIGURE 10.13   Abstract of a research study in motor learning.

Wulf, G., Shea, C. H., and Whitacre, C. A.
Physical-guidance benefits in learning a complex motor skill.
Journal of Motor Behavior, Vol. 30(4), 367–380, 1998.

The effects of physical guidance on learning to perform slalom-type movements on a ski-simulator were examined in 22 participants (18 in Experiment 1, 4 in Experiment 2). In Experiment 1, one group of participants practiced the task with ski poles, whereas another group practiced without poles. Retention tests without poles were performed at the end of each of the 2 practice days and 1 day later. Although the use of poles produced more effective performance in terms of movement amplitude during practice, both conditions led to similar amplitudes in immediate and delayed retention. With regard to the efficiency of the movement pattern, the pole group demonstrated a more efficient coordination pattern than the no-pole group did, not only during practice but also in immediate (Day 2) and delayed retention. In Experiment 2, how the poles functioned to enhance the learning of a more efficient movement pattern was examined more closely. The results suggest that physical guidance can have beneficial effects not only on performance during practice but also, under certain conditions, on the learning of motor skills.

Source: Wulf, G., Shea, C. H., and Whitacre, C. A. Physical-guidance benefits in learning a complex motor skill. *Journal of Motor Behavior,* Vol. 30(4), 367–380, 1998.

The next theory of motor learning appeared in 1975 when Schmidt published his paper on schema theory (37). Schmidt's main dissatisfaction with Adams's theory was that it implied that a distinct perceptual trace and memory trace needed to be learned for every action that one could perform. If you wanted to learn to shoot a basketball, for example, you would have to practice shooting from each and every point on the court to be prepared for a game situation. This did not make sense to Schmidt and others in the field. Instead, Schmidt proposed that learners acquired rules (that is, schemas) for producing movement and for evaluating performance that could be used in situations where novel movements were required. The recall schema was the rule used for producing movement, and the recognition schema was used to evaluate one's performance. The recall schema is developed by learning the relationship between the parameter (for example, force or amplitude) used with the generalized motor program and the outcome of the action provided by KR. The recognition schema is developed by acquiring the relationship between the sensory feedback from the movement and the outcome of the action.

How might the recall schema, for example, develop with practice? Let's say that you want to teach basketball shooting to a novice. On each practice trial, the learner chooses the force parameter that they think will be required to get the ball to go the appropriate distance. If the ball is short or long, the performer adjusts the force parameter appropriately to correct the error on the previous trial. When moving to different positions on the court, different force parameters are required for the different distances involved. This is called *variable practice,* and Schmidt believes that it is the best way to strengthen the recall and recognition schemas relative to constant practice. With variable practice, a wide range of force parameters is used, so the relationship between the parameter and the outcome is strong and can be used to estimate the parameter needed for a novel distance. Constant practice does not allow for a strong rule to be formed since only one parameter is used. In fact, the major prediction of schema theory is that novel variations of the movement can be produced more effectively following variable, as opposed to constant, practice. In the next section we will see if these theories are still viable today.

Future Directions and Issues

Now that you know about some of the theoretical approaches taken in motor control and motor learning, what are some of the current issues in both subdisciplines? Do we favor one theoretical approach over another? Are the theories of learning still viable? What are the current areas of contention between scientists in the area?

In motor control research, Rosenbaum (34) has identified four main questions that provide much of the research direction for current researchers. The first deals with the degrees-of-freedom problem. Movements are very complex and involve many muscles and joints. How does the nervous system coordinate and control all the components? Is the control achieved by a motor program or by some other controlling structure? Or do dynamic principles play a large role, with little involvement of the higher centers? This is probably the hottest topic in the area right now, and many people do not see it dying down anytime soon (42). A second main question deals with the serial-order problem; that is, how are long sequences of our actions controlled? The motor program theory states that movements of 500 to 800 milliseconds might be controlled by a single program, but how about longer sequences of actions? Dynamic systems theory can explain shifts in coordination patterns, but little is said about how the actions are actually controlled. A third issue deals with the perceptual–motor integration problem. Here the issue is how information from the environment is used to plan and adjust our movements. How does sensory information influence an ongoing motor program or the stability of a coordination pattern? Finally, how does a coordination pattern change with learning? What are the changes in the nervous system that underlie the change in the coordination pattern? These questions clearly indicate the strong link between motor control and motor learning and the difficulty in trying to study one subarea without considering the other.

In motor learning, two major findings in the past 10 years have shaken the once solid beliefs of many researchers in the area and have provided a huge stimulus to reexamine some older issues. The first finding, in 1990, was that by reducing the amount of KR given during practice one could actually improve the long-term retention of a task relative to a 100% KR schedule (48). This finding flew in the face of Adams's closed-loop theory and Schmidt's schema theory, which both held that KR should be provided on every trial to strengthen the perceptual trace, memory trace, recall schema, and recognition schema. Since 1990, a number of researchers have investigated the generality of the original finding and explored the optimal KR frequency schedule for a number of tasks. The issue is still raging, but it is clear that KR must not be given so often that learners become dependent on it for error detection, rather than focusing on their own intrinsically based error-detection mechanism.

The second main issue deals with how to organize a practice session when multiple motor programs must be acquired (for example, forehand, backhand, and volley in tennis). For many years, drills were designed that used *blocked practice,* where one skill was repeated over and over again until it was stamped in, before moving on the next skill. However, research since 1979 has indicated that *random practice,* in which a different program is required on each trial, is more effective for learning that blocked practice (39). Current research deals with whether this finding generalizes to all tasks and learners of different levels (27). Figure 10.14 is an abstract of a research study in motor learning that involves random practice.

Also, the area of observational learning has finally become an important issue in motor learning research. Long ignored by the theories of motor learning, the processes by which we learn by watching someone else perform motor skills has finally been recognized as an important part of the motor learning process. Based on Bandura's social learning theory (4), current work has shown that we can learn motor skills even when KR or KP (*knowledge of performance*) is not given (29). This finding also has shaken confidence in closed-loop theory and schema theory, both of which hold that KR is required during practice for learning to take place.

Educational Preparation and Career Opportunities

There are two main vocational avenues for people with expertise in motor control and motor learning. First, if one is interested in expanding the knowledge base in the academic subdiscipline in motor learning and motor control, one should pursue a doctoral degree and

FIGURE 10.14   Abstract of a research study in motor learning.

Sherwood, D. E.
The benefits of random variable practice for spatial accuracy and error detection in a rapid aiming task.
Research Quarterly for Exercise and Sport, Vol. 67(1), 35–43, 1996.

The role of blocked and random variable practice in the development of a spatial error-detection mechanism in two experiments was investigated in the present study. Twenty-four (Experiment 1) college-aged participants made either 20, 40 or 60° quick lever reversal movements in the sagittal plane. During acquisition in both experiments, blocked practice resulted in less spatial absolute constant error (|CE|) relative to the random group. The blocked practice group showed a smaller mean absolute objective–subjective difference than the random practice group during acquisition (Experiment 1). On no-knowledge of results retention tests in both studies, the random practice group showed a smaller |CE| and a smaller mean absolute objective–subjective difference than the blocked practice group, even on a novel amplitude (Experiment 2). The study demonstrated the advantage of random variable practice over blocked variable practice on retention tests for spatial performance in developing a spatial error-detection capability.

Source: Sherwood, D. E. The benefits of random variable practice for spatial accuracy and error detection in a rapid aiming task. *Research Quarterly for Exercise and Sport,* Vol. 67(1), 35–43, 1996.

aim for employment at the college or university level. Most doctoral students take classes in motor learning, motor control, neurophysiology, cognitive psychology, and exercise and sport psychology, but their research emphasis is usually in either motor learning or motor control. Most programs are housed in kinesiology or exercise science departments, except for those teaching neurophysiological techniques, for which the program is in a biology or physiology department or a medical facility.

The second vocational avenue for others with interest in motor learning and motor control is to use their knowledge in some applied field. Many students pursue a masters in kinesiology or exercise science with an emphasis in motor learning and motor control and then go on for training in another related area. Some students might be interested in applying their knowledge about human learning in an industrial setting by continuing their work in human factors. Those in human factors help to design workplace environments to increase productivity and minimize the possibility of injury. Others may go on for a master's or doctorate in physical therapy, for which the background knowledge in motor learning and motor control is invaluable for those rehabilitating injuries and reteaching motor skills. In addition, many current teachers and coaches take graduate classes in motor learning and motor control to advance their own careers and to keep up to date on the rapidly expanding knowledge base in the field.

Professional Associations

American Alliance for Health, Physical Education, Recreation, and Dance (AAHPERD)

Canadian Society for Psychomotor Learning and Sport Psychology (CSPLSP)

North American Society for the Psychology of Sport and Physical Activity (NASPSPA)

Psychonomic Society

Society for Neuroscience

Prominent Journals

Brain Research
Experimental Brain Research
Human Movement Science
Human Performance
Journal of Experimental Psychology (Human Learning and Memory)
Journal of Experimental Psychology (Human Perception and Performance)
Journal of Human Movement Studies
Journal of Motor Behavior
Motor Control
Neuroscience
Perceptual and Motor Skills
Quarterly Journal of Experimental Psychology
Research Quarterly for Exercise and Sport

Summary

Motor control and motor learning are different, yet very closely related. Motor learning deals primarily with how one learns to control the proper muscles and coordinate the limbs to execute a movement. Motor control, however, involves understanding how actions are produced by the nervous system.

It is important for exercise science students to study motor control and motor learning because they are related to physical activity in both healthy individuals such as athletes and injured or ill patients such as those in rehabilitative settings. For example, a strength and conditioning coach can use the principles of motor control and motor learning to teach the proper techniques for olympic lifting. A physical therapist, however, may use related principles to help a stroke patient regain mobility. Motor control and motor learning have applications in many areas of exercise science.

STUDY QUESTIONS

1. What are the differences between motor learning and motor control?

2. How was the idea of animal spirits as a controlling factor in movement control finally disproved?

3. What is the law of effect?

4. How are the following structures involved in movement control: motor cortex, cerebellum, basal ganglia, spinal cord, muscle spindle?

5. What is the difference between open-loop and closed-loop control?

6. What are the two main vocational avenues for people in motor learning and motor control?

GLOSSARY

Basal ganglia   A collection of subcortical nuclei that is responsible for movement initiation.

Blocked practice   The type of practice in which the learner repeats practice trials using one motor program before the acquisition of a different program.

Cerebellum   A structure located at the base of the brain that is involved in the regulation of coordination and the control of fine movements.

Closed-loop control   A type of motor control through which sensory feedback from the limbs is used to correct errors in the initial movement plan or program.

Deafferentation   A surgical technique by which the afferent nerves are severed to prevent sensory information from reaching the central nervous system. Usually only performed on animals.

Generalized motor program   A stored set of movement commands that activates the proper muscles in the correct sequence with the correct timing without the influence of sensory feedback. Variables such as overall duration and force can be varied from trial to trial with a parameter modification.

Knowledge of performance   A source of feedback that indicates errors in the learner's movement pattern, not the outcome.

Knowledge of results   A source of feedback that indicates whether the outcome of the practice trial was successful in reaching or achieving the goal.

Motor control   An area of study that deals with how the nervous system controls movement.

Motor cortex   A cortical brain region responsible for movement initiation and where most of the upper motor neurons originate.

Motor learning   An area of study that deals with how we acquire and retain motor skills.

Muscle spindle   A sensory receptor located in parallel with the main (extrafusal) muscle fibers that is sensitive to the amount of muscle stretch.

Open-loop control   A type of control whereby the entire movement is controlled by the higher centers without the influence of sensory feedback from the lower centers.

Random practice   A type of practice schedule in which the learner performs a different motor program on each trial (for example, tennis forehand, tennis backhand, and tennis volley).

Reflex arc   A neurological circuit that produces an automatic response to a stimulus and involves a sensory receptor, a sensory (afferent) neuron, a motor neuron (efferent), and an effector (that is, a muscle fiber).

Supplementary motor cortex   A brain area anterior of the motor cortex responsible for the planning of movement.

Variable practice   Practice involving the use of different program parameters (for example, force or overall duration), instead of only one parameter (constant practice).

SUGGESTED READINGS

Christina, R. W. Motor learning: future lines of research. In: M. J. Safrit and H. M. Eckert (Eds.), *The Cutting Edge In Physical Education and Exercise Science Research.* American Academy of Physical Education Papers No. 20, pp. 26–41. Champaign, IL: Human Kinetics, 1987.

Christina, R. W. Whatever happened to applied research in motor learning? In: J. S. Skinner, C. B. Corbin, D. M. Landers, P. E. Martin, and C. L. Wells (Eds.), *Future Directions in Exercise and Sport Science Research.* Champaign, IL: Human Kinetics, 1989, pp. 411–422.

Christina, R. W. Concerns and issues in studying and assessing motor learning. *Measurement in Phys. Edu. Exercise Sci.* 1:19–38, 1997.

Rose, D. J. *A multilevel approach to the study of motor control and learning.* Boston: Allyn and Bacon, 1997.

Schmidt, R. A. *Motor Learning and Performance: From Principles to Practice.* Champaign, IL: Human Kinetics, 1991.

REFERENCES

1. Adams, J. A. Response feedback and learning. *Psycholog. Bull.* 70:468–504.

2. Adams, J. A. A closed-loop theory of motor learning. *J. Motor Behavior* 3:111–149, 1971.

3. Adams, J. A. Historical review and appraisal of research on the learning, retention, and transfer of human motor skills. *Psycholog. Bull.* 101:41–74.

4. Bandura, A. *Social Learning Theory.* Englewood Cliffs, NJ: Prentice Hall, 1977.

5. Bartlett, F. C. The measurement of human skill. *Occupational Psychol.* 22:83–91, 1948.

6. Bernstein, N. *The Co-ordination and Regulation of Movements.* New York: Pergamon Press, 1967.

7. Book, W. F. *The Psychology of Skill.* New York: Gregg Publishing, 1925.

8. Bryan, W. L., and N. Harter. Studies in the physiology and psychology of the telegraphic language. *Psycholog. Review* 4:27–53, 1897.

9. Bowditch, H. P., and W. F. Southard. A comparison of sight and touch. *J. of Physiology,* 3:232–254, 1882.

10. Craik, K. J. W. The theory of the human operator in control systems: II. Man as an element in a control system. *Brit. J. Psychol.* 38:142–148, 1948.

11. Cratty, B. J. *Movement Behavior and Motor Learning.* Philadelphia: Lea and Febiger, 1964.

12. Evarts, E. V. Contrasts between activity of precentral and postcentral neurons of the cerebral cortex during movement in the monkey. *Brain Research* 40:25–31, 1972.

13. Feldman, A. G. Once more on the equilibrium-point hypothesis (lamda model) for motor control. *J. Motor Behavior* 18:17–54, 1986.

14. Fleishman, E. A. Testing for psychomotor abilities by means of apparatus tests. *Psycholog. Bull.* 50:243–262, 1953.

15. Gibson, E. J. A systematic application of the concepts of generalization and differentiation to verbal learning. *Psycholog. Review* 47:196–229.

16. Grillner, S. The role of muscle stiffness in meeting the changing postural and locomotor requirements for force development by the ankle extensors. *Acta Physiolog. Scand.* 86:92–108, 1972.

17. Henry, F. M. Physical education: An academic discipline. *Proceedings of the 67th Annual Conference of NCPEAM*, 6–9, 1964.

18. Henry, F. M., and D. E. Rogers. Increased response latency for complicated movements and a "memory drum" theory of neuromotor reaction. *Research Quart.* 31:448–458, 1960.

19. Hollingworth, H. L. The inaccuracy of movement. *Arch. Psychol.* 13(whole No. 13):1–87, 1909.

20. Hull, C. L. *The Principles of Behavior.* New York: Appleton-Century, 1943.

21. Hunter, W. S. Learning: II. Experimental studies of learning. In C. Murchison (Ed.), *The Foundations of Experimental Psychology.* Worcester, MA: Clark University Press, 1929, (pp. 564–627).

22. Jeannerod, M. *The Brain Machine.* Cambridge, MA: Harvard University Press, 1985.

23. Keele, S. W. Movement control in skilled performance. *Psycholog. Bull.* 70:387–403, 1968.

24. Kelso, J. A. S. *Dynamic Patterns: The Self-organization of Brain and Behavior.* Cambridge, MA: MIT Press, 1996.

25. Kelso, J. A. S., K. G. Holt, P. Rubin, and P. N. Kugler. Patterns of human interlimb coordination emerge from the properties of nonlinear, limit-cycle oscillatory processes: Theory and data. *J. Motor Behavior,* 13:226–261, 1981.

26. Kincaid, M. A study of individual differences in learning. *Psycholog. Reviews* 32:34–53, 1925.

27. Magill, R. A., and K. G. Hall. A review of the contextual interference effect in motor skill acquisition. *Human Movement Sci.* 9:241–289, 1990.

28. Matthews, P. B. C. Muscle spindles and their motor control. *Physiolog. Reviews* 44:219–288, 1964.

29. McCullagh, P., and J. K. Caird. Correct and learning models and the use of model knowledge of results in the acquisition and retention of a motor skill. *J. of Human Movement Studies* 18:107–116, 1990.

30. McGeoch, J. A. The acquisition of skill. *Psycholog. Bull.* 26:457–498, 1929.

31. McGeoch, J. A. The acquisition of skill. *Psycholog. Bull.* 28:413–466, 1931.

32. Merton, P. A. How we control the contraction of our muscles. *Scientific Amer.* 226:30–37, 1972.

33. Neisser, U. *Cognitive Psychology.* New York: Appleton-Century-Crofts, 1967.

34. Rosenbaum, D. A. *Human Motor Control.* New York: Academic Press, 1991.

35. Sabbatini, R. M. E. The discovery of bioelectricity. *Brain and Mind* 2:1–4, 1998.

36. Salmoni, A. W., R. A. Schmidt, and C. B. Walter. Knowledge of results and motor learning: A review and critical appraisal. *Psycholog. Bull.* 95:355–386, 1984.

37. Schmidt, R. A. A schema theory of discrete motor skill learning. *Psycholog. Review* 82:225–260, 1975.

38. Schmidt, R. A. *Motor Control and Learning.* Champaign, IL: Human Kinetics, 1982.

39. Shea, J. B., and R. L. Morgan. Contextual interference effects on the acquisition, retention, and transfer of a motor skill. *J. Experimental Psychol.: Human Learning Memory* 5:179–187, 1979.

40. Sherrington, C. S. The integrative action of the nervous system. New York: Charles Scribner and Sons, 1906.

41. Taub, E. Movement in nonhuman primates deprived of somatosensory feedback. In: J. Keogh and R. S. Hutton (Eds.), *Exercise and Sport Sciences Reviews,* 1976. Santa Barbara, CA: Journal Publishing Affiliates, pp. 335–374.

42. Thomas, J. R. Motor behavior. In: J. D. Massengale and R. A. Swanson (Eds.), *The History of Exercise and Sport Science.* Champaign, IL: Human Kinetics, 1997, pp. 203–292.

43. Thorndike, E. L. *Educational Psychology.* New York: Columbia University, 1914.

44. Thorndike, E. L. The law of effect. *Amer. J. Psychol.* 39:212–222, 1927.

45. Thorndike, E. L., and R. S. Woodworth. The influence of improvement in one mental function upon the efficiency of other functions. *Psycholog. Review* 8:247–261, 1901.

46. Van Rossum, J. H. A. The schema notion in motor learning theory: Some persistent problems in research. *J. Human Movement Studies* 6:269–279, 1990.

47. Wallace, S. A. The dynamic pattern perspective of rhythmic movement: a tutorial. In: H. N. Zelaznik (Ed.), *Advances in Motor Learning and Control.* Champaign, IL: Human Kinetics, 1996.

48. Winstein, C. J., and R. A. Schmidt. Reduced frequency of knowledge of results enhances motor skill learning. *J. Experimental Psychol.: Learning, Memory, Cognition,* 16: 677–691, 1990.

49. Woodrow, H. Factors in improvement with practice. *J. Psychol.* 7:55–70, 1939.

50. Woodworth, R. S. The accuracy of voluntary movement. *Psycholog. Review,* 3(Supplement 2), 1899.

51. Wozniak, R. H. Mind, brain, and adaptation: The localization of cerebral function. In *René Descartes and the Legacy of Mind/Body Dualism* (on-line). 1996. Available:http://serendip.brynmawr.edu/Mind/Descartes.html.

INDEX

AAHPER Youth Fitness Test, 236
Abbas, Ali, 49, 59
Abilities, 102, 222, 223, 233, 25
Ability grouping, 227
Absorption, of food, 157, 201
Academic exercise and sports psychologist, definition, 204–205
Academic preparation. *See also* Curriculum; Graduate program; Undergraduate program
  curriculum, 5
  in dietetics, 176–180
  for athletic trainers, 70, 84
  for exercise and sport psychology, 204, 205–207
  growth of, 3–5
  in exercise physiology, 142–145
  in nutrition, 185
  NATA guidelines, 82, 83
  options, 74, 83
Academy of Kinesiology and Physical Education, 101
Academy of Physical Education, 101
Acceleration
  use of accelerometer, 109
  use of digitizer, 107
Accelerometer, definition, 109, 119
Accidents, biomechanical consequences, 105
Accreditation procedure, for athletic trainer, 84–86, 87, 91, 92
Accredited graduate, as education option, 74
Achievement tests, 239, 250
Achievement to norms, 227
Achilles tendon, 56, 57
Acidosis, 162
Acquired immunodeficiency syndrome (AIDS), 139
Acupuncture, history of anatomy and, 42
Adams, J. A., 258, 260, 269
Adam's apple, 57
Adam's closed-loop theory, 269, 271
Adaptations, physiological, 215, 216, 223
Adderson, John, 209
Adenosine triphosphate (ATP), 128, 137
  definition, 128, 152
Adipose tissue, 141, 160
Aerobic exercise, 134, 203
  definition, 152
  determining fitness, 140
  fitness movement, 3
  testing standards for, 8
  use of in rehabilitation, 128, 131, 132, 139
Aerobic fitness scoring system, 22
Aerobics, 19, 22, 161, 162
  definition, 34
  father of, 18
Aerospace physiology, 24
Aescalapias, 59
Affective domain, 231, 232, 240–241, 244
  definition, 231, 250
Afferent neuron, 266, 267, 269, 274, 275
  group 1A, 264, 265

group 2, 264, 265
Africanus, Constantinus, 49, 59
Age levels, biomechanical analysis at, 102
Aggression, 203, 220
Agility, 233
Aging
  free radicals and, 162
  life-style practices and, 168
  physiology of, 18, 19, 24, 32
  sports medicine clinics and, 77
Agonist muscles, 268
Alarm stage, 215
Alcmaeon, 44, 59, 66
Alcohol, use of, 14, 159, 166, 174
Aldini, Giovanni, 255
Alexander the Great, 45, 46
Alexandrian library, 45–47, 59
Allied health, 3
  definition, 10
Allied health profession, 70, 83
Allopathic medical school, 144
Alpha motor neurons, 262, 264
Altitude, exercise and, 136
Alzheimer's disease, 61
Amar, Jules, 100, 102
Amenorrhea, 163
American Academy of Family Physicians, 81
American Academy of Pediatrics, 81
American Alliance for Health, Physical Education, Recreation and Dance (AAHPERD), 26, 64, 81, 146, 273
  Biomechanics Academy of, 101, 102
  definition, 7, 10
  Measurement and Evaluation council of, 247
  Sport Psychology Academy, 220
American Association of Anatomists, 64
American Association of Cardiovascular and Pulmonary Rehabilitation (AACVPR), 146
American College of Obstetrics and Gynecology (ACOG), exercise guidelines, 135
American College of Sports Medicine (ACSM), 18, 24, 124, 146, 221
  certification program, 4, 146–147, 148, 189, 197
  definition, 10, 34
  description, 14–15, 125, 145
  as major professional organization, 33, 64, 220
American Dietetic Association (ADA), 177, 178, 179, 180, 185, 190, 199
  certification by, 197
American Heart Association, 199
American Institute of Nutrition (AIN), 167, 199
American Medical Association (AMA), 96
  athletic training recognition, 70, 80, 83, 84
  Council on Medical Education (CME), 83
American Physiological Society (APS), 145

American Psychological Association's (APA) Division 47 (Exercise and Sport), 205, 207, 210, 220
  accreditation, 206, 221
  formation of, 209, 213
American Public Health Association, 73
American Society for Nutrition Science, 167
American Society of Biomechanics (ASB), 101, 102, 113
American Society of Exercise Physiologists (ASEP), 125, 145
Amino acids, 160, 169, 171
Ammons, Carol, 259
Ammons, Robert, 259
Amphetamines, 137, 164, 169
Anabolic steroids, 130, 137, 164, 169
  definition, 152
Anabolism, definition, 201
Anaerobic enzyme, 128
Anaerobic exercise, 162
Anaerobic metabolism, 19, 30, 129
Anatomy, 1, 82, 86, 100, 123
  definition, 34, 36–37, 66
  employment opportunities, 63–64
  and exercise science, 13, 14, 37–39
  father of, 46, 59, 67
  future trends, 65
  history of, 39–58
  present-day, instrumentation and techniques, 58–63
  professional associations, 64
  professional journals, 65
  purpose of study, 38–39
  "Reformer of," 52, 53, 60, 67
  subspecialties, 37, 64, 65, 66
Anderson, William G., 207, 210, 234
Anemia, 164
Animal electricity, 255
Animal experimentation, 253, 256, 265, 274
Animal spirits, 254–255
Anorexia athletica, 205
Anorexia nervosa, 205
Antagonist muscles, 268
Anthropometric measurement, 17, 234, 235
Anthropometry, 64
Antiinflammatory compounds, 161
Antioxidants, 129, 162, 165, 166, 169
  definition, 200
  multiple, 164
  role in disease, 158
Antonelli, Ferruccio, 211
Anxiety, 203, 205, 214, 217
  adverse effects on competition, 207, 211
  assessing, 240, 241
  definition, 222
Aorta, 45
Applied research, 237
Applied sport psychologist, 204, 205, 208, 209, 212
  definition, 205, 222
Appreciations, development of, 250
Apprenticeship, 73

Apprenticeship (*continued*)
  as educational option, 74, 82, 83
Arabs, history of anatomy and, 47, 49, 59
The Arbeitsgemeinschaft für Sportsycholo-
    gie (ASP), 212
Archimedes, 46, 99
Aristotle, 45, 49, 57, 59, 66
  biomechanics and, 99, 102
Arteriosclerosis, 52
  definition, 66
Artificial electric stimulation, 131–132
Asclepiades, 48
Asmussen, Erling, 19, 22, 31
Aspartame, 174
The Association for the Advancement of Ap-
    plied Sport Psychology (AAASP), 205,
    213, 220, 221
  certification, 213
Association Suisse de Psychologie du Sport
    (SASP), 211
Associazone Italiana di Psicologia dello
    Sport (AIPS), 212
Asthma, exercise-induced, 127
Astrand, I., 32
Astrand, Per-Olaf, 20, 32, 168
Astrand-Rhyming Nomogram, 32
Astrology, 50
Atherogenic processes, 166
Atherosclerosis, 133, 148, 165, 201
  definition, 126, 152
Atherosclerotic lesions, 166
Athletes, 16, 70
  specialized needs for, 2
Athletes heart, 15
  definition, 34
Athletic Badge Tests, 235
Athletic equipment, anatomy and design of,
    38
Athletic performance, 12, 137, 220
  applied sport psychologist, 204, 205, 222
  dietary supplements and, 169, 170, 199,
    200
  endurance, 30, 31–32, 162–163, 171, 239
  ergogenic aids, 137–138, 152–153,
    168–169, 199, 201
  ergogenic aids, definition, 137, 153, 164
  evaluating, 270
  exercise nutrition and, 157, 158–164, 168,
    199, 201
  impairment, 153, 159
  level of skill and, 215, 253
  sport psychology and, 208, 209, 222
  sports physiology and, 150
  staleness, 203, 215–216, 223
  use of software to record, 249
Athletic Research Laboratory, 207, 208, 210
Athletic Trainer Certified (ATC). *See* Certi-
    fied Athletic Trainer (CAT)
Athletic trainers, 2, 4, 70
  definition of, 72–73, 95, 96
  role of, 70, 71, 86, 95
  state regulation, 75–76
Athletic training profession, 69–97
  academic training, 82
  AMA recognition, 83
  CAAHEP accreditation, 84–92
  definition of trainer, 72–73
  employment opportunities, 92, 93, 95
  employment settings, 76–80
  future trends, 92–94

history of National Athletic Trainers' As-
    sociation (NATA), 70–72
history of NATA professional education
    committee, 83
NATA Board of Certification, 73–76
NATA today, 80–82
professional journals, 94
Athletic training techniques, 82
Atrioventricular valves (AV valves), 45
Atsushi, Fujita, 212
Attentional focus, 253
  definition, 222
Attitudes, 226, 250
  assessing, 240, 241
Attribution theory, definition, 222
The Australian Applied Sport Psychology
    Association (AASPA), 213
Autonomic nervous system, 127–128, 153
  definition, 127, 152
Avicenna, Avenzoar, 49, 59

Balance, 262
Balke, Bruno, 18, 24
Bandura's social learning theory, 272
Bartlett, F. C., 259
Basal ganglia, 260, 261, 262, 267
  definition, 274
Basal metabolic rate (BMR), definition, 200
Basketball, 235
  psychology of, 207
Bates, Barry, 101, 109, 113
Beckman, Peter, 25
Behavior, science of, 203, 222, 223
Behavioral orientation, 216, 217
Behnke, Robert, 83
Bernstein, N., 260
Bernstein, Nicholas, 100
Beta-carotene, 162, 165, 166
Beta-hydroxy beta methylbutyrate (HMB),
    169
Bicarbonate, 164, 169, 172
Biddle, Stuart, 213
Biochemistry, 13, 32, 64, 123
  definition, 158
Biodex, 71
Bioelectrical impedance analysis (BIA), 141,
    176
Bioelectricity, 254, 255
Bioenergetics, 126, 128–129
Biographical tradition, 216
Biology, definition, 158
BIOMCH-L (Biomechanics' List), 101, 112,
    117
Biomechanical analysis, 100, 102
Biomechanical instruments
  complex, 106–109
  simple, 106–109
Biomechanical research, 100, 102
Biomechanics, 38, 86, 98–118, 253
  as academic foundation course, 8, 142
  advanced expertise in, 109–112
  definition, 98–99, 100, 101, 119
  developmental, 102–103, 118
  employment opportunities, 112–113, 118
  of exercise and sport, 103–105, 110, 118,
    150
  four areas of inquiry, 101–106, 118
  history of, 14, 32, 99–101, 102, 237
  professional associations, 113–116
  professional journals, 116–118

techniques and technology used, 101–106,
    118
Biomechanics Academy of AAPHERD,
    101, 102
Biomechanist, 2
Biomedical Engineering Network, 118
Biophysics, 13, 32
Black bile, 45
Blackie, William, 234
Blanz, Friedrich, 212
Bleeding ulcers, 216
Blocked practice, 253, 272
  definition, 274
Blood, as "humor," 45
Blood analysis, 171, 173
Blood characteristics, 21
Blood clotting, 166
Blood doping, 138, 164, 169
Blood pressure, 127, 150
  decreased, 166
  high, 159
  norms for, 235
Board of Medicine, state regulation, 75–76
Bock, Arlie, 21, 26
Body builders, protein intake, 160, 161
Body composition, 134–135
  changes in, 38, 39, 159
Body composition assessment, 142,
    175–176, 177, 195, 239
  field techniques, 175–176
  testing standards, 8
  two-component model, 140–141
Body fat, 162, 218
  obesity and, 134
  percentage in elderly, 131, 134
  percentage of body weight, 218, 230, 239
Body image, 208, 209
Body mass, measuring, 170, 175, 201
Body temperature, 214
  regulation, 164
Body volume, measuring, 201
Boise State University, 5, 6
Bo Jackson Fitness Center, 115
Bomb calorimeter, 172
  definition, 171, 200
Bond, Jeffrey, 212
Bone mass
  effect of exercise on, 130, 138
  microgravity and, 130
Bone mineral content, DEXA assessment,
    141
Bone mineral density (BMD), 130, 201
  osteoporosis and, 153
  pediatric, 138
  postmenopausal, 165
Bones, form and function, 30
Bone tissue, estimation of amount of, 67
Book, W. F., 259
Boredom, 216
Borelli, Alphonso, 100, 102
Boston Bruins, 195
Bowdich, H. P., 259
Bracing, 76
  as psychomotor skill, 96
Bradycardia, definition, 123
Brainstem, 262
Braune, Christian Wilhelm, 19, 30, 100
The Brazilian Society of Sport Psychology,
    Physical Activity and Recreation (SO-
    BRAPE), 212

Breakfast eating, 14
Breathlessness, 133, 150
British Association of Sports, 211
British exercise scientists, 19, 26, 30
The British Society of Sports Psychology, 211
Bruising, 164
Bryan, W. L., 259
Bulgarian Union for Sport and Physical Culture, Committee for Sport Psychology, 211
Bulimia nervosa, 205
Buoyancy, principle of, 46
Burnout, 215, 216, 220
Buskirk, Ellsworth, 21
Bypass surgery, rehabilitation, 133

Cadavers, 36, 37, 52, 64
  history of anatomy and, 36, 37, 52, 64
Caffeine, 137, 162, 164, 169, 174
  possible health problems and, 159
Calcium, 158, 159, 163, 166, 174
  as electrolyte, 164
  skeletal system and, 130
Calorie, 140, 160, 174
  definition, 201
Calorimetry, 171, 173
  definition, 200
  direct, 171, 172
  indirect, 172
Canadian Association of Health, Physical Education and Recreation (CAHPER), Psychomotor Learning and Sport Psychology Committee, 211, 212
The Canadian Mental Training Registry (CMTR), 213
The Canadian Registry for Sport Behavioral Professionals (CRSBP), 213
The Canadian Society for Psychomotor Learning and Sport Psychology (CS-PLSP), 212, 220, 273
Cancer
  dietary habits and, 2, 158, 159, 166
  free radicals and, 162
  obesity and, 134
Canon Law, 48
Carbohydrate loading, 137, 160, 168
  definition, 201
Carbohydrates, 31, 137, 174, 201
  oxidation, 162, 172
  sports performance and, 158–160, 162, 169–170, 195–196, 199
Carbon dioxide, 126, 153
  production of, 126, 172, 173
  role of in control of breathing, 19, 30
  as waste product, 126, 129
Cardiac rehabilitation, 5, 144
  employment opportunities, 4, 5, 147
  in-patient service, 133, 149–150
  outpatient services, 133
Cardiac rehabilitation program, 24
  exercise adherence and, 214
  exercise component, 124, 126, 133
  nutrition counseling, 196
  phase II exercise program, 196
  phase III exercise program, 196
Cardiac surgery, rehabilitation from, 133
Cardiopulmonary, psychology and rehabilitation, 204, 205
Cardiopulmonary resuscitation (CPR), 8, 75

certification, 8, 147
Cardiovascular accidents, 14
Cardiovascular degeneration (CVD) study, 168
Cardiovascular disease, 17, 126
  effect of exercise on, 143
  exercise testing, 138, 148
  morbidity risk decrease, 26, 126
  mortality risk decrease, 26, 126
  primary prevention of, 196
  risk factors, 131, 228
  secondary prevention of, 196
Cardiovascular endurance, 8
  assessment of, 227, 239, 244, 248
Cardiovascular exercise physiology, core curriculum courses, 143
Cardiovascular system, 2, 126, 127
  exercise benefits, 123, 126
Career opportunities. See Employment opportunities
Carnitine, 162
Case study approach, 216
Catabolism, 160
  definition, 201
Catalase, 162
Catell, James K., 235
CAT scan. See Computerized tomography
Cauterization, 40
Cell, historical understanding of, 58
Cell assembly ignition, 267
Cell theory, historical development of, 57, 60
Cellular biology, physiology and, 123
Celsus, Aulus, 48, 59
Center for Nutrition Policy and Promotion, 198
Central monoamine neurotransmitters, 214
Central nervous system (CNS), 274
Central pattern generator concept, 264
Cerebellum, 261, 262
  definition, 274
Cerebral cortex, 262, 263, 267
Cerebral localization, 254, 256–257
Cerebro-cerebellar loop, 261
Cerebrovascular accident (CVA), 132
Cerebrum, 256, 257
Certification. See Professional certification
Certification laws, 181
Certified Athletic Trainer (CAT).
  continuing education units (CEU), 75
  employment settings, 76–80
  licensing, 76
  salary projections, 78
Certified Consultant of the Association for the Advancement of Applied Sport Psychology (CC, AAASP), 213, 221
  certified Personal Trainer, 147
Certified nutritionist (CN), 181
Certified personal trainer, 197
Certified sport nutritionist, 184
Certified Strength and Conditioning Specialist (CSCS), 147, 197
Character development, 220
Chemistry, 64
  definition, 158
Chicago Cubs, 208, 211
Child abuse, sport-related, 220
Children
  as athletes, 218
  exercise and sports psychology, 203, 204, 205, 210, 220

pediatric exercise physiology, 138–139
China, history of anatomy and, 42–44, 59
The China Society of Sport Psychology, 212
Chiropractics, 5
  career opportunities, 4
Chiropractic schools, 144
Chloride, 164
Cholesterol, 166, 174
  blood (serum) levels, 126, 158, 166, 168, 201
  definition, 152, 201
  possible health problems with, 135, 159, 165
  reduction, 126, 190
Chordae tendinae, 45
Christensen, E. H., 31, 32, 159, 168
Chromium picolinate, 169
Chronic disease, 162, 168
  definition, 201
  prevention, 157, 158, 196, 201
Chronic disease rehabilitation program, exercise adherence, 214
Chronic obstructive pulmonary disease (COPD), 127, 150
Cinematography, 106
  definition, 107, 119
  high-speed, 103, 104, 106, 107
  movement and use of serial pictures, 100, 102
Circle of willis, 57
Circulatory system, 235
  historical description of, 56, 60
Civil Aeromedical Research Institute, 24
Classification system, 227, 230, 231, 250
Client education, in cardiac rehabilitation, 133
Clinical dietitians, 184, 189
Clinical exercise physiology, 21, 147–148
  employment opportunities, 147–148
Clinical Exercise Specialist, 149
Clinical exercise testing, 133, 148
Clinical instruction, 86–87
  definition, 96
Clinical psychology programs, 206, 208
Clinical rehabilitation, 9
  definition, 10
Clinical sport psychologist, 221
  definition, 205, 222
Closed-loop control, 264–268, 272
  definition, 274
"The Closed-Loop Theory of Motor Learning," 258, 260
Clysters, 167
Coaching, 4, 32, 38, 273; see also Strength and conditioning coach
  assessing skills, 240
  sports conditioning, 150
Coaching educators, 206
Code of Hammurabi, 42, 59, 67
Cognition, 208, 215, 216, 220, 233
Cognitive-behavioral orientation, 216, 217
Cognitive domain, 232, 233, 238–239, 241, 244
  definition, 231, 250
Cold War, 236
Collegiate athletic program
  athletic trainers and, 72, 73, 79, 94, 95
  employment opportunities, 209, 221, 273
  historical evolvement, 236

Colombian Society of Applied Sport Sciences, 213
Columbia Assessment Service (CAS), 70, 74
Commercial health club, 3, 4, 196, 197; *see also* Private health club
Commission on Accreditation/Approval for Dietetics Education (CAADE), 177, 180
CAADE-accredited dietetic internship (DI), 177, 178, 180
definition, 179
CAADE/ADA Commission on Accreditation/Approval for Dietetics Education of the American Dietetic Association, 180, 181, 193
CAADE-approved preprofessional practice program (AP4), 177, 178, 179, 180
Commission on Dietetic Registration (CDR), 177, 179, 180, 181
Committee on Accreditation of Allied Health Education Programs (CAAHEP), 74
curriculum accreditation process, 84–92
definition, 96
Committee on Allied Health Education and Accreditation (CAHEA), 84
professional accreditation process, 84
Communication skills, 8, 195
Community fitness/wellness facility, 3–5, 9, 10, 196–197, 200
Community referral services, 8
Comparative anatomy, 59, 66
definition, 37, 67
Competencies, 86, 87
Competition, 210
use of mental preparation techniques, 223
Competitiveness, definition, 222
Computer, as measurement tool, 237, 244–245, 247
hardware, 244
software, 173, 244–245, 249
Computer-assisted performance analyzers, 140, 237
Computerized tomography (CT scan, CAT scan), 61, 142
definition, 66
Conant, James B., 21
Concentration, assessing, 241
Concentric contraction, definition, 152
Conditioning programs. *See* Strength and conditioning programs
Conferences, CEU requirements, 75, 81
Confidence, assessing, 241
Confucianism, 43
Construct validity, 243–244
definition, 250
Consultants
employment opportunities as, 205–206, 209, 221, 245, 247
private, 3, 4, 10
Consumer Information Center, 198
Content validity, 243–244
definition, 250
Continuing education, 81
Continuing education unit (CEU), 75, 92
definition, 96
Contractile protein, 128
Contrast x-rays, 61
Cooling down, 16
Cooper, John, 101
Cooper, Kenneth H., 18, 22, 23
Cooper, Mildred, 22

Cooper Institute, 4, 22
Coordinated Program (CP), 177–181, 185, 188
definition, 179
Coordination, 260, 261, 274
patterns of, 269, 270, 271
Coronary artery disease, 126, 134, 148
definition, 126
Coronary heart disease (CHD), 158, 162, 196, 200, 228
definition, 201
risk factors, 2, 165, 166
Corporate or agency fitness, 3, 5, 77, 196–197, 200
career opportunities, 3–5, 9, 150, 246, 247
definition, 10
Correlation coefficient, 242, 244
Cortical cell assemblies, theory of, 267
Cortisol, 129, 171
Couch potato, 23
Council on Education Division of Education Accreditation/Approval, 179
Counseling centers, 209
Craik, K. J. W., 259
Cramer Products, Inc., 81
Crampton's Blood Plosis Test, 235
Cratty, Bryant, 211, 260
Creatine, 164
Creatine kinase, 171
Creatine monohydrate, 169, 170
Creatine phosphate, 137
Creatine supplementation, 137–138
Creativity, measuring, 250
Creighton University, 5, 6
Criterion validity, 243, 244
definition, 251
Cross-country skiing ergometers, 140
Cross-cultural sport, 220
Cross education, 207
Cultural factors, 166
Cummins, Robert A., 207, 210
Cureton, Thomas K., 18, 23, 24, 27
Curriculum programs, 14, 237; *see also* Academic preparation; Graduate program; Undergraduate program
biomechanical sample, 110
CAAHEP accreditation, 84–92
CAAHEP guidelines, 74, 92
division of, 13
emphasis on science, 237
for dietetics, 179, 182, 183
for exercise and sport nutrition, 185–188
for exercise physiology, 123, 124, 142–143
historical changes in, 235
NATA approval, 74, 82, 92
Cut-off points, determining, 227
Cybex, 71
Cycle ergometer, 30, 139–140, 148
Czechoslovakian Union of Physical Education and Sport, 211

Dance, 163
history of exercise science and, 14
The Danish Society of Sport Psychology, 212
The Danish Sport Federation, 213
Darwin, Charles, 45, 135
Data collection methods, 219
David, Michelangelo's, 52, 54
Davis, Howard, 13

Deafferentation, definition, 265, 274
Decision making, 228
Degenerative diseases, evolution of exercise science and, 14
Degrees of freedom, 271
Dehydration, 164, 168
Dehydroepiandrosterone (DHEA), 169
Delforge, Gary, 83
Dellamary, Guillermo, 213
della Torre, Marcantonio, 52
Delsarte, Francois, 234
Densitometry, 175, 176
definition, 175, 201
Dentistry, 4, 145
study of anatomy and, 38, 66
Depression, 203, 210, 216, 223
chronic, 204
role of exercise in, 205, 214, 241
Descartes, René, 254, 256
Deuterium (^{2}H), 172
Deutsche Hochschule für Leibesubungen, 210
Developmental anatomy, 37, 66
definition, 37, 67
Developmental biomechanics, 102–103, 118
Developmental motor skills, 102
Dewey, John, 235
Diabetes, 124, 126, 166
definition, 152
diet, exercise and, 135, 165, 166, 171
exercise and sport psychology, 204
insulin-dependent, 135
Type I, 135, 152
Type II, 134, 135, 152
Diabetic foot evaluation, 109
Diagnosis
measurement techniques, 228, 250
use of goniometers and, 108
Didactic Program in Dietetics (DPD), 177, 178, 179, 180, 185
definition, 179
Diem, Carl, 210
Diet
athletic performance and, 158
deficiencies/excesses, 173
disease risk factors, 2, 159
recall and analysis, 173–174
Dietary analysis, 173, 174
Dietary fat. *See* Fat
Dietary intervention program, 171, 175
Dietetic internship (DI), 177, 178, 180
definition, 179
Dietetics, 167
definition, 158, 176, 201
Dietetics professionals, 189
accreditation, 176, 177
Dietetic technician, 178, 180, 189, 190, 192
definition, 176, 179
Dietetic Technician Program (DTP), 180, 183
Dietetic Technician, registered (DTR), 176, 178–180, 195, 197
definition, 179
Dietitians, 184, 189, 190
definition, 176
Digestion, of food, 157, 201
Digitizer, 107, 108
definition, 107, 119
Dill, David B., 18, 20–22, 31, 167
Dillman, Charles, 100–101

Diphtheria, 14
Direct calorimetry, 171, 172
Direction, dimension of, 222
Disabled, exercise and sports psychology, 204
Disease
  occurrence and prevalence of, 165, 166, 199, 201
  risk factors, 2, 3
  treatment machines, 96
Disordered eating, 163
Displacement, use of digitizer for, 107
Dissection
  computer simulation, 37
  definition, 36
  history of anatomy and, 43–49, 51–53, 55, 60, 64
  techniques, 53–54, 60
Dissertation, 144, 246
Distance running, 130, 150, 163
Distance-run tests, 244
Distraction hypothesis, 214
Dizzy Dean, 208
Doctor of Chiropracty (D.C.), 144
Doctor of Education (Ed.D.), 143
Doctor of Medicine (M. D.), 144
Doctor of Osteopathy (D. O.), 4, 144
Doctor of Philosophy (Ph.D.), 143, 189, 206
Dopamine, fatigue and, 127
Dorsal root ganglion, 266
Douglas, Claude G., 19, 30
Douglas Bag, 19, 30
Drinkwater, Barbara, 21
Drug laws, anabolic steroids and, 137
Drugs, 164; see also Ergogenic aids
  abuse of, 203, 205
  performance and, 158
  weight-loss, 166
Dual-energy x-ray absorptiometry (DEXA, DXA), 61, 63, 64, 141, 175
  definition, 67
  use of in study of anatomy, 61, 63, 64, 66
The Dutch Psychological Association, 213
Dutch Society for Sport Psychology, 213
Dynamic pattern theory, 260, 268–269, 271
Dynamics, definition, 99, 119
Dynamography, definition, 108, 119
Dynamometer, 17, 243
Dyspnea, 150

Early Middle Ages, history of anatomy and, 48, 49
Eating Attitudes Test (EAT), 218
Eating disorders, 195, 205, 209
Eccentric contraction, definition, 136, 152
Education, importance of measurement in, 235
Educational philosophy, 235, 237
Educational sport psychologist, 208, 221
  definition, 222
Educational Task Force, 18 recommendations, 87, 91–92
Education programs. See academic preparation
Educator dietitian, 190, 191
Effect, Law of, 257, 259
Efferent neuron, 261–262, 265–267, 269, 275
Efficiency studies, 257
Egypt

history of anatomy and, 42, 50, 59
history of dietetics, 167
Elderly
  bone mass, 130
  exercise and quality of life, 131, 152
  osteoporosis, 163
  physical conditioning myths, 15, 16
  testing standards for, 8
  use of anabolic steroids, 130
Electrical stimulation, 257
Electrocardiogram (ECG), 133, 143, 148, 228
Electroencephalography, 217
Electrogoniometer (elgon), 108
Electrolytes, 138, 158, 164, 169, 199
  definition, 164
Electromechanical device, 108, 120
Electromyography (EMG), 31, 100, 128, 141–142, 217
  definition, 108, 119, 152
  in motor learning and motor control, 253
  intramuscular measurement, 141
  surface measurement, 141
Electron microscope, 13, 58, 64, 66
Electrotherapeutic devices, 71
  definition, 96
Elements of performance, 16
Elgon, 108
Elite athlete, 214, 252
Elite Athlete Project, 208
Embryology, 13, 64, 66
  definition, 37, 67
Emergency Medical Technician (EMT),
  CEU requirements, 75, 81
Emotional problems, 222
Empedocles, 44, 47, 59
Emphysema, 127
Employment opportunities, 3–5, 9, 38
  collegiate, 77, 79, 93, 95
  for athlete trainer, 92, 93, 95
  for exercise physiologists, 124, 147–150
  for measurement specialists, 245, 246, 247
  in anatomy, 38, 63–64
  in biomechanics, 112–113, 118
  in dietetics, 189–192
  in exercise and sport psychology, 205–207, 209, 221
  in exercise nutrition, 31, 150, 193–197, 200
  in motor control and motor learning, 273
  in private practice medical setting, 93
  in professional sports, 79–80, 93–94, 95
  in secondary education, 79, 95
  in sports medicine, 77, 92, 95
  world-wide web listings, 82
Employment settings, 76–80
  of athletic trainers, 72, 76–80, 95, 96
Endocrine gland, 153
  definition, 129, 153
Endocrine system, 123, 129–130, 138
Endorphins, 214
Endurance, taxonomy of, 233
Endurance exercise, 15–16, 128
  altitude and, 136
  during space flight, 131
  for pulmonary rehabilitation, 134
Endurance performance, 16, 162, 171, 239
  athlete's potential for, 30, 31–32
Endurance testing, 248
Endurance training, 30

protein requirements, 160
unhealthy diet practices, 163, 164
Enemas, 167
Energy expenditure measurement, 153
Energy metabolism, 128, 172–173
Enjoyment, definition of, 219
Entrepreneurs, 150
Environmental exercise physiology, 136–137, 167
Environmental heat and cold, 164
Enzyme concentration, 128
Ephedrine, 169
Epidemiological research, 163, 165
Epidemiology, 168
  definition, 201
Epinephrine, 129
Eponyms, 56, 57, 58
Equilibrium-point model (EP), 260, 268, 269
Equivalence method, 243
Erasistratus, 46, 47, 59, 67
Ergogenic aids, 130, 137–138, 152
  definition, 137, 153, 164, 201
  effect on performance, 161, 162, 168–169, 195, 199
Ergolytic, definition, 137, 153
Ergometers
  arm crank, 131, 140, 207
  cross-country skiing, 140
  cycle, 30, 139–140, 148
  hand-cranked, 207
  rowing, 140
Ergonomics consultant, 4
Eristratus, 256
Error in performance
  detecting/correcting, 268, 269, 271, 272
  evaluating, 253
  in movement pattern, 140, 274
  of measurement, 242, 253
Erythopoietin, 138
"Essentials and Guidelines for an Accredited Educational Program for the Athletic Trainer," 86
Essing, Willi, 212
Estimating sample size, 248
Estrogen, 166
  osteoporosis and, 130
Ethics, 8
Ethnic factors, 166
Ethnographic tradition, 216
Euclid, 46
Euphoria, 214
European Federation of Sport Psychology, 211
Eustachian tube, 57
Eustachio, Bartolomeo, 57
Evaluation, 229
  definition, 228, 251
Evarts, E. V., 260
Exercise, 2, 15, 16, 96
  acid-base balance during, 23
  adaptations to, 123–124, 126–129, 131, 136
  age and, 17, 19
  definition, 1, 10
  during space flight, 131
  effects of heat on, 31
  effects of high altitude on, 31
  high-intensity, 12, 15, 137–138, 214, 218
  immune function and, 17
  lean muscle loss, 162

Exercise (*continued*)
  myths, 15
  prolonged, 169
  research, 20
  response to, 123–124, 126, 128–129, 131
  self-monitoring, 133
  submaximal, 130
Exercise addiction, 208, 220
  definition, 223
Exercise adherence, 209, 214–215, 220
  definition, 214, 223
  factors in, 215
Exercise and sports nutrition, 157–199
  academic training and certification,
    176–189
  areas of study and research, 158–166
  employment opportunities, 189–197
  historical aspects, 167–170
  professional journals, 197–199
  related disciplines, 158
  technology used, 170–176
Exercise and sport psychology, 203–222
  academic preparation, 205–207
  activities of, 204–205
  areas of study, 209–216
  certification, 221
  definition, 203
  employment opportunities, 205–207, 221
  future research, 220
  history of, 207–209
  parent disciplines, 204
  professional journals, 221–222
  professional organizations, 220
  theory and research methodologies, 216,
    217–219
Exercise and Sport Sciences Review, 145
Exercise and sports nutrition specialists,
    194–195
Exercise capability, muscle adaptation and,
    128
Exercise capacity, measuring, 133
Exercise epidemiologists, 2
Exercise equipment, 103, 104
Exercise-induced asthma, 127
Exercise intervention, 124, 171, 175
Exercise machines, biomechanics and de-
    signing, 103
Exercise nutrition, 158, 192–197
  definition, 157, 201
Exercise physiologist, 1–2
Exercise physiology, 8, 15, 122–152
  academic training, 142–145
  areas of applied study, 123, 130–139
  areas of basic study, 125–130
  certification, 146–147
  definition, 123, 124, 151
  employment opportunities, 124, 147–150
  "father" of, 20
  and gerontology, 131
  history of, 124–125, 237
  important leaders in, 24, 26, 30
  nutrition contributions, 167–170
  parent disciplines of, 123–124
  pediatric, 138–139
  professional journals, 151
  professional organizations, 145–146
  research tools used, 139–142
Exercise prescriptions, 17, 65, 108, 143, 246
  for bradycardia, 123
  for cardiac rehabilitation, 196

  for quadriplegia, 132
  pediatric, 139
  testing standards for, 8
Exercise programs
  designing, 150, 151
  for cardiac rehabilitation, 126, 133, 149
  for prevention of cardiovascular disease,
    126
  for pulmonary rehabilitation, 133, 149
  home-based, 196
Exercise psychology, 209, 214–215, 222
  definition, 204
Exercise science
  athletic programs, 3–5, 185
  definition, 1, 10
  history of, 12–33
  present/future trends, 32–33
  professional standards for programs,
    5–9
Exercise science researcher, 38
Exercise scientist, areas of study, 2–3
Exercise Specialist (ES), 38, 147, 196, 200
Exercise techniques, biomechanical develop-
    ment of, 103, 118
Exercise testing, 133, 138, 143, 144, 148
Exercise Test Technologist (ETT), 147
Exercise tolerance, in cardiac rehabilitation,
    133
Exercise training, as disease intervention,
    135, 148
Exhaustion stage, 215
Exogenous hormone supplementation, 130,
    135
Experimental Brain Research, 273
Expert witness work, 105
Extrafusal muscle fibers, 264, 275
Extrapyramidal tract, 262
Eye movement response patterns, 217

Failure, 217
  attribution theory, 222
Fallopian tube, 57
Fallopius, Gabriele, 57
Falls, biomechanical evaluation of, 103
Fat, 174
  blood levels, 201
  distribution, 142, 166, 175
  estimation of amount, 67
  facilitating loss, 134, 137, 141
  intake and performance, 31, 160–162, 195,
    196, 199
  monosaturated, 174
  oxidation, 162, 172
  polysaturated, 174
  possible health problems, 126, 158, 159,
    166
  saturated, 174
Fatigue, 17, 30, 127, 134, 142
  definition, 34
  ergogenic aids and, 164
  mechanisms of, 128, 142
  psychological aspects of, 208, 209, 214
Fat patterning, 166
Fat substitutes, 166
The Federation Espanola de Asociaciones de
    Psicologia de la Actividad Fiscia y el De-
    pote, 212
The Federation Europeenne de Psychologie
    des Sports et des Activites Corporelles
    (FEPSAC), 211

Feedback loops, 267–268; *see also* Sensory
    feedback
Feldman, A. G., 260
Female athlete triad, 163
Femininity culture, 219
Fenn, W. O., 100, 102
Fensterheim, Herbert, 209
Ferrier, David, 257
Fiber, 166, 174
  role in disease, 158, 159
Final common path, 259
The Finnish Society of Sport Psychology, 212
First aid, 8, 75, 82, 86
First International Seminar on Biomechan-
    ics, 101, 102
First International Society of Sport Psychol-
    ogy (ISSP) Congress, 211
First-order neurons, 262, 263
Fischer, Otto, 19, 30, 100
Fitts's Law, 259
Fitz, George W., 18, 20, 207, 210
Fleishman, E. A., 259
Flexibility, 16, 233
  testing standards, 8
Flexibility exercise, for pulmonary rehabili-
    tation, 134
Flourens, Marie-Jean-Pierrre, 256, 257
Fluid balance, 136, 164, 168, 169
Food, 171
  deterioration of, 158, 201
  nature of, 158, 201
  processing/preparing, 158, 201
Food and Drug Administration, 198
Food and Nutrition Board, 201
Food and Nutrition Information Center, 198
Food science, 185
  definition, 157, 158, 201
Food Technology, 197
Foot and Ankle International, 116
Football, 207
  ergogenic aids, 137
Foot-ground impact, 118
Force parameter, 270, 271, 275
Force platforms, 103, 104, 108, 109
  definition, 120
Force transducers, 108, 109
Forearm flexion, 268
Fracture, 164
  bone density and, 130, 138
  osteoporosis and, 153
Framingham Heart Study, 168
Free-fatty acids (FFA), 160, 161, 162
Free radicals, 162
  damage from, 162
Fritsch, Gustav, 257

Gait patterns, 102, 264, 269; *see also*
    Walking
  analysis of, 93
  pathological, 109
Galen, Claudius, 46, 48–49, 59, 67, 100, 254,
    256
  history of anatomy and, 51, 52, 53
Galilei, Galileo, 100
Gall, Franz Josef, 256
Galvani, Luigi, 255
Galvanic skin response, 217
Galvanic stimulators, 71, 96
Gamma motor fiber, 265
Gas analyzer, 172

Gastric emptying, role of, 169
Gastrocnemius muscle, 94
Gastrointestinal distress, 138
Gatorade, 81, 168
Gatorade Company, 168
Gatorade Sports Science Institute (GSSI), 168, 169, 199
Gender difference, 16, 134, 219, 220
Geneology of leadership, 26, 27–29
General adaptation syndrome, 216
Generalized motor program, 267, 270
  definition, 274
General learning theories, 258
General psychological theories, 222
Gene therapy, 166
Genetic engineering, 166
George Williams College, 18, 23, 33
German exercise scientists, 19, 23, 25, 30–31
Geron, Ema, 212
Gerontology, 21, 124, 126, 131
Gibson, E. J., 259
Global assessment, 241, 248, 253
Glucagon, 171
Glucose, blood concentrations of, 129, 135, 153
Gluthione peroxidase (GPX), 129, 162
Gluthione reductase (GR), 129
Glycerol supplementation, 162
Glycogen, 160, 168
  definition, 201
Goal setting, 209, 227, 274
  definition, 223
Goddard, Henry H., 235
Goniometer, definition, 108, 120
de Graaf, Regnier, 57
Graafian follicle, 57
Graduate assistantships, 79, 91, 112
Graduate education program, 5–8, 9, 32
  biomechanics specialization, 100–101, 109–110
  CAAHEP accreditation, 84, 87, 91, 92
  doctorate, 195
  doctorate, biomechanics, University of Oregon, 111–112, 118
  doctorate, dietetics, 181, 184
  doctorate, exercise and sports psychology Track I, II, III, 206, 221
  doctorate, exercise physiology, 143–144
  doctorate, exercise science, 246
  doctorate, motor control and motor learning emphasis, 272, 273
  doctorate, nutrition, 188, 189
  doctorate, University of Virginia sample, 87, 90–91
  in exercise and sports psychology, 205–207
  in exercise science and/or nutrition, 185, 188–189
  in physical education, 237
  in psychology of physical activity, 259
  masters, 195
  masters, biomechanics, University of Oregon sample, 110, 118
  masters, dietetics, 181
  masters, exercise and sports nutrition, 188, 189
  masters, exercise and sports psychology, 206
  masters, exercise physiology, 143, 189
  masters, motor learning and motor control emphasis, 273

masters, nutrition, 188, 189
masters, University of Oregon sample, 87, 89
Graduate Record Examination (GRE), 79, 90, 110, 111, 188
Graduate School Foreign Language Test (GSFLT), 111
Grave robbing, 52
Gravity, limb movement and, 100
Gray, Henry, 57, 60
Gray's Anatomy, 57, 60
Greeks
  origins of anatomy, 41–42, 44–49, 59
  origins of athletic trainers, 69
  origins of biomechanics, 99, 100
  origins of dietetics, 167
  origins of exercise and sport psychology, 207
  origins of exercise physiology, 124
Griffith, Coleman R., 207, 208, 210, 211
Grillner, S., 260
Gross anatomy, 63, 66, 109
  definition, 37, 67
  historical development of, 57, 58, 64
Gross movement, 261
Grounded theory tradition, 216
Group dynamics, 209, 215
Group Ia afferent fiber, 264, 265
Group II afferent fiber, 264, 265
Growth and development, 17, 37, 38, 139
Growth hormones, 129, 161, 171
Growth patterns, measurement of, 234
Growth plate injury, 138
"Guidelines for Professional Preparation in Exercise Science," 5
Guillain-Barré syndrome, skeletal muscle, 128
Gulick, Luther, 235
Guttman, Giselher, 212
Gymnastic movement, 14, 163, 233–236
  German system, 234
  pediatric exercise physiology and, 139
  Swedish system, 234
Gyri, 42

Hahn, Erwin, 212
Haldane, John S., 19, 30
Haldane method, 19, 30
Hall, G. Stanley, 207, 210, 235
Hall, K. G., 260
Hammurabi, 42, 59, 67
  code of, 42, 59, 67
Hanson, Ole, 31, 159, 168
Harmon, John M., 211
Harter, N., 259
Hartwell, Edward M., 234
Harvard Alumni Study, 168
Harvard Fatigue Laboratory, 26, 32–33, 125, 167
  historical contribution of, 18, 20–23
Harvey, William, 43, 56, 60, 67
Havers, Clopton, 57
Haversian canal, 57
Haversian system, 57
Hay, James, 101
Hayford, Scott, 149
Healing rates, 164
Health and fitness, 14, 239
  methodology for developing optimal, 16–17

Health and fitness industry, employment opportunities, 148–150
Health care reform, trends, 92–94
Health Fitness Director (HFD), 147
Health Fitness Instructor (HFI), 147
Health Fitness Leader (HFL), 147
Health insurance, 4, 93
Health maintenance organizations (HMOs), 189
Health promotion, 8, 196
  diet and exercise, 165, 166
Heart, neurological control of, 126
Heart attack, 14, 126
  aerobic exercise and, 128
  atherosclerosis and, 152
Heart disease, 15, 26, 133
  as diabetes complication, 135
  dietary habits and, 134, 159
Heart rate (HR), 2, 132, 217, 235
  measuring, 229
  monitoring, 150
  response, 20, 31, 164
  resting, 123
Heart Rate Reserve (HRR), 218
Heart strings, 45
Heat exchanged, 126, 136, 200
Heat stroke, 136
The Hellenic Society of Sport Psychology and Applied Neurophysiology (HESPAN), 212
Hematocrit (Hct), 218
Hemenway Gymnasium, 17, 18, 20
Hemiparesis, definition, 132, 153
Hemoglobin (Hgb), 163, 164, 218
  definition, 136, 153
Henderson, Lawrence J., 18, 20
Henry, Franklin, 208, 211, 258, 259, 260
Herodotus, 42
Herophilus, 46, 47, 59, 67
Hetherington, Clark W., 235
Hettinger, Theodor, 19, 30
Hick's Law, 259
High blood pressure, 135, 159
High-density lipoprotein cholesterol (HDL), 165, 166
Higher education, 9
  definition, 10
High School Victory Corps, 236
Hill, Archibald V., 19, 26, 30, 100
Hippocrates, 44–45, 59, 67, 100, 256
  history of anatomy and, 47, 48, 49, 59
Histology, 13, 64, 66
  definition, 37, 67
History of measurement in U.S., 233–238
Hitchcock, Edward, 234
Hitzig, Edward, 257
Hohwu-Christensen, Erik, 20, 22, 31
Hollingworth, H. L., 259
Hollmann, Wildor, 19, 31
Holt, K. G., 260
Homer, 41
Home study courses, 75
Hooke, Robert, 56, 60
Hop-skip-jump, 235
Hormone, 130, 171
  definition, 129, 153
Horvath, Steven, 21
Hospital based clinics, 77, 78, 95
HR/VO$_2$ relationship, quadriplegia, 132
Huang Ti, 43, 59

Hubbard, Alfred, 258
Hull, C. L., 258, 259
Human immunodeficiency virus (HIV), 139
Human Nutrition Information Service, 198
Humidity, exercise and, 136
Humoral theory of the body, 45, 48
Hydraulic model, of muscle inflation, 254, 255
Hydrogen 2 (^{2}H), 172
Hydrometry, 175, 176
Hydrostatic weighing technique, 141, 175, 201
Hyperglycemia, 135
Hyperlipidemia, 165, 166, 171
    definition, 201
Hypertension, 14, 158, 165, 166, 201
Hypobaric chamber, 136
Hypoglycemia, 135
Hypohydration, 164
Hypokinetic disease, definition, 34

Iceberg profile, 214
Imagery, 205
    definition, 223
Immune system, 2, 130
Immunology, exercise and, 139
Immunosuppression, exercise and, 130, 139
Incentive to act, 223
Independent *t*-test, 245
Index of reliability, 243
India, history of anatomy and, 42–44, 59
The Indian Association of Sport Psychology (IASP), 212
Indirect calorimetry, 128, 148, 172
    definition, 129, 153
Inducement to act, 223
Industrial biomechanics, 110
Industrial design and safety, 100
    biomechanics, 105–106
Industrial Revolution, 233
Inertia wheel, 26
Infectious diseases, 14
Information processing approach, stages in, 258
Ingestion, of food, 157, 201
Injuries, 70, 76, 103
    immediate care of, 71, 76, 86, 95
    nutrition and rehabilitation, 164
    prevention of, 2, 8, 71, 76, 86, 95
    product liability, 106
    recovery from, 162, 164, 204, 205
    reduction, 103
    rehabilitation and reconditioning, 71, 76, 93, 95, 273–274
Institute for Environmental Stress, 21
Insulin, 152, 171
    definition, 135, 153
    resistance, 135
Insurance companies, employment opportunities, 246, 247
Intellectual skills, development of, 250
Intelligence quotient (IQ), 244
Intelligence tests, 235
Interactional approach, 215
Intercollegiate athletic programs, 70, 235
    CAT career opportunities, 77, 78, 79
Intercollegiate Strength Test, 234
Interests, objective of, 250
Interferential electrical muscle stimulation, use of in treatment, 71, 96

International Center for Sports Nutrition, 199
International Congress of Anatomists, 58
International Olympic Committee rules, 138
International Society for Biomechanics in Sport (ISBS), 101, 102
International Society of Biomechanics (ISB), 101, 102, 114
International Society of Sport Psychology (ISSP), 211, 213, 220
Internet, 185
    nutrition information sources, 199
Internships, 9
    dietetic, 177, 178, 180
    as educational option, 74, 91, 92
Interpersonal attraction, 223
Interscholastic athlete, sports medicine clinics, 77
Intersegmental reflexes, 232
Interval measurement, 230, 250
    definition, 251
Intervention techniques, 206, 208
Intestinal absorption, role of, 169
Intraclass method, 243
Intrafusal muscle fibers, 264
Intrinsic feedback, 269
Introspective research methodology, 217
Involuntary response, 264
Iron, 163, 174, 218
    supplements, 164
Ischemic heart disease, 18, 25
    definition, 34
Isokinetic machine, 71
    definition, 96
Isokinetics, 103
Isometric training, 30
Isotonic machine, 71
    definition, 97
Isotopes, 173
    definition, 172
The Israeli Association of Sport Psychology, 212
Iwao, Matsuda, 212

Jackson, C. O., 210
Jacobs, Andrew, 209
Japan, history of anatomy and, 42–44
Japanese Society of Sport Psychology (JSSP), 212
Jewish Community Centers, career opportunities, 3, 4
Job market, present and future trends, 4, 33; *see also* Employment opportunities
Jogging, 22
Johnson, Warren R., 211
Johnson and Johnson, Inc., sponsorship of NATA, 81
Joint Review Committee-Athletic Training (JRC-AT), 80, 84–85
    definition, 97

Karpovich, Peter V., 18, 23
Keele, S. W., 260
Kellor, Frances A., 210
Kelso, J. A. S., 260, 268
Kennedy, John F., 236
Ketone bodies, 162
Keys, Ancel, 18, 21, 167
Keys (K)-rations, 167
Kilocalories, 171, 172
    definition, 171, 201

Kincaid, M. A., 259
Kinematic data, 106, 108, 109
Kinematics, 100
    definition, 99, 120
Kinesiology, 82, 86, 101, 185
    definition, 13, 34, 98–99, 101, 120
    evolution of exercise science, 13–14, 32, 33, 237
Kinesiology Academy of AAPHERD, renamed, 102
Kinesthetic awareness, 244
Kinetic data, 106, 108, 109
Kinetics, 100
    definition, 99, 120
Knipping, H. W., 19, 31
Knowledge
    cognitive domain and, 250
    recall or recognition of, 226, 228, 233, 238, 246
Knowledge of performance (KP), definition, 272, 274
Knowledge of results (KR), 259, 260, 270, 271, 272
    definition, 269, 274
Knute Rockne, 208
Korean conflict, 236
Kranidiotis, Pantelis, 212
Kraus, Hans, 19, 25, 26, 236
Krogh, August, 19, 22, 32
Kroll, Walter, 258
Kugler, P. N., 260
Kwan, Michelle, 252

Laboratory for Physiological Hygiene, 18, 21
Lacerations, 164
Lactate, blood levels of, 170, 217
Lactic acid, 19, 30
Landers, Dan, 209
Lane, Dennis, 169
Lateral corticospinal tract, 262, 263
Latin grammar school, 234
Lawn Tennis Association, 235
Lawther, John, 208, 211
Leaders in exercise science, 18–20
    contributions, 22–23
Lean tissue loss, 162
Learning, maximizing, 258
Learning curve, plateaus in, 257, 259
Learning process, three phases of, 253, 254
Lecithin, 162
Leeuwenhoek, van, Antony, 13, 56, 60
Lesgaft, Peter F., 210
Less than information, 230
Lewis, Dio, 234
Licensed dietitian (LD), 181
Licensed medical nutrition therapist (LMNT), 181, 189
Licensing, of athletic trainers, 75–76
Licensure, 180–184, 195
Life cycle, anatomical changes during, 37, 67
Life span, 134, 139
    essential movement patterns, 102
Life style, 14, 16
    active, 2, 4
    "good life" practices, 168
    role of exercise in, 3, 23
    sedentary, 2, 31, 218
Lindhard, J., 31
Lipids, 196, 201
Little Leagues, 195

Liver disease, 159
Locomotion control center, 264
Locomotor movement, 232
Low-density lipoprotein (LDL) cholesterol, 165, 166
Lower motor neurons, 262, 263, 264, 265
Luft, Ulrich, 18, 24
de'Luzzi, Mondino, 51, 52, 60

McCurdy, J. J., 235
McGeoch, J. A., 259
Macrominerals, 164
Magill, R. A., 260
Magnetic resonance imaging (MRI), 106, 128–129, 142, 175, 237–238
  definition, 67, 108, 120
  noninvasive testing, 106, 108
  use of in study of anatomy, 61, 62, 64, 66
Mahoney, Michael, 209
Malignancies, 14
Malondialdehyde, 171
Malpighi, Marcello, 56, 60
Management dietitians, 190
Manipulative movement, 232
Marathon running, 130
Marey, Étienne Jules, 100
Margaria, Rodolpho, 22
Marketing strategies, 8
Marteniuk, Ronald, 258
Martins, Rainer, 209
Massage, 69
Master of Science degree (M. S.), 188, 189
Mastery hypothesis, 214, 239
Mathews, P. B. C., 260
Maximal oxygen consumption (VO2 max), 30, 140, 164, 244
  age changes, 31
  definition, 153
Maximum work times to exhaustion, 164
May, Jerry, 209
Meal planning, 195, 196, 197
Meals, regularity of, 14
Measurement, 226–250
  accuracy of, 226, 227, 230, 241–244, 250
  applications of, 238–241
  definition, 228, 251
  domains of human experience, 231–233
  evaluating the accuracy of, 226
  global, 241
  history of, 233–238
  levels of, 230
  of motivation, 227
  nature of, 228–231
  physical self-description questionnaire, 248
  precision of, 230
  procedures for developing, 226
  professional journals, 247–250
  refining practices, variables and, 226
  sport-specific, 241
  uses of, 227–228, 229
  versus evaluation, 228, 229
Measurement apparatus, 243
Measurement specialist, 227, 237, 244–247
Mechanical analysis, theory of, 100
Medical imaging techniques, 58
Medicine, 5, 124
  allopathic (M.D.), 4, 144
  anatomy as branch of, 38, 39, 41, 66
  osteopathic (D.O.), 4, 144

Medium-chain triglycerides (MCT), 160, 161, 162
Medulla, 262
Megadoses, 162
Memory
  long-term stores, 258
  short-term stores, 258
Memory drum theory, 259
Memory trace, 269, 270, 271
Menarche, delayed, 139
Meninges, 42
Menopause, estrogen levels and, 130
Menstruation, 218
  irregularity, 130, 138
Mental health, 205, 208–209, 214, 220, 241
  mood states, 203, 214, 218
Mental health model, 214
Mental illness, 204
Mental preparation techniques, 205, 206, 223
Mental processes, science of, 210, 223
Merton, P. A., 259
Metabolic diseases, 166, 171
Metabolic hormones, 171
Metabolic measurement, 30, 140, 171–173
Metabolic measurement carts, 140, 172, 173
Metabolic rate, 30, 131
Metabolic responses, 208
Metabolism, 126, 137, 167, 169
  bioenergetics and, 128–129
  definition, 201
  of food, 157, 201
Metabolites, 126, 141, 142
3-methylhistidine, 171
The Mexican Society of Sport Psychology, 213
Meyerhof, Otto, 19, 26, 30
Michelangelo, 52, 54 Micrographs, 58
Microgravity, Space Flight and, 130–131
Microminerals, 164
Microscope, 13, 37, 58
  development of, 55, 56, 60
Microscopic anatomy, 63
Microscopy, 58
Microwave diathermy, 71, 96
Midbrain, 264
Middle Ages, history of anatomy and, 47, 49–51
Middle level neurons, 264
Military conditioning, 12, 236, 257–258
Miller, Doris, 100
Miller, Sayers "Bud," 83
Milo of Crotona, 44
Mind-body dyad, 207
Minerals, and performance, 162, 163, 199
Minimum Muscular Fitness Test, 236
Minnesota Starvation Study, 167
Minnesota Vikings, 195
Mitsuo, Matsui, 210
Modeling techniques, 109
Model of muscle activation, 254
Molecular biology, evolution of exercise sciences and, 13, 32, 33
Monoamine hypothesis, 214
Monosynaptic stretch reflex, 264, 266
Montoye, Henry J., 26, 27
Mood states, 203, 214, 218, 240, 241
More, Kelli, 163
Morgan, R. L., 260
Morse code, 259

Motivation, 204, 206, 208–209, 215–217, 219
  assessing, 240, 241, 250
  definition, 223
  external motivars, 227
Motivational techniques, 8
  learning process and, 253
Motor abilities, assessment of, 239, 240
Motor behavior, 253, 260
Motor control, 127, 252–254
  academic training, 272–273
  applications, 273, 274
  chronology of events, 259–260
  definition, 252, 274
  employment opportunities, 272–273
  future directions, 271–272
  history of, 237, 254–258
  issues across learning process, 253
  multilevel, 260–264
  professional associations, 273
  professional journals, 273
  research in, 269
  theoretical approaches, 258–271
Motor cortex, 257, 260, 261, 262
  definition, 275
Motor homunculus, 261
Motor learning, 127, 142–143, 204, 252–254
  academic training, 272–273
  applications, 273, 274
  chronology of events, 259–260
  definition, 252, 253, 275
  employment opportunities, 272–273
  future directions, 271
  historical studies, 207, 208, 210
  history of, 254–258
  issues across learning process, 253
  professional associations, 273
  professional journals, 273
  theoretical approaches, 258–271
  theoretical developments, 257–258
  theories of, 257, 269–271, 272
Motor neuron, 261, 266, 275
Motor program, 267, 271, 274, 275
Motor program theory, 267, 268, 269, 270, 271
Motor skills, 267, 270, 272, 273
  acquiring/retaining, 252, 253, 257, 275
  historical research, 257–258
  reteaching, 273
Mountain sickness, 136
Movement, human, 106, 108, 264
  anatomical aspects, 98, 99
  control of fine, 261, 274
  initiation, 260, 261, 269, 274
  mechanical aspects, 98, 99, 100, 101
  nondiscursive, 233
  nonlocomotor, 232
  patterns, 105, 269, 270
Müller, Erich A., 19, 30
Multiple sclerosis, 128
Multitrait-multimethod (MTMM) data, 248
Mummification, 42
Muscle, estimation of amount of, 67
Muscle activation, 108, 142
Muscle biopsy technique, 128, 129, 141, 142, 170–171
  role of diet and exercise and, 160, 168
Muscle bound, 15
Muscle contraction
  eccentric, 152

Muscle contraction (*continued*)
historic theories of, 254, 255
Muscle damage, 162, 168, 171
Muscle fatigue, 138, 142
mechanism of, 128
research on, 18, 19, 31
Muscle fiber type, 141, 142
Muscle glycogen, depletion and resynthesis, 168, 171
Muscle mass, 130, 131, 138, 139, 162
Muscle physiology, 26
Muscle soreness, 16, 136, 162, 216, 231
causes of, 31
Muscle spindle, 259, 264, 265, 266, 268
definition, 275
Muscle strength/endurance, 8
role of protein in, 160, 161
Muscle tone, excessive, 132, 153
Muscle work, 128
German exercise scientists, 30
Scandinavian exercise scientists, 19, 31
Muscular hypertrophy, 30
Muscular system, adaptation to exercise, 123, 128
Musculoskeletal function, 239
Muybridge, Edweard, 100, 102
Myocardial infarction, 133

National Association for Sport and Physical Education (NASPE), 7, 10
National Association of Intercollegiate Athletics (NAIA), 81
National Athletic Trainer's Association (NATA), 76, 79, 97
administrative and leadership structure, 80–81, 82, 92
associate membership, 72
certified membership, 72, 73, 78
current activities, 80–82, 92
history of, 70–72
international membership, 72
membership categories, 72–73, 78
-mission statement, 80, 81
on worldwide web, 81–82
student membership, 72, 73
National Athletic Trainer's Association Board of Certification (NATABOC), 73–76, 96, 97
certification, 72, 79, 82–85, 87, 91–92
continuing education unit (CEU) requirements, 75
examination, 73, 74–75, 92
National Athletic Trainer's Association Educational Task Force (ETF), 87, 91–92
National Athletic Trainer's Association Fax-on-Demand, 82
National Athletic Trainer's Association Professional Education Committee (NATA-PEC), 91
curriculum guidelines, 83, 84
history of, 83
National Athletic Trainer's Association Research and Education Foundation (NATA-REF), 81
National Center for Nutrition and Dietetics, 199
National Collegiate Athletic Association (NCAA), 81
Division I university, 194

National Commission for Certifying Agencies, 147
National Dairy Council, 199
National Federation of State High School Associations, 81
National Football League, 80
National Health and Nutrition Examination Survey (NHANES III), 166
The National Institute of Physical Education, Tokyo, 210
National Organization of Competency Assurance (NOCA), 74
National Strength and Conditioning Association (NSCA), 4, 138, 146, 199
certification, 147, 189, 197
-certified Personal Trainer, 147
National Strength Coaches Association, 146
Near-infrared interactance spectrophotometry, 177
Near-infrared reactance (NIR), 141
Near-infrared spectroscopy, 176
Neff, Joseph, 234
Neissen, U., 258, 260
Nelson, Richard, 100, 102
Nervous system, 252, 253, 258, 274
autonomic, 127–128
control of respiration, 125–126
motor control and, 254, 264, 269, 271
open and closed loop control, 264–268
voluntary, 127
Neuroanatomy, 64
Neuromuscular disease
intramuscular EMG measurement, 141
muscle soreness, 136
Neuromuscular electrical stimulation (NMES), use in treatment, 71, 96
Neuromuscular rehabilitation, 127, 128
Neuromuscular system, levels of, 260
Neuroses, 14
New England Patriots, 195, 196
Newsletters, nutrition, 198
Newton, Sir Isaac, 100, 102, 109
mechanical laws, 100
New York Giants, 195
New York Nets, 195
The New Zealand Sport Psychology Interest Group, 212
Nideffer, Robert, 209
Nielson, Marius, 22, 32
Nigg, Benno, 109, 117
Nike, 114, 115
Nike Sport Research Laboratory (NSRL), 114
Nitrogen metabolism, 160
Nominal measurement, 230, 250
definition, 230, 251
Nonlinear dynamics, 269
Nonparametric statistics, 231
Norms
constructing, 227
use in program assessment, 228
Norske, Arno, 212
North American Society for the Psychology of Sport and Physical Activity (NASPSPA), 205, 211–212, 220–221, 260, 273
Nuclear bag, 264, 265
Nuclear chain fibers, 264, 265
Nuclear magnetic resonance spectroscopy (NMR, MRS)), 128, 142

Nursing, study of anatomy and, 38, 66
Nutrients
as ergogenic aids, 169, 200
essential, 158, 164–167, 173, 201
Nutrition, 8, 133, 166, 249
classical studies, 19, 21, 31
consultants, 195, 196, 200
counseling, 180, 194, 195, 196, 197
curriculum requirements, 82, 86, 143, 185, 188
definition, 157, 167, 201
as element of performance, 16, 150
exercise and sport psychology and, 205, 216
historical perspective, 69, 167, 237
patient education, 150, 196
pediatric, 139
Nutritional supplements, 169, 170, 171, 174, 200
Nutrition Laboratory at the Carnegie Institute, 167
Nutrition science, 167–170

Obesity, 129, 142, 166, 200
definition, 134
Objectivity, 244
definition, 251
Observational learning, 272
Occupational biomechanics, 105–106, 118
Occupational therapy, 4, 38, 66
The Oesterreiche Arbeitsgemeinschaft für Sport Psychologie, 212
Office of Disease Prevention and Health Promotion, 198
Ogilvie, Bruce, 208, 209, 211
Olympic athletes, biomechanical analysis of, 2
Olympic Games, 12, 212, 235
1992, 137
Olympic-level sports, 227, 274
Olympic Training Center, career opportunities, 4
Omega-3 fatty acids, 160, 161
100-yard dash, 235
Open-loop control, 264–268
definition, 264–265, 275
Operation Everest II, 136
Optometry, 4, 145
Ordinal measurement, 230, 231, 250
definition, 230, 251
Orthopedics, 204
Orthostatic hypotension, 131
Osteopathic medical school, 144
Osteoporosis, 130, 158, 201
definition, 153, 201
dietary habits and, 159, 163, 165, 166
Ostrow, Andrew, 213
Outcome goals, process of setting, 223
Outreach services, 77
Overload principle, 30
Overtraining, 203, 215–216
Oxygen, 129, 152
consumption, 31, 126, 153, 172
exchange of, 126
role in control of breathing, 19, 30
transport of, 126, 153, 163
Oxygen debt, 22
Oxygen 18 (^{18}O), 172
Oxygen saturation, 150
Oxygen uptake (VO$_2$), 132

Paidotribi, 69
Pain, strategies to control, 205
Paleolithic cultural period, 39–40
cave painting, 39, 40
Pancreas, insulin hormones, 153
Papal Bull, 51, 60
Papyruses, 42, 59
Paralysis, 131, 262; *see also* Paraplegia,
Quadriplegia
Parametric statistics tests, 248
Paraplegia, 131, 132
use of arm-crank ergometer, 140
Parasympathetic nervous system, 127–128
definition, 127, 153
Parthenogenesis, 46
Patellar tendon, 264
Patient education, 196
Pathological anatomy, 66, 109
definition, 37, 67
Patrick, G. T. W., 207, 210
Pechlat, Augustin, 210
Pediatric exercise physiology, 138–139
Pentathlon, 235
Perceptual abilities, 232
Perceptual-motor template, 268, 271
Perceptual trace, 269, 270, 271
Performance-enhancement specialist, 206
Performance, human, 65, 164
applied exercise physiology and, 123, 151
biomechanics to improve, 103, 104
exercise scientists and sport, 2–3
hormones influencing, 129, 130
inactivities of daily living, 134, 151, 152
in special conditions, 136
measuring, 240
pediatric sport, 38
special aids to, 16, 138
Peripheral artery disease (PAD), 133
Peripheral vascular disease, 133
Personal injury, expert-witness, 105
Personality, 203, 208, 210, 215
assessing, 241
definition, 223
Personality disorders, 222
Personality traits, assessing, 240, 241
Personal trainer, 4, 150, 196
certified, 197
Pestalozzi, Johann Heinrich, 234
Pharmacology, definition, 158
Phenomenological research methodology,
216, 217
Phlegm, 45
Phosphorus, 174
Photography, 106, 107
Photon absorptiometry, 175
Physical chemistry, 13, 14
Physical education, 32, 146, 245
academic program, 3, 9
development of exercise science and, 12,
14, 233, 234
exercise and sport psychology and, 204,
205, 207, 210
as parent of exercise physiology, 123
pediatric exercise physiology, 138–139
programs, K–12, 205
Physical fitness, 1–2, 14, 167, 222, 226–227
assessing, 150, 196, 228, 230, 239–240
classic studies, 20, 21
definition, 34
history of exercise science, 12, 20, 236

need for testing, 17
need of definition, 16
societal lack of, 3, 4
Physical fitness movement, 18, 23
Physical fitness testing, 236
Physical inactivity, 166, 168
Physical Self-Description Questionnaire
(PSDQ), 248
Physical therapists, 127, 274
Physical therapy, 4–5, 38, 66, 124, 144
Physical training programs, historically, 235,
236, 237
Physician extender, 93
Physician's assistant, 4, 145
Physiological dependence, 203, 205, 223
Physiology, human, 32, 64, 82, 86, 100
definition, 13, 34, 123
father of, 47, 59, 67
as parent of exercise physiology, 123
Piezoelectric elements, 108
Plagenhoef, Stanley, 101
Plan strategies, use of software and, 249
Plaque forming, 165, 166
Plateaus, learning curve, 257, 259
Platelet aggregation, 166
Plato, 45, 46, 256
Play, and psychology, 210
Plyometrics, 103
Pneuma, 44, 59
Poliomyelitis, 14
Pollution, exercising in, 136
Polybus, 45
Polyunsaturated fatty acid, 161
Pope Boniface VIII, 51
Pope Sixtus IV, 51, 60
Positron emission tomography (PET) scan,
61, 66, 253
definition, 67
Postpolio syndrome, 128
Posture, 134, 262
Potassium, 164, 174
Potentiometer, 108
Power output (PO), 132
Power sports, 274
use of ergogenic aids, 137, 152
Practical experience, 9
Practice session, 253, 270
blocked, 253, 272, 274
constant, 269, 271, 275
learning process during, 253, 272
random, 253, 272, 275
Practice trial, 269, 274
Practicums, 9
Prediction, using measurement techniques
to, 227–228, 250
Pregnancy, exercise and, 13, 135–136
Preprofessional schools, 4, 144–145
Prescientific period, 39–41
President's Council on Physical Fitness, 26
President's Council on Youth Fitness, 236
Pressure platform/pressure insole, 109
definition, 109, 120
Preventive reconditioning centers, European/
USA comparison, 25
Primary motor area, 263, 265
Prince of Physicians, 48, 59, 67
Private consulting, 3, 4
definition, 10
Private health club, 148, 150, 151, 209; *see
also* Commercial health club

Private practice, 93, 206
Probability, determining, 245, 250
"Proceedings: Mild Brain Injury in Sports
Summit," 81
Product liability, 106, 114
Professional associations/organizations, 9,
64
of exercise and sport psychology, 220
for athletic trainers, 70
for exercise physiologists, 145–146
for motor control and learning, 273
for nutrition, 199
Professional certification, 4, 24
continuing education unit, 75, 92
for dietetics, 176, 180–184, 193, 195
for exercise and sport psychology, 221
NATABOC definition, 70
NATABOC examination process, 73,
74–75, 92
Professional development, 9
role of athletic trainer, 71, 95
Professional Examination Service (PES),
73
Professional journals
anatomical, 65
for athletic training, 70, 94
for biomechanics, 116–117, 118
for exercise and sports psychology,
221–222
for exercise physiology, 125, 151
for motor control and learning, 273
for nutrition and exercise nutrition,
197–198
of measurement specialists, 247
Professional sports teams, 195, 196, 200
career opportunities, 72, 78–80, 93–95
consulting for, 206, 208, 221
Professional standards, 5–9
Profile of Mood States (POMS),
questionnaire, 214
Program Director (PD), 147
Program evaluation, measurement tech-
niques and, 228
Proprioception, 259
Prosthesis, development of, 100, 105
Proteases, 164
Protective devices, 104
Protein, 164, 169, 171, 172, 174
and athletic performance,160, 162, 195,
196, 199
Protein supplements, 160
Psyche, 46
Psychological dependence, 223
Psychological domain, 240–241
definition, 250
Psychological intervention, 216
Psychological refractory period, 259
Psychological skills training (PST), 220
Psychological well-being, 204, 222
Psychology, 82, 86, 204, 205, 235
definition, 223
Psychometrics, 206, 209
Psychomotor domain, 96, 231–233,
239–241, 244
definition, 231, 251
Psychonomic Society, 273
Psychophysiological orientation, 216, 217
Public Health Service, 168
Pull-ups, 239
Pulmonary disease, testing for, 138, 148

Pulmonary rehabilitation, 124, 127, 133–134, 149–150
employment opportunities, 4, 147–148
program, exercise adherence, 127, 214
Pulmonary system, 2, 126–127
Pulmonary ventilation rate, 126
Pulmonologists, 127
Puni, A. Z., 210
Pyramidal motor tract, 262, 263, 267
Pythagoras, 256

QSR NUD•IST, 217
Quadriceps muscle, 264
Quadriplegia, 131, 132
Qualitative research methodology, 216, 219
Quality control, state regulation, 75–76
Quality of life, 3, 26, 139
applied exercise physiology and, 123, 134, 151
exercise and the elderly, 131, 152
Quantitative research methodology, 216–217, 218
software technologies, 217

Raab, Wilhelm, 18, 19, 25, 26
Racial groups, body composition assessment, 141
Radiography, 175
Radioisotopes, 172
Random practice, 253, 272
definition, 275
Range of motion exercises, 97, 131
Ranking procedure, 230
Raphael, 52
Rating of perceived exertion (RPE), 132, 150
Ratio measurement, 230, 231, 250
definition, 231, 251
Ray, Richard, 91
Reaction time, 207, 210
Recall schema, 270, 271
Reciprocal innervation, 259
Recognition schema, 270, 271
Recommended Dietary Allowances (RDA), 162, 173
definition, 201
Record keeping, 96
Recovery time, 160, 162
Recreational athletes, 77
Red blood cell count, 164
Red Grange, 208
Redundant degrees of freedom, 99
Reentrant loops, 267
Reference mechanism, 268
Reflex, 127
Reflex arc, definition, 275
Reflexive control of movement, 232, 259, 264, 266
Regional anatomy, definition, 37
Registered dietitian (RD), 176–178, 180–181, 184–185, 188, 195
definition, 179
as requirement, 193, 196, 197
salary levels, 190
Registration, as state regulation, 76
Registration Examination for Dietitians, 177, 178, 179, 180, 181
Rehabilitation/reconditioning, 2, 95, 127, 132, 144
clinical instruction, 96
devices/machines, 71, 108

in secondary school setting, 76
nutrition and, 164
Rehabilitative biomechanics, 105, 118
Rehydration beverages, 169
Reinforcement/punishment strategies, 203
Reliability of measurement, 239–245, 250
definition, 241, 251
Religious belief, history of anatomy and, 42, 48–49, 51
Remedial exercise, as NATA curriculum requirement, 82
Renaissance
history of anatomy and, 51–55
history of biomechanics during, 100
Reproduction, history of anatomy and, 46
Research, 4, 5, 143
applied, 237
employment opportunities in, 112, 124, 193, 200
in exercise and sport psychology, 205, 206, 208
in motor learning, 271
use of measurement in, 228, 237, 245–246, 250
Research and Education Foundation (REF), 81
Research dietitians, 190, 191, 200
Research methodologies, 216–219, 220
Research sport psychologist, 208
Resistance training, 131, 134, 138, 149, 215
Resistive devices, 96–97
Respiration, control of, 125, 126
Respiratory gas analysis, 19, 30
Respiratory gas analyzer, 30, 172
Respiratory physiology, 24, 30, 31
Respiratory therapists, 127, 150
Response programming, 258
Response time, measurement of, 230
Resting blood pressure, 126
Resting heart rate, 123, 127
Resting metabolic rate, 131, 134
Retention, 253, 270
long-term, 257, 259, 271
Retention tests, 270, 272
Rhinoplasty, 44
Rieger, C., 207
Risk-factor concept, 168, 196
Robinson, Sid, 18, 21
Rodahl, Kaare, 20, 32
Roentgen, Wilhelm, 58, 60, 67
Roentgen rays, discovery of, 58, 67
Rogers, D. E., 259
Role delineation study, 70, 75
Roman empire, history of anatomy and, 47, 49, 59, 167
Romanian National Committee for Physical Culture and Sport, Sports Psychology Committee, 211
Rowing ergometers, 140
Rubin, P., 260
Running high jump, 235

Safety equipment, 70
biomechanical development of, 105
Saliva analysis, 173
Salmoni, A. W., 260
Salvini, Alessandro, 213
San Francisco Bay to Breakers run, 22
Sargent, Dudley Allen, 17, 18, 20, 234
Sargent Jump Test, 17

Sargent's Universal Test for Speed, Strength, and Endurance, 235
Scale weight, 175, 201
Scandinavian exercise scientists, 19–20, 31–32
Scanning electron microscope, 58
"A Schema Theory of Discrete Motor Skill Learning," 258, 260, 269, 270–271, 272
Schilling, Guido, 211
Schleiden, M. J., 57, 60
Schmidt, Richard A., 258, 260, 267, 270
Scholander, Peter F., 22
Scholar-practitioners, 32
Schrader, John, 83, 91
Schwann, Theodor, 57, 60
Schwann cell, 57
Science, 1
definition, 10
Scientific period, 41–49
Scientific skepticism, 41
Scientist scholar-educator, 206
Scoring
observed, 242
true, 242
variability, 251
Scouting statistics, use of software and, 249
Scripture, E. W., 207, 210
Secondary schools, 209, 219, 236
athletic trainer in, 72–73, 76–79, 92–93, 95
conditioning programs, 150
Second International Society of Sport Psychology (ISSP) Congress, 211
Second-order neurons, 262, 263, 265
Segmental reflexes, 232
Self-confidence, 217, 220
Self-defense, 236
Self-efficacy, 217
definition, 223
Self-esteem, 203, 205, 208, 217, 241
Self-monitoring of exercise, 133
Semilunar valves, 45
Seminars, CEU requirements, 75, 81
Semistarvation, 167
Sensory cortex, 257
Sensory feedback, 253, 261, 265–270, 274, 275; see also Feedback loops
Sensory neuron, 266, 275
Sensory receptors, 261, 275
Serial-order problem, 271
Serotonin, fatigue and, 127
Service responsibilities, 247
Shea, J. B., 260
Sherrington, C. S., 259
Shoe design research, biomechanical, 103–104, 106, 109, 113–114, 117
Shorten, Martyn, 114–115
Shortwave diathermy, 71, 96
Shot put, 235
Siebert, Werner W., 19, 30
Simonson, Ernst, 18, 25
Simulation technique, 109
Single-channel hypothesis, 259
Sit and reach, 239
Situational approach, 215
Sit-ups, 239
Skeletal muscle, 127, 137, 141
changes during exercise, 128, 129
Skeletal system, 130
Skilled movement, 233
Skills, 222

acquiring specific, 250, 257
assessment of, 102, 239, 240
definition, 99
sport, 209, 215, 223
teaching, 233, 253
Skinfold measurement, 141, 170, 176, 218, 239
reliability, 244
Slater-Hammel, Arthur T., 208, 258
Sleep, 14, 208, 216
Slip and fall accident, 103
Slow positioning movements, 269
Smith, Alan A., 83
Smith, Murray, 213
Smoking, 14, 165, 168
Social cognitive theory, 218
Social cohesion, 203, 209
definition, 223
Social learning theory, 215
The Sociedad Columbiana de Ciencias Aplicadas al deporte, 213
The Societa Italiana di Psicologia (SIPS), 213
La Societe Francaise de Psychologie du Sport (SFPS), 212
Society for Neuroscience, 273
Sodium, 164, 169, 174
Sodium bicarbonate, 138
Sodium chloride, 159, 166
"The Soft American," 236
Somatosensory cortex, 261, 262
Somatotopically organized, 261
Southard, W. F., 259
Space Flight, microgravity and, 130–131
Spasticity, definition, 132, 153
Special Olympics, 204
Speed, as element of performance, 16
Speed-accuracy trade-offs, 257, 259
Spinal cord, 262, 263, 264
Spinal cord injury (SCI), 131–132
Spinal feedback loop, 267–268
Spinal level, 262, 265, 266
Split halves method, 243
Sport, definition, 223
Sport biomechanics, 110
Sport psychology, 215–216, 222, 237; see also Exercise and sport psychology
definition, 203, 204
Sport Psychology Advisory Board, 212
The Sport Psychology Association of Australia and New Zealand (SPAANZ), 213
The Sport Psychology Association of India, 212
Sports and Cardiovascular Nutritionists (SCAN), 199
Sports anemia, 164
Sports drinks, 168, 169
Sports equipment, biomechanical design of, 103, 104
Sportsmanship, measuring, 250
Sports medicine, 77, 92, 95, 164
Sports medicine clinics, 71, 206, 209
athletic trainers in, 72, 73, 95
hospital-based, 77, 78
state licensing, 76
Sports nutrition. See Exercise and sports nutrition
Sports nutritionist, 2, 194–195
Sports physiology. See Exercise and sports physiology

Sport-specific measurement, 241
Sport-specific psychological tests, 206
Sport-specific theories, 204, 222
The Sports Psychology Association of Nigeria, 212
Sport techniques, biomechanical development of, 103, 118
Sprains, 164
Springfield College, 18, 23, 33
Sprint cycle training, 129
Sprint running, cinematographical analysis of, 100, 102, 106
Sputnik I, 237
Stair-stepping machines, 104
Staleness, 203, 215–216
definition, 223
Stamina, 168
Standards and Guidelines for an Accredited Education Program for the Athletic Trainer, 84
Starvation, research on effects of, 167
State Department of Health, 184
State regulation/licensing, 75–76, 92, 180–184
Statics, definition, 98–99, 120
Statistical tests, 231, 245
Statistics
as measurement tool, 228, 244, 245, 247
nonparametric test, 231
parametric test, 248
Stearns, William, 234
Steele, Bill, 211
Steinhaus, Arthur H., 18, 23
Stelmach, George, 258
Stimulus-response (SR) approach, 258
Strain gauges, 108
Strains, 164
Strength, 233
as element of performance, 16
use of anabolic steroids, 152
Strength and conditioning coaches, 2, 4, 146, 194, 274; see also Coaching
in secondary schools, 150
Strength and conditioning programs, 147, 150
Strength and conditioning specialist, certified, 197
Strength and flexibility programs, testing standards for, 8
Strength athletes, protein intake and, 160
Strength training, 147, 234, 235
ergogenic aids, 130, 137
for specific conditions, 131, 132, 134, 139
muscle adaptation to, 128
neurological adaptations to, 127
pediatric risk, 138
sport nutritionists and, 160, 194
use of MRI, 142
Stress, 159
athletic performance and, 208, 209, 211, 215–216
Stress management, 8, 133, 139
Stressors, exercise as, 123
Stress testing, 148
Strokes, 14, 61, 132, 135, 152
regaining mobility, 274
Submaximal exercise, 130
Substance abuse, 8
Substance-abuse specialist, 206
Substitution devices, development of, 105

Substrate utilization, 171, 173
Success, 214
attribution theory, 222
Sudden death, neurological risk, 128
Sugar, 32, 174
Sugito, Genpaku, 43
Suinn, Richard, 209
Summative evaluations, 227
Superoxide dismutase (SOD), 129, 162
Superstition, history of anatomy and, 40, 42
Supplementary motor cortex, 261, 262
definition, 260, 275
Supplement devices, development of, 105
Supplier NATA membership, 73
Suprasegmental reflexes, 232
Surgery, history of anatomy and, 51
Surveys, as evaluation tool, 228
Survival prediction, 148
Susruta, 43, 59
Sweating, 136
The Swedish Association for Behavioral Sport Science, 212
Sylvius, Jacobus, 48
Sympathetic nervous system, 127–128, 132
definition, 127, 153
Symposium on Footwear Biomechanics, 114, 115
Symposiums, CEU requirements, 75, 81
Systemic anatomy, definition, 37

Tackle football, sports injuries, 70
Taping, 76, 96
as psychomotor skill, 96
Task cohesion, definition, 223
Taxonomies, domains of human experience, 231–233
Taylor, Henry Longstreet, 21
Teacher/athletic trainer, 77–79, 93
definition, 77, 97
Teacher preparation, 32, 63–64, 123
Teaching, 4–5, 112, 118, 146, 273
exercise nutrition, 193, 200
in exercise and sport psychology, 205, 206, 208
measurement specialists and, 245, 246
Team Danmark, 213
Temporal analysis, 106
definition, 99, 120
Terman, Lewis M., 235
Test construction, 238, 240
Testing, 8, 228; see also Measurement
field, 248
noninvasive, 108, 120
reliability, 251
validity, 238, 240
Test of English as a Foreign Language (TOEFL), 110, 111
Testosterone, 129, 130, 170, 171
drugs derived from, 137, 152
Test-retest method, 243
Thalanus, 262
Theory of motor learning, 254
Theory of perceptual learning, 259
Therapeutic effects of exercise, 220
Therapeutic modalities, 86
application of, 96
Thermal adjustments, 136
Thermogenic hypothesis, 214
Thermoregulatory system, exercise as stimulus, 123

Thesis, 189, 246
Thomas, J. R., 260
Thorndike, E. L., 235, 257, 258, 259
Thrombotic processes, 166
Time-motion studies, 257
Tissue biomechanics, 110
Tissue perfusion, 161
Tools, mechanically efficient, 105
Total body electrical conductivity, 175
Total iron binding capacity (TIBC), 218
Tournament scheduling, use of software for, 249
Tracer techniques, 172
Training camp, 196
Training rooms, 96
Training table, 195, 196
Traits, 203, 210, 215, 223; *see also* Personality traits
Trait theory, 215
Transcutaneous electrical nerve stimulation (TENS), 71, 96
  use in treatment, 96
Transducers, 108–109
  definition, 108
Transgene technology, 166
Transportation modules, improving the design of, 105
Treadmills, 109, 139–140, 238, 264, 269
  stress testing, 24, 30, 148, 228, 244
Trephining, 40, 41
Triglycerides, 160, 162
Triplett, Norman, 207, 210
True variance, 242, 243, 244
Tuberculosis, 14
Tutko, Thomas, 208, 211
Type I diabetes, definition, 135, 152
Type II diabetes, 134
  definition, 135, 152

Ulrich, Celeste, 208, 211
Ultrasound sonography, 63, 64, 142
  definition, 67
  therapeutic, 71, 94, 96
  use in study of anatomy, 63, 64, 66
Undergraduate education program
  CAAHEP accreditation, 84–87, 88
  curricula, 6–7, 9, 32
  in dietetics, 181, 185, 186
  in exercise and sport nutrition, 184–185
  in exercise physiology, 142–143
  in nutrition, 185, 187, 188
  in physical education, 204, 237
Underwater weighing, 61, 141, 175, 201, 239
USSR Sports Psychology Federation, 210
U.S. Air Force, 24, 257
United States Bureau of Labor Statistics, 189
U.S. exercise scientists, 18–19
  trained abroad, 18–19, 23–26
United States Golf Association, 235
United States government agencies, 198
U.S. Olympic Committee (USOC), 208, 212, 213, 221

Sport Psychology Committee, 212
U.S. Olympic teams, 208
Universal education, 234
University counseling center, 206
University of Bologna, 51, 60
University of Florida Gator football players, 168
Upper motor neurons, 262, 263, 264, 275
Upper respiratory tract infection, 130
Urine analyses, 171, 173

Validity of measurement, 239, 240, 241, 245, 250
  construct, 243, 244
  content, 243–244
  criterion, 243, 244
  definition, 241, 251
Values, objectives of, 250, 252
Vanek, Miroslav, 211
Van Rossum, J. H. A., 260
Variable practice, 270, 271
  definition, 275
Variables, 268
  in generalized motor progrm, 274
Variance (s^2), 242, 243, 250
Vascularization, 128
Velocity, 107, 264
Ventilitory rate, 2
Ventral corticospinal tract, 262, 263
Verbal feedback, 253, 269
Vesalius, Andreas, 52–56, 60, 67, 100
Video, high-speed, 107, 120
Videography, 106, 107
  definition, 107, 120
Videotape, 107, 120, 253
Vietnam War, 237
Vinci, da, Leonardo, 52, 53, 60
  biomechanics and, 100, 102
Virchow, Rudolph, 57, 60
Virgin birth, 46
Vitamin deficiency, 162
Vitamins, 162, 199
  A, 174
  C, 162, 166, 174
  E, 162, 165, 166
  multiple, 164
  as supplementation, 162
Vivisection, 46
Voluntary movement, 259, 262, 264, 266, 267
VO$_2$ max. *See* Maximal oxygen consumption

Walking, 1–2, 16, 102; *see also* Gait patterns
  biomechanical aspects of, 19, 30
Walter, C. B., 260
Warming up, 16, 31
Washburn, Richard, 26
Water
  intake and athletic performance, 136, 158, 164, 168–169, 199
  use of isotonically labeled, 172

Weber, Sonya, 236
Weber brothers, 100
Weight, 14
Weight-bearing exercise
  during space flight, 131
  pediatric, 138
Weight lifting, 137, 138, 160, 236
Weight management, 8, 17, 133–135, 196
  gaining techniques, 195
  loss, 134, 166, 190, 195
  unhealthy diet practices, 163
Weight training, 15
Wenz, Betty, 209
Western Medicine, Father of, 44, 59, 67
Wheelchair exercise, 131
Width, dimension of, 222
Widule, Carol, 101
Width, dimension of, 222
Wilberg, Bob, 211
William of Saliceto, 51, 60
Willis, Thomas, 57
Wilmore, Jack, 21
Winship, George, 234
Withdrawal symptoms, 223
Wolff, Julius, 19, 30
Wolff's law of bone transformation, 19, 30
Wood, Thomas D., 235
Woodrow, H., 259
Woodworth, R. S., 259
Work force, physical fitness and, 4
Work physiology, 20, 32
Workplace environment design, 105, 273
World's Fair, 1933, in Chicago, 234
World War II, 236, 257, 259
  nutrition and, 167, 168
Worm, Olaus, 57
Wormian bones, 57
Wrestling, pediatric exercise physiology and, 139
Wrigley, Philip, 208, 211
Written examination, 238, 239, 243
  five requirements of construction, 238, 239

X-rays, 58, 60, 61, 66, 67

Yellow bile, 45
Yin and yang, 43, 45
YMCA, 3, 4, 17, 34, 234
  leaders and exercise science, 18, 22, 23, 33
YMCA/YWCA, employment opportunities, 148, 150
Youth sport, 206, 220
YWCA, 3, 4
  career opportunities, 3, 4

Zodiacal man, 50